Praise for *A Life in Psychiatry*

"A fascinating account of the history of psychiatry and the personal and professional journey of one of Canada's leading psychiatrists. Dr. Garfinkel's attention to detail and his superb storytelling skills allow readers to appreciate how the tensions between psychotherapists and those offering pharmacologic approaches to treatment have impacted not only patient care but also the establishment and day-to-day operations of some of Canada's most prominent hospitals and teaching institutions. His vivid experiential recollections lead to sage advice for clinicians, teachers, researchers, and leaders—of value not only to psychiatrists but also to family physicians, other medical specialists, and health care professionals, and anyone with administrative or government responsibilities related to mental health care. Most importantly, this book opens the door for all to an enhanced understanding and increased sensitivity to the challenges faced by those with mental illness. A riveting read."

Calvin Gutkin, former executive director and chief executive officer, The College of Family Physicians of Canada

"A basic book for any young psychiatrist. This engaging autobiography shows how a good psychiatrist is formed. Excellent studies are only part of the picture. It takes a wide variety of life experiences to forge a professional and enable him to see the complexity of psychiatric illnesses. Perhaps this is why, at a time when traditional psychiatry was building barriers between the disciplines, Paul Garfinkel understood the need for a multidimensional approach."

Beatrice Bauer, professor of organization and human resources management, Bocconi University, Milan, Italy

"An honest and insightful account of the coming-of-age of a profession as seen through the evolving career of one of its foremost and successful practitioners. It will be an interesting read for those who practice the profession and those who are served by it; for those fascinated by the profession and those wary of it—because it speaks the engaging stories of patients and the institutions that try to serve them. The blend of science and humanity that has defined Paul's career shines through this book."

Shitij Kapur, dean and head of school, Institute of Psychiatry, King's College, London

"A great history of the ebbs and flows in psychiatry leading to the current balance between analysis and evidence-based medication treatment. As a layman, I found it a very interesting read. Particularly enjoyed the section on the CAMH merger."

Michael Wilson, chairman of Barclays Capital Canada Inc., former Canadian minister of finance

"Paul Garfinkel's book is a rare book that should be read by anyone with an interest in the history of psychiatry in Ontario, the evolution of the Clarke Institute to CAMH, leadership, and organizational politics. Paul manages to integrate these themes with his personal journey in a biography that combines science with scholarship, history with personal reflection, as well as critical analysis of who psychiatry should and does serve and professional boundary issues, including sexual relations with clients. Such a wide-ranging tome could make for difficult reading, but instead I found it very hard to put down!"

Steve Lurie, executive director, Canadian Mental Health Association, Toronto Branch

"Paul Garfinkel has changed the landscape for mental health and addictions, not only in Toronto but internationally. His vision to end the stigma on mental health; his work as a world-class clinician, and his leadership in creating CAMH—one of the most important health sciences centres in the world—has changed the lives of many people. His book will be of great interest to those who care about this important issue."

Don Tapscott, bestselling author of 15 books, most recently Macrowikinomics

"With impressive breadth and wisdom, Paul Garfinkel describes his career as an international leader in psychiatric research and administration. His description provides novel and important insights on the personal and professional challenges encountered along the path to his landmark accomplishments."

B. Timothy Walsh, professor of psychiatry, Columbia University

A Life in Psychiatry

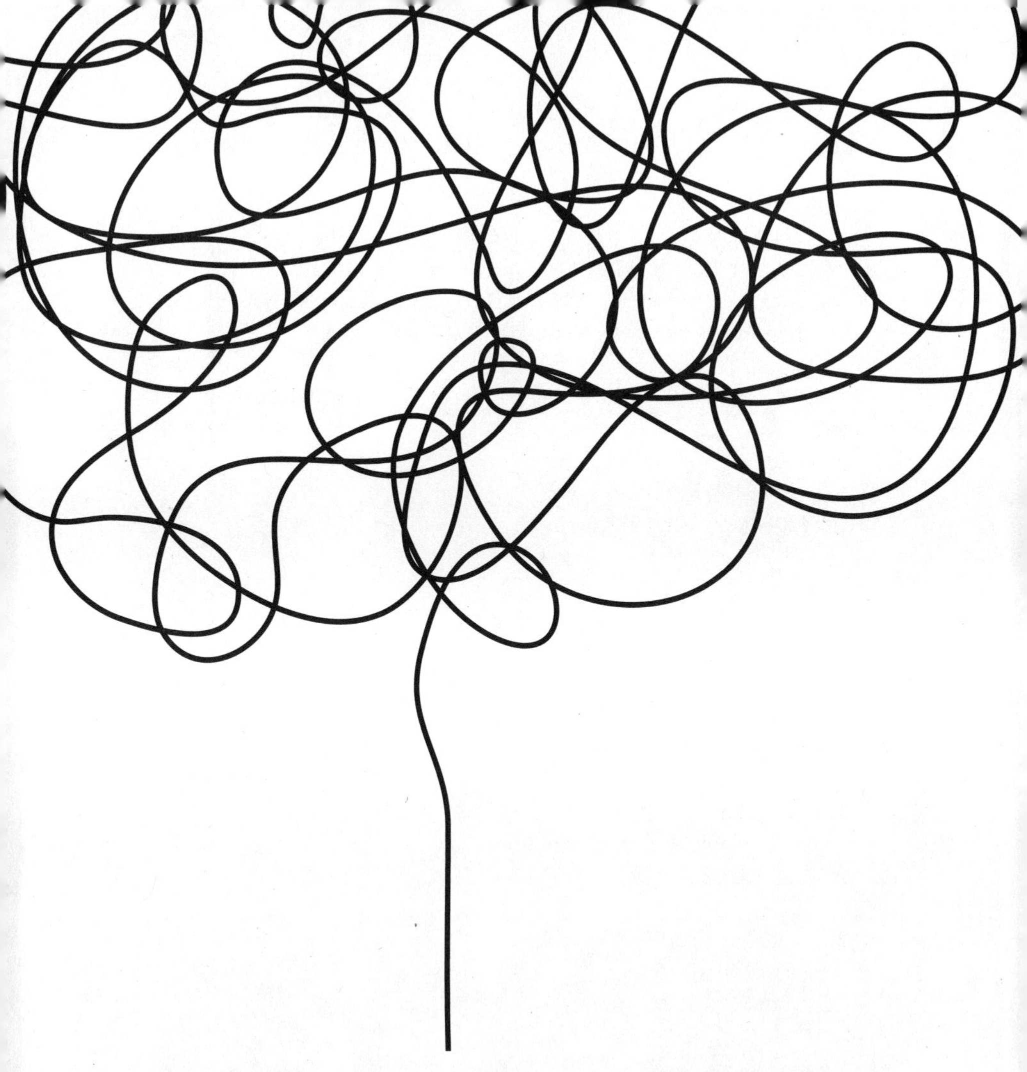

A Life in Psychiatry

Looking out, Looking in

Paul Garfinkel MD

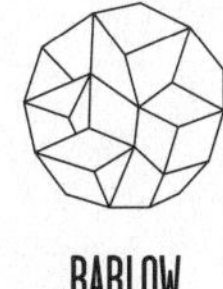

BARLOW

Copyright © Paul Garfinkel, 2014

All rights reserved. No part of this publication may be reproduced, stored in a retrieval system or transmitted, in any form or by any means, without prior written consent of the publisher.

Library and Archives Canada Cataloguing in Publication data available upon request.

ISBN 978-0-9917411-7-5 (print)
ISBN 978-0-9917411-8-2 (ebook)

Printed in Canada

ORDERS:
In Canada:
Jaguar Book Group
100 Armstrong Avenue, Georgetown, ON L7G 5S4

In the U.S.A.:
Midpoint Book Sales & Distribution
27 West 20th Street, Suite 1102, New York, NY 10011

SALES REPRESENTATION:
Canadian Manda Group
165 Dufferin Street, Toronto, ON M6K 3H6

Cover and interior design: Luke Despatie
Page layout: Kyle Gell Design
Production/Editorial: At Large Editorial Services

For more information, visit **www.barlowbookpublishing.com**

Barlow Book Publishing Inc.
96 Elm Avenue, Toronto, ON, Canada M4W 1P2

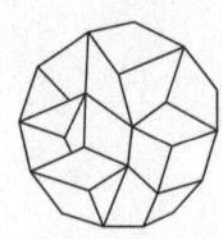

BARLOW

For my patients

Contents

FOREWORD

The Man Down the Hall

Almost 30 years ago, as a green but curious senior resident in psychiatry, I attended a special lecture at McGill University given by a visiting professor from Toronto—a person I had never heard of, talking about a condition I had never seen in my four years of psychiatric training. Paul Garfinkel gave a one-hour overview of anorexia nervosa; it was thoughtful, rich in perspective, and supported by evidence. It was the most synthetic and intriguing lecture in psychiatry I had ever heard. It was a "sliding doors" moment for me, where a chance encounter with an individual changed the trajectory of my life.

A few weeks later, I visited Paul in Toronto, at his suggestion to "come see what we're doing." He introduced me to a group of young, enthusiastic clinicians and researchers from multiple disciplines—psychiatry, psychology, nursing, social work, occupational therapy, and nutrition—who were all collaborating in advancing understanding and treatment of people with eating disorders. I was hooked.

Less than a year later, I found myself working at Toronto General Hospital as a Medical Research Council fellow under the supervision of Paul. His office was down the hall from mine, and I made frequent pilgrimages each week to his corner suite for teaching and mentoring about research, clinical care, collegiality, and life in general. He was 40 years old and I was 31, but unlike me, his nose-to-the-grindstone dedication to his academic career in medicine had propelled him a generation ahead; he was already an internationally recognized scholar in the eating disorders community and a galvanizing leader in the hospital community. Nevertheless, as a supervisor (much as a therapist must do), he had the capacity to make me feel that, for the time we were together, I had his attention, interest, and concern. He taught me how to review grants, how to write papers, how to give talks, and, ultimately, how to think as an academic physician.

Paul is that *rara avis* in our field who successfully fuses the roles of clinician, researcher, teacher, and administrator. In all four roles, he has been a generous mentor, committed to bringing along the next generation and sharing opportunities. Although his own research career is over, he sits on the Governing Council of the Canadian Institutes of Health Research because he wants to promote the chance for others to benefit from the kind of support he received. He takes pride in the teams he built. At the same time, he describes in this book the inevitable antipathy and isolation that leaders must endure if they wish to be effective and make change.

Now, as he approaches the end of his sixties and I approach the beginning of mine, we are once again a couple of doors apart—greyer, likely wiser as well as more scarred, and our relationship has evolved. What began in 1985 as teacher-student then became boss-lieutenant and continues now as both colleagues and close friends. We cover each other's clinical practices during absences, confide in each other about our personal and professional lives, and celebrate the accomplishments (and commiserate over struggles) in our families.

Thus, any perspective I can provide on Paul requires this lengthy disclaimer. But it is counterbalanced by the advantages of working very closely with and knowing someone for 30 years. The intimacy of our connection is reinforced when I hear people who know him less well describe him as aloof or intimidating; those are qualities I haven't experienced with him, but I can understand what might make people see him that way.

Tall, olive-skinned, and with a trim beard that he sometimes cups meditatively, drawn to darker clothing, he at times wears his sense of responsibility like a heavy weight. It emanates from being a classically studious and conscientious "good boy," as well as from the early leadership roles he assumed. He has a strong moral code, which both leads to being judgmental and causes some trepidation among those to be judged. This, coupled with his insistence on standards in work and behaviour, makes some people fear him. He is also careful. He weighs his words and even worries about them, and his talks as a leader are typically written out on index cards or slides and are considered rather than extemporaneous. Neither shy nor ebullient, he nevertheless has a reserve that can be misinterpreted as distance—except by those who make the effort to get to know him.

He has a reverence for history and a preoccupation with the future. Both of these are reflected in this book. Over the years, he acquired leather-bound reproductions of the classic textbooks in psychiatry, as well as obscure journal articles unknown by the current generation of psychiatrists. At the same time, he agitated for change in each of the three clinical settings in which I worked with him, and got angry when he encountered resistance.

When I first met him, he was driven along classical academic physician lines—get research grants, publish peer-reviewed articles and books, give formal lectures, and lead teaching hospitals. Apart from a fondness for unusual beers and fine cigars and a love of his young family, he seemed to have little interest in the world beyond. A trip to another city to give a lecture was an opportunity to get some work done in a hotel room rather than to explore new horizons.

Something changed for him in his 50s. He outlived his parents, who had both died young; his marriage ended, a new relationship began; and the exigencies of leadership broadened. Paul broadened also, taking new-found interest in music, art, Italy, wine, and politics. It seemed like a delayed voyage of discovery. His own brushes with a grave accident and a serious illness had not extinguished him but perhaps gave him new licence to live in new ways. And while challenges continued to emerge, he displayed more equanimity and took the blinkers off his focused curiosity. No longer on the treadmill of professional advancement, he returned to the thing that drew him into his profession in the first place: a profound curiosity about and concern for people with mental illness and their families. So now he is once again the man down the hall, seeing patients, and wandering into my office to share a perplexing clinical issue or just shoot the breeze.

This book reflects the many components of a complex person, from the influence of formative years both personally and professionally to his evolution as a leader both academically and administratively. But the book is also reflective of what is enduring about Paul—inquisitive, mindful of detail, committed to standards, and respectful of evidence. After 40 years in the field, he is able to take the long view of his profession in both directions.

I was fortunate to have him as a mentor and always felt supported by him as a colleague; I am lucky and proud to call him my friend.

David Goldbloom

INTRODUCTION

In 1975, just a few months after I completed my psychiatric residency, the brilliant film adaptation of Ken Kesey's 1962 novel One Flew Over the Cuckoo's Nest was released. It depicted the mental institution as a nightmarish place where the authoritarian Nurse Ratched squeezed the humanity out of the souls locked up inside. That dark portrait of the asylum and, by extension, of psychiatry itself was just one of a barrage of critical grenades being launched at my chosen profession. Through the media, we saw a whole variety of abuses: In New York there was horrendous patient overcrowding and abuse at the famous Willowbrook State School—a "snakepit," Robert Kennedy famously called it. In the United Kingdom in the early 1970s, nurses were murdered at Tooting Bec, a mental hospital in south London. In Quebec, orphans were falsely diagnosed with mental illness or intellectual disabilities and confined in asylums as part of a corrupt scheme to extract money from the government. In the 1960s, famed author Pierre Berton had exposed the horrible conditions and overcrowding at Ontario Hospital School, Orillia—overcrowding so severe that patients were sleeping head to head.[1] This was the public face of modern psychiatry, and it was in crisis.

Then asylums emptied; their patients were dispatched to the community—or, given the lack of resources to care for them, to the streets and city parks. In Toronto, the great Victorian edifice that was once the Toronto Lunatic Asylum fell to the bulldozer, to be replaced by banal concrete blocks, a campus that was supposed to erase the memory of what took place inside.

It was the end of the asylum, and that was supposed to be a good thing, according to anyone who cared to comment. It is easy to forget, though, that the asylum was the beginning of modern psychiatry. It was a genuine attempt on a large scale to treat people with mental illness humanely, as people who were sick, and not as animals or wretched sinners, as they had been viewed by most people in Europe for centuries. The asylum was, in fact, a revolution that would leave its imprint on psychiatry right up to the time when I began taking care of patients.

The idea that people with mental illness should be treated with kindness and respect began in the late 1700s when a new generation of humanitarian leaders removed the chains that restrained them in the cruel madhouses and called for a new regimen of kindness. This was the beginning of the lunatic asylums, a place where people who were "mad" could be cared for and treated.[2] It was a new way to look at mental illness, and it lay the groundwork for psychiatric practice as we know it today; that is, as a relationship between someone who is ill and another who cares for him or her, a doctor. This represented, at least at the beginning, a tangible hope for the mentally ill.[3]

By the time I started my psychiatric career, the asylum had degenerated into something far less noble, but it wasn't just the asylum that was under attack. Psychoanalysis, the other pillar of modern psychiatry, had also fallen out of favour. By the 1970s, North Americans had become disillusioned by what they considered its false promise and were far more willing to embrace scientific evidence and faster cures.

The father of psychoanalysis, Sigmund Freud, famously said that his talking cure to probe the unconscious could not be tested by conventional scientific means, and that attitude still prevailed in psychoanalytic circles when I began studying psychiatry in 1970. By then, Freud's disciples, who thought mental illness was all about the internal drives—sex and aggression, and how we unconsciously dealt with them—dominated the academic centres in the

United States. These psychoanalysts had an aggrandized sense of the method's power, even though there was no empirical proof of its effectiveness.

They didn't have much to worry about as long as psychiatry was not considered a scientific practice. But science was finally moving in. New drugs, developed in the 1950s and tested according to conventional scientific means, were proven to ease depression and some psychotic illnesses. These drugs could have terrible side effects, especially neurological ones, or extreme and rapid weight gain, but they could end the hallucinations and delusions that made the life of a person with schizophrenia so difficult to endure. Depression could now be treated with medicines as well as shock treatments.

With the development of new drug therapies, mental illness was no longer defined as hidden demons in the unconscious, but rather as chemical problems. Psychiatrists became prescribers of pills. The heyday of psychoanalysis was at an end. Science and medicine took over the practice; the human touch was not considered to be important, especially for the institutions funding the bills.

It was at this formative moment in psychiatry, with its widening, deepening rift between the role of science and the human touch, that I began my career. I have spent it, in my clinical as well as in my administrative roles—trying to bridge that divide, to bring science and caring together.

In my role as a researcher, teacher, practising physician, and founding CEO of Canada's largest mental health and addictions facility, the Centre for Addiction and Mental Health in Toronto, I have been both participant and observer as psychiatry has swung from an obsession with psychoanalysis to its fixation with the chemistry of the brain. Essentially, psychiatry has exchanged one single-minded fixation for another.

When I began in my career, many psychiatrists were psychoanalysts. What they cared about was the unconscious sexual development, the drives, and the transference that evolved in therapy; some even believed that the drug revolution was a form of resistance to treatment. They clung rigidly to a model of human behaviour, just as their forebears had. Now the scientific white coats who dominate the profession are making the same mistake; they are sweeping aside the profound insights of Freud's intellectual descendants to prescribe a pill. Psychiatry, for them, has become just chemistry.

This single-minded thinking ignores how exceedingly complex mental illness is, with no single root cause. Many factors may contribute to the development of illness, including genetic makeup; disorders of chemistry and hormones; and our relationships, personality, attachments to others, life experiences, and sense of meaning or purpose. As well, socioeconomic issues play a role in who becomes ill, and in the course of the illness. Even infectious organisms can cause mental disease: the spirochete bacterium that causes syphilis was responsible for at least 15% of male cases in mental hospitals 100 years ago.

Some mental diseases, which we currently define by their symptoms, may actually be clusters of several diseases. Schizophrenia—a term first used by the Swiss psychiatrist Eugen Bleuler in the early 1900s—is such an example.[4] Characterized by auditory hallucinations, delusions, and a breakdown of thought processes, schizophrenia is very likely a syndrome, made up of several illnesses, rather than a single disease. We just have not yet been able to tease apart or fully understand its underlying causes.

It's as if we were studying jaundice 100 years ago. Doctors then knew that the skin turned colour and that the liver was involved. What they didn't know was that liver disease could be caused by many things—alcoholic cirrhosis, cancer, and infection, for instance—that were later discovered to cause the clinical symptoms of jaundice. In other words, there are many routes to a person displaying the clinical state. This is as true for mental illness as it is for medical conditions such as jaundice. Schizophrenia appears to have a strong biological base, whereas other conditions that we treat are more related to the person's temperament, personality, or life events—some forms of depression, personality disorders, and posttraumatic stress disorder are examples of these.

Many factors, physiological and psychosocial, can contribute to mental illness. These variables interact differently in different patients. No two people, even those suffering from the same mental illness, are the same, so a treatment that works for one patient may not work for another. We do need scientific evidence to help determine not only what the best treatments are but also how to tailor these to each specific person.

Fortunately, we now have powerful and proven treatments for mental illness, such as medications, electroconvulsive therapy, specific forms of psychotherapy, and rehabilitation. We also know that medicines combined with psychotherapy are often better than either one alone. The clinician has a range of theoretical models and treatments to apply to people who are ill. The issue is what mix of approaches works for any specific patient. The effective clinician will select the model that will be most beneficial to the patient, rather than trying to fit the patient to the model. (Like visitors of Procrustes, of Greek legend, who had to stretch or cut off their legs to fit his bed, our models are never perfect, but we must be guided by the patient's needs, not our own.)

There was a time when psychiatry did not hold itself accountable for the outcomes of therapy. Some practitioners were just not interested; others held themselves above the rules of science. Some argued it was just too difficult to measure outcomes from such complicated treatments. Yet now we can prove that powerful new drugs can improve the lives of many people with mental illnesses. Even with talk therapy, we can measure outcomes to tell whether therapies are effective or not—and they are, when applied well and for the right disorders. Clinical research on outcomes has been changing the practice of psychiatry. Yet it seems, in my experience, that many private psychiatrists aren't listening to the evidence. They continue to use therapies that don't work, rather than ones that do. All too often, the type of treatment they offer depends on their training and their ideas about what mental illness is, rather than on the needs of the patient. One psychiatrist might think it's a chemical problem; another swears it's something hidden in the unconscious; still another blames the parents or conditioning. Changes are needed in both understanding and accountability. Our patients deserve better than a simplistic, one-model approach.

Fads come and go, but one thing in the doctor-patient relationship never changes: the need for a patient to connect on a human level with the therapist. No matter what combination of approaches a psychiatrist chooses, we can never overlook the real therapeutic value of empathy, or sitting and being with a person through a very difficult moment. In a world fixated on the extraordinary power of drugs to cure or relieve mental illness, it's easy to forget the human side of therapy. Psychiatrists can become primarily drug dispensers, and if this happens, a significant part of therapy is lost. In other words, science is necessary, but it's not enough. A relevant modern psychiatry must fuse the scientific method with caring.

• • •

This book is a memoir of a life's work, focusing on key moments that have contributed to my understanding and advocacy of the mentally ill and my vision for their care. I was initially drawn to psychiatry by the plight of severely ill patients. But then, as a student, I came under the influence of several outstanding mentors, who guided me in developing an individualized, multifaceted understanding of each person, combining all data based on enquiry. The treatment approaches that followed from this have involved a fusion of the science with a caring humanism that involves increased accountability outside the profession. During my career I have been able to apply this approach to people who are suffering, to programs of care, and to academic departments and hospitals. These varied experiences have permitted me to examine what is good about my profession and what is currently profoundly off track.

CHAPTER I
A Naive Beginning

I grew up in Winnipeg, one of three sons of Jewish immigrant parents scrambling to make a living after World War II. I was an unlikely candidate for psychiatry. In school, I spent more time on the basketball court than in the library. In fact, my overwhelming obsession in high school was trying to figure out how our Hebrew School basketball team could beat the Mennonites, who all seemed like giants to me. (We never did beat them.) I was an ordinary teenager at St. John's High School, and I showed no special affinity to anyone who was different or socially awkward. It was ironic in many ways, because my family, as immigrant Jews, knew what it was to be excluded.

My home was in the north end of the city, where immigrant, working-class Jews, Slavs, Scandinavians, and Germans set up small houses and struggled to make new lives. North Enders were outsiders to start with, as far as the city's Anglo-Saxon Protestant establishment was concerned, but Jews were doubly affected, excluded not only by the establishment but also by the other Eastern European immigrants in the neighbourhood. As children, we were taught to be careful on the streets, and to ward against possible anti-Semitic acts, which did occur from time to time. When I was seven or eight, I was the target of taunting on my way to school. This double dose of prejudice formed the backdrop for the Jewish community where I grew up. We could feel the painful tinge of prejudice every day: it was us versus them, and it only made us more eager to belong.

My mother, Jenny, arrived in Canada as a toddler during World War I. She had been born in 1913 in Mezrich, a Jewish community about 90 kilometres north of Lublin, in what is now eastern Poland

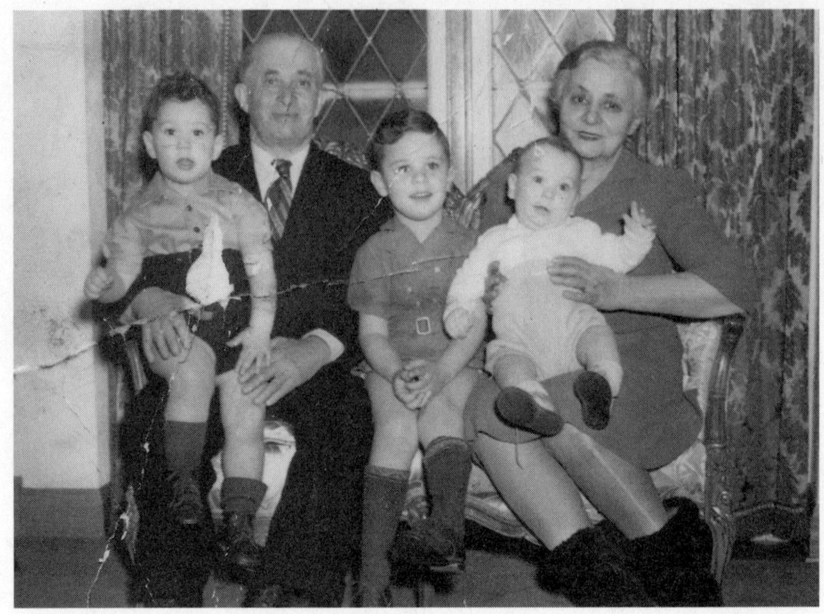

Paul on his grandfather's knee, Barry on his grandmother's, and Marvin in the middle (circa 1950).

but was then Russia. Her father, Yehoshua (Sam), an officer's aide in the Russian army, had moved with his wife, Eda, and young daughter to Canada to avoid a second term of duty. Once he landed in Winnipeg, Sam became a junk peddler. In his horse-drawn cart, he drove out to the farms and towns around Winnipeg, buying things from the farmers and townspeople, loading them into his cart, and bringing them back to Winnipeg to sell. The horse, along with some chickens, lived beside the abundant vegetable garden of Sam and Eda's house on Alfred Avenue.

After finishing high school, my mother went to secretarial college and worked as a stenographer at a law firm that would one day help remove the quota system from the University of Manitoba's Faculty of Medicine. She also taught piano and played a big community role as president of the Young Women's Hebrew Association. As an only child, Mother remained devoted to her parents, who often called on her to help negotiate their complicated new life in Manitoba.

My father, Saul, moved to Winnipeg in 1927 from Gac, a very small shtetl northeast of Warsaw. He had apprenticed as a barrel maker in Poland and, after moving to Winnipeg at age 20, found work as an upholsterer, eventually setting up his own small business.

My parents met through a young adults' group and they had three sons: my older brother, Marvin; my younger brother, Barry; and me. Jewish tradition was an integral part of our family life. Most Friday evenings and every Jewish holiday were spent at my grandparents' Alfred Avenue home, where we would feast on my grandmother's delicious meals: melt-off-the-bone chicken with potatoes, smothered with huge amounts of chicken fat and onions, or cabbage rolls, *varenickes*, and *varnishkes*. I remember Babba as an expansive woman—both physically large and with a big personality, with a real flair for drama.

Babba never lost her love of a theatrical response. Later in life, when she was in her late 80s and she could no longer care for herself, it fell to my brother Marvin, the only one of us boys living in Winnipeg, to tell her she was moving to a nursing home. Marvin took her to Kildonan Park, her favourite spot, to break the news. When he started to explain what was to happen, she threw herself onto the ground and started screaming, "Look what my grandson is trying to do to me! He's killing me!" Eventually, she did move and she thrived in the Sharon Home.

Religion was important to our grandfather, our zaidy. He attended daily services at his beloved shul, a small, orthodox synagogue on Manitoba Avenue, and there he had a place of honour, facing the congregants. Zaidy ruled the roost, at shul and at home, largely with kindness and compassion, and he loved to indulge his grandsons. If, for example, we wanted to play football on the Sabbath when we really shouldn't, he would bend the rules for us.

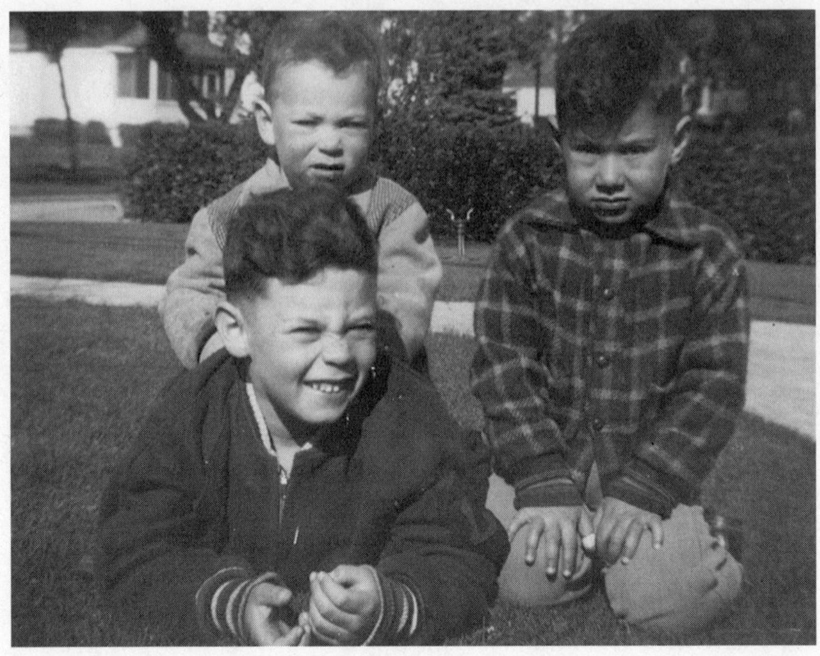

Garfinkel brothers: Barry on Marvin, and Paul to the right (Winnipeg, 1953).

We adhered to the rules of kashruth, the Jewish dietary laws, and keeping kosher was important to our family. I took it so seriously that the first time I ate nonkosher food, with friends at a Chinese restaurant, I threw up in the sink when I got home—an early marker for me of culture's profound effects on our bodies.

Smoking was an issue. Both my parents were heavy smokers, but smoking was forbidden during the two-day Rosh Hashanah holiday or on Yom Kippur. But these holidays had a hierarchy, with Yom Kippur being the holiest day. So the family found a compromise: smoking would be allowed on the New Year's days but not on Yom Kippur. At age 12 or 13, to assert my allegiance to my parents—or just for the joy of breaking a rule—I started to smoke on New Year's, even though I didn't smoke the rest of the year.

My father strongly identified with being Jewish—he rooted for great Jewish baseball players like Al Rosen, the "Hebrew Hammer." Rosen was a four-time all-star and was a tough amateur boxer who took on anyone who insulted his religion. In elections, Father always followed the Jewish candidate, which in North Winnipeg usually meant supporting the socialist Co-operative Commonwealth Federation (CCF) or, later, the left-leaning New Democratic Party. The exception to Father supporting the Jewish candidate was if the Jewish candidate represented the Communist Party; he would never vote for the Communists.

But my father wasn't observant. He didn't keep kosher out of the home. He attended synagogue with us only on the High Holidays, not on the Sabbath. He quietly participated in the Passover Seders, led by my grandfather, but he would try to speed things up so we could watch the Stanley Cup playoffs. Zaidy, being indulgent with his grandsons, would hurry through the last half of the Seder ritual so we could get to our hockey game.

A humble man, my father loved the underdog, especially when it came to the Brooklyn Dodgers, the perennial losers until they won the World Series in 1955. For me, the love of the underdog encapsulated what it felt like to be Jewish in North America, at least in the way we were brought up in that era. The message was that, even when you're up against a tough opponent, you fight hard. It's about persistence in the face of adversity, and about honour and dignity as much as it is about winning and money.

My father was proud to provide for the family, and although he splurged occasionally, he watched his budget carefully. One time he bought a maroon Ford Mercury without a radio so he could have a cheaper American one installed the next time we drove to Fargo, North Dakota. On the way home from that trip, the customs officer at the border asked whether we had bought anything. No, Father answered. From the back seat, I piped up: "What about the car radio?" My father had to pay the duty, and I was not allowed to use my new baseball mitt for a week. I was only seven and didn't understand why I had been punished; we had been taught to always be honest.

My father was a kind man, but he didn't show much emotion, except when he was watching sporting events. Maybe that's why I loved watching our local football team, the Blue Bombers, with him. Sports connected us. When I was in grade three, the school needed bases for baseball games. As Father was an upholsterer, he volunteered to make them. I was proud to play on those bases throughout public school, and Father was thrilled to receive a letter from our class thanking him.

Providing for the family, though, was hard for him. The upholstery business hurt his back, and after a couple of unsuccessful stints in business, he spent four years without a job. I later learned he supported our family by playing poker, a game where his cool demeanour came in handy. Eventually, he and a friend bought a small hotel in a seedy part of town. It included a "beer parlour" for men only, a "beverage room" for "ladies and escorts," and a small restaurant. It probably rented rooms by the hour. Business was good—until my father discovered that his friend had betrayed him: he was stealing from the business. They sold the hotel at a profit, and the next year Father bought another hotel with a different partner, and turned it into a success.

My mother never complained, even when my father was unemployed; I only saw her cry once about this, when I was about 15. She worked hard to keep up appearances. The house was spotless, and she covered the furniture in plastic to keep it that way. The plastic came off only when we had company. She made sure we ate properly and dressed reasonably well, even if it was in hand-me-downs or clothes with patches.

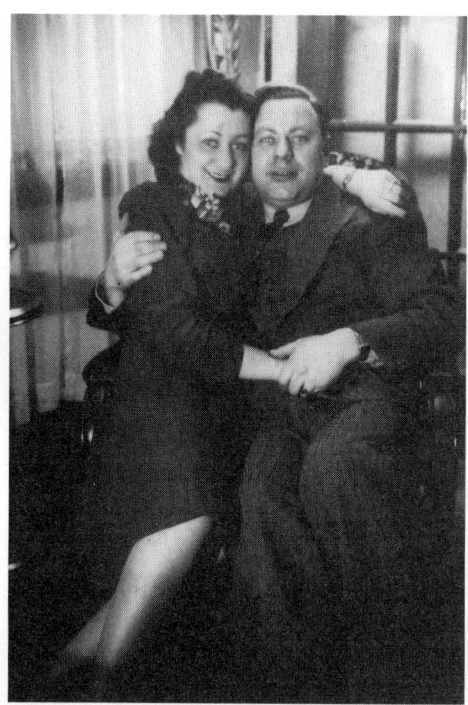

Paul's parents, Jenny and Saul Garfinkel (Winnipeg, early 1940s).

We were overprotected, even by the standards of Jewish North Winnipeg. We weren't even allowed to go to overnight camp. I think my mother was determined to protect us from anything unsafe in the world.

We were a tiny family, but my grandmother Eda's sister, Molly, and her husband, Nathan, lived close by with their two children, Eadie and Gedalyia (Gerry). They were our extended family. Gerry was a real role model for me. He had been the first in our family to go to university, and he had taken a master's degree in agriculture so that he could be of use when he emigrated to Israel, which he planned to do over the coming few years.

The summer I was 13, our family suffered a terrible loss. As I was getting ready to go with my friends to the local public golf course one morning—golf had become my passion, and I even

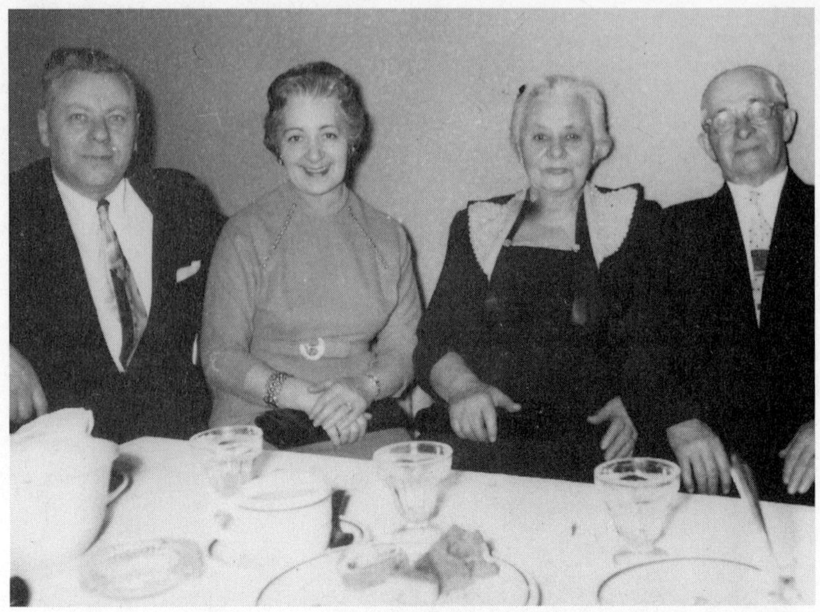

Saul and Jenny Garfinkel with Paul's maternal grandparents, Eda and Sam Cohen (Winnipeg, late 1950s).

caddied in the Canadian Open two years later when it came to Winnipeg—my mother received a telephone call. Her cousin Gerry had been killed in a motor accident when his car was struck head-on on the highway by a drunk driver in a pickup truck coming off a side dirt road.

Gerry's death shook the entire family. We had all been close to Gerry, particularly my mother. He was at every Passover Seder (and it was Gerry who encouraged me to get drunk for the first time at a Seder, when I was nine). This was my first experience with death. Until then, death was an abstract thing, somewhat vague. Death became very real after Gerry was gone, forever.

It must have been a terrible time for my mother. She was in her early 50s, working hard to please parents, husband, and children. With my father out of work, money was tight, and along with Father's back problems, he had high blood sugar, cataracts, and glaucoma. He spent a few nights each week playing poker, then worked the other evenings at the hotel. My brothers and I were all adolescents by then, and beginning to pull away from our mother. Then, in all this, her closest cousin was struck down. I don't know if she became depressed in a clinical sense, but she definitely lost some of her sparkle. Often I felt so sad for her but didn't know how to help.

We were Jews in a city dominated by Anglo-Christians. The student population at school was a mix of nationalities and religions, mostly Ukrainian and Jewish, but our teachers were Anglo-Canadians, often of Scottish descent. So, at gym in grade nine, my Jewish classmates and I practised the schottische, a dance of Romanian origins adapted by the Scottish, along with the other students. We mouthed the Lord's Prayer every morning, and Christmas carols in December. Occasionally, a classmate would remind us that it was the Jews who had killed Christ, but as disconcerting as the accusation was, we tended to shrug it off. It had no meaning to me.

There were some things we didn't do, such as join certain fraternities or, as adults, join social clubs or golf clubs. But that was just the way it was. The Jewish community had evolved its own set of facilities, but outside of the Jewish Community Centre, our family didn't belong to those either. Discussions of firms that restricted employment for Jews were frequent; it was said, for example, that it was hard for Jews to break into Eaton's, a Toronto-based department store chain, or to rise to any prominence at the large central banks. Some law firms and medical clinics were entirely without Jews. We knew of anti-Semitism in the professional schools at the university and in some law firms and group medical practices, but these were disappearing. And all this anti-Semitism did was make me and my brothers try harder.

Naturally, our parents wanted my brothers and me to succeed. And the key to success was education. As children of immigrants, particularly Jewish immigrants, our education was prized not just as a way to cultivate our minds. We were expected to become professionals. Professions were financially secure and highly esteemed, more so than professional sports or the uncertain life of the artist, musician, or teacher. So my older brother, Marvin, was steered to law, and I, as the second son, was directed toward medical school. Marvin eventually became a provincial court judge, a position he filled with distinction. He remained in Winnipeg and with his wife, Merle, raised their three children in a similar manner to our own upbringing. My brother Barry, the real talent in the family, was not only as smart as his brothers but could also play piano, as our mother did. He could dance and paint and draw as well. It was decided that Barry should go into architecture, an honourable profession. But instead, Barry followed me into medical school, specializing in child and adolescent psychiatry. After a period in Toronto, he moved to Brown University in Providence, Rhode Island, and later settled in Minneapolis, Minnesota, where he and his wife, Lili, brought up three daughters.

The only question I really had to concern myself with was what kind of doctor I wanted to be. I got the answer early. My mother used to play mah-jong twice a week with friends, something she looked forward to partly because it gave her an opportunity to boast about her sons. One day when I was eating tinned salmon, I found a tiny bone in it; I removed it, looked it over, then put it on my plate. "Paul is so interested in medicine," I later overheard Mother tell her friends, "he even examined the salmon bone from a clinical point of view. He's just fascinated by these things." I was all of 11 years old. Similarly, when I needed a skin graft to close a wound on my thigh after falling off Marvin's bicycle, which I had taken against instructions, Mother described to her friends how

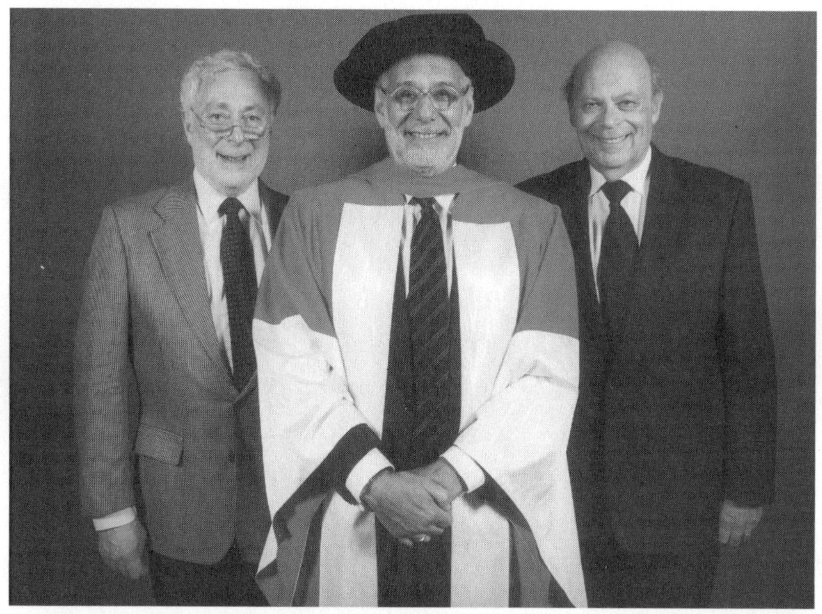

Barry (left) and Marvin (right) with Paul, who is receiving an honorary Doctorate of Science from the University of Manitoba in 2012.

I had asked for a local anesthetic only, so I could watch the surgery. I don't remember it that way, and I'm fairly certain I had no interest in watching.

Still, I accepted my parents' plans for me. I definitely wanted to please them, and I was genuinely interested in how the body worked. And, I wanted to be of use to others. After skipping a grade, I graduated from high school at age 16 and enrolled in a bachelor of science program at my hometown university. I didn't even consider a school away from home—it wasn't in my frame of reference, either emotionally or financially, and I didn't know anyone who had gone away to university.

By the end of my first year, my grades had improved dramatically. It was the first time that grades were important to my future: the competition to get into medical school was intense, and only those with top grades would be admitted—and for me, getting admitted was now all that mattered. The career choice I had initially accepted with mild interest was closer to becoming reality, and I had to deliver. Not only did I study hard to get the grades I needed, I learned that science was the door to admission: it was easier to get a 90% in physics than in literature or philosophy, where the "right" answer is often nebulous.

In retrospect, I can see that the goal-directed culture of premed has a deep flaw. It's too narrowly focused on grades and science. I missed out on studying English and humanities after first-year university, something I consider as a big hole in my education. Particularly for a psychiatrist, a deep appreciation of Shakespeare would be far more valuable than a smattering of knowledge of physics and mathematics. The practice of medicine is a social interaction, an art based on scientific knowledge, so it's important to study both science and the arts. But educators didn't think like that then and many still don't today. The need for top grades sometimes gets in the way of a real education.

Having been an overprotected boy, I had, perhaps unsurprisingly, a narrow view of the world, even by the standards of Jewish Winnipeg of the early 1960s. It wasn't until I got a summer job at Molson Brewery that I saw what "real" life was about. My work mates were mostly uneducated men in their 30s and 40s whose aim seemed to be getting the day's work done, and battling authority by drinking on the job instead of waiting for the break. They whistled at women, cheered for the local baseball team, and had a lot of fun. They took care of their families, especially the one year when they all prepared for a looming strike.

Those men showed me how most people lived. They were about fun, doing the day's work, and not having to always please others and better yourself—they were more about living in the present than the people I knew. They also made me feel, for the first time, that I could belong in a broader world, playing crib and drinking at break or at a baseball game together, and not just in the Jewish cocoon in which I grew up. In many ways, these men were more important to me than the students and teachers at university. Certainly, they taught me a lot more about people than I ever learned in the undergraduate classroom.

CHAPTER 2
Falling for Psychiatry

When it came time to apply to medical school, I had the grades but needed a reference letter. The only practising physician I knew was my family doctor, Dr. Phil Goldstein, a general surgeon and busy clinician. I didn't know much about him, until the day I went to ask him for a letter of recommendation. Just that day he had been given the job of assistant professor at the University of Manitoba's medical school. We had a long chat, and he told me about how, in the 1930s, he had had to leave Winnipeg to study medicine at the University of Saskatchewan, in Saskatoon, because of the quota on the number of Jews who could attend medical school in Manitoba in any given year. Under the rules of the time, the first-year class of 60 students at the University of Manitoba could have a total of four Jews, Eastern Europeans, and women—no more, no matter how qualified they were. It was a humbling story, and a valuable reminder about the challenges an earlier generation of Jews had faced.

I was accepted to the University of Manitoba, and at medical school, I dived into my studies, memorizing every bone in the body and learning about the biochemical pathways. I even won a scholarship in anatomy. I liked anatomy; it was so definite, and that says something about me: I like clarity and order. I was also intrigued by endocrinology, the study of hormones. By then, endocrinology was becoming the study of orderly feedback loops. Cortisol, for example, was known to be a stress hormone, part of the fight-or-flight mechanism that evolved in humans over thousands of years. By the time I was studying medicine, these hormones were being measured and understood. That is not to say that endocrinology didn't have its mysteries. Although endocrinologists could measure hormone levels, they often weren't sure what varying levels meant. For example, what effect did mild but chronic elevation of these stress hormones have on organs? Why did some people with thyroid insufficiency develop a mental illness, the so-called myxedema madness, but not others? What impact did these hormones have on brain function? It was a fascinating line of inquiry, but from a practical point of view, I thought family medicine might be a better bet, especially since a general practitioner could run his own office, without interference from other practitioners. I wasn't in any way oriented to teamwork.

There was one area of medicine that was not on my list: psychiatry. My first exposure to psychiatry, in my second year of medical school, was an introductory lecture on obsessive-compulsive disorder by Dr. Philip Katz, an excellent psychiatrist with an interest in youth. Katz described one woman who was so "obsessional" that she planned in advance her family's meals for each day of the week. I was taken aback. My mother had a weekly meal plan: Monday night was liver, Tuesday was fish, Wednesday meat, Thursday hamburger, Friday chicken, and so on. How could this be an illness? I could not take seriously any line of thinking that would suggest my unsuspecting mother was mentally ill. Rather than being intrigued, I came away from that lecture a skeptic.

At the end of the 1960s, when I was in medical school, psychiatry was still a new branch of medicine, and it was under attack both from within and from without the medical profession. The brain was still a black box. We didn't know much about what was going on inside; the brain imaging we know today hadn't yet been invented. Psychiatrists were just beginning to use seemingly effective drugs or therapies to treat conditions like depression and schizophrenia, but much of what was practised was not based on scientific evidence. Some of the psychological therapies were not proven to be effective; others would be confirmed by scientific studies, but only years later. The field was in a furor.

The psychoanalysts who dominated US academia were under attack because their theories sounded so unusual, so outside the frame of reference of medicine. People were always asking, "Does psychotherapy work?" There was no answer at that point; good studies didn't exist. We were far from the gold standard of randomized controlled trials for psychotherapies. On the other side of the medical spectrum were those psychiatrists who were interested in medication, brain surgery, and heavy doses of insulin to induce comas, often with unpredictable effects. Both groups were looked down upon by their medical colleagues.

Meanwhile, psychiatrists in Winnipeg seemed to have little interest in researching the new drugs that were being developed, though they did use them in treatments. Rather, they saw their role as describing what they saw and helping people cope with illnesses the other doctors didn't understand and could not cure.[1]

Psychiatry, from my point of view, was a profession that appeared to be going nowhere. Most of my fellow medical students saw it the same way. In the late 1960s, only 5% of medical students chose psychiatry as a specialty (a figure that hasn't changed much since then). It was the outcast of the medical profession.[2]

Only in my third year of medical school would my attitude toward psychiatry begin to shift. The previous summer I had married Dorothy, my high-school sweetheart. To earn extra money, I did physical examinations at the local mental hospital, the Psychopathic Institute (PI), earlier known as the Winnipeg Psychopathic Hospital, which opened in 1919 in response to the casualties of World War I.[3] Two evenings a week I would go in for four hours and examine the new patients. But because it was a relatively long-stay site, "business" was slow; so slow that I had lots of time just to be with the patients. These people, suffering with psychoses or severe depression, made an indelible impression on me.[4]

On my second night at the PI, a 19-year-old man, just two years younger than me, was admitted. Tall and extremely thin, with significant acne, he had been subdued with heavy doses of chlorpromazine. The patient's auditory hallucinations had been telling him to run off and harm himself so he could reach a better world. As I listened to him, I was stunned by how closely he reminded me, in physical appearance and in his speech, of Bobby, an old high-school classmate.[5] Bobby was a brilliant but introverted boy who was absent from school for months at a time, institutionalized at the asylum. I never tried to befriend him or even get to know him, nor did I protect him when classmates teased him; I even joined in. I was comfortable with what I knew, and uncomfortable with anything and anybody I didn't understand. Now that I saw how genuine and severe an illness schizophrenia was, I shuddered with embarrassment at my teenaged ignorance, and at how cruel I had been to tease and exclude my classmate at school.

Many of the women who came to the PI were suffering from depression. The Mennonite communities around Winkler, about an hour's drive southwest of Winnipeg, contributed their share of cheerless, hard-working women struggling to cope. Emily came to the PI when she was almost 50 years old, after one of her sons had been killed in a farm accident. She had once had a lively spirit, loving to create with her hands and imagination, but she now seemed old and worn out, broken. Still, Emily read a great deal in spite of a busy household of six children and a husband who viewed life as a hard task to be silently endured. To fight her depression, she was given electroconvulsive therapy (ECT) rather than antidepressant drugs, which at that time had many side effects. Gradually, she responded to ECT; over several weeks, her depression lifted. She was still sad and grieving, Emily told me, but she could distinguish this from depression, which involved the loss of will, motivation, and energy, and her body slowing completely. I was struck by her differentiation of the two states, which, I thought, spoke to her intelligence and sensitivity. Nevertheless, I wondered what long-term benefit we provided Emily by curing her depression, only to send her home to an aloof, angry husband who didn't believe in counselling. Emily shook me up: in that period of the 1960s, there was tremendous antagonism toward ECT. I saw first-hand and for the first time how powerful ECT could be in removing depressive symptoms, but also how worrisome it is to treat just the symptoms and not the whole person in her environment.

Another woman who made a big impression on me was not a patient but a nurses' aide. Lisa was in her late 20s, slight and frail, with long, straight hair. We used to chat in the evenings, and she was clearly ill: she hallucinated and often heard voices commenting on her activities. These voices began in a very frightening manner when she was in her teens, living with her chaotic, abusive family in the southern United States. The voices had been so upsetting that she had cut her wrists and landed in a state hospital. But Lisa hated her experience there and the psychotropic drugs that made her sluggish and heavy. So she avoided further treatment. When I met her, almost a decade later, she had developed not only insight into the nature of her hallucinations but also an equanimity—she had learned to live with them, to not be bothered by them, and even at times to enjoy their company.

Lisa taught me a valuable lesson: that not everyone with symptoms needs treatment. At some point in our lives, we all have some symptom or other. Problems often go with strengths. Only when the symptom or symptoms impair the quality of a person's life does he or she need treatment. It is the task of the psychiatrist, then, to help a patient live a rich life, a life of dignity, in spite of chronic illness. In the final analysis, we all have to play the hand we are dealt.

By the fourth year, during my clinical clerkship, I began to seriously consider psychiatry as a career, largely because of the patients and the doctors I'd met at the PI. The PI had been a part-time job. Now I had to spend a few weeks on psychiatry as a clinical clerk. My friend Calvin Gutkin and I were assigned to the local veterans' hospital, Deer Lodge, where our patients were veterans of World War II, many of whom could be described as shell-shocked or as having neurasthenia, a disorder characterized by fatigue and weakness. (Today we would label these conditions as posttraumatic stress disorder.) These men had often served Canada with dignity, yet paid a huge price, suffering from depression, family breakup, and alcohol misuse.

One of our patients was Ben, a war veteran in his early 50s. Ben had been unable to speak for 20 years. When he tried to talk, words came out in a faint whisper. Physicians could find nothing physically wrong with him. Calvin and I were determined to get Ben speaking again. We decided to interview Ben with the aid of sodium amytal, the so-called truth serum. In theory, the drug, once injected, would disinhibit Ben, overcoming the conflict that kept him from speaking and thereby permitting his normal voice to return.

Once we had convinced the attending doctor, Gordon Lamberd, that this was a reasonable trial, we assembled the syringe, the medication, and all the accompanying equipment. As we approached Ben in his hospital bed, Calvin directed me to take the syringe. Too late did I realize that I had never administered a medication by needle, nor did I know how to find the vein. I awkwardly started jabbing around. Unfortunately for Ben, I kept missing the mark. Calvin started to giggle, then laugh, and soon had to remove himself from the room. I was left alone with Ben.

At that point, Ben began to speak in a normal voice; he spoke of his great appreciation for what we were doing and for helping him return to a normal life. Ben continued to speak normally for the next seven hours. He went to sleep that evening and when he awoke, he fell back into the hysterical conversion disorder that prohibited his normal speech.

Calvin and I were both very excited. None of the sodium amytal had gone into Ben's vein, yet his voice had returned to normal. What was the potential if the medicine had actually worked? The next day, Calvin successfully administered the medication intravenously. Imagine our confusion—and disappointment—when this had no effect on Ben's speaking voice; he continued speaking only in a whisper.

This was amazing to me. We had had two trials in two days. In one, the medicine did not reach the man's brain, but Ben could speak for a while. In the other, the medicine did reach the brain, with no benefit. It was an aha moment for me. Ben could temporarily respond to hope, as well as to the significant attention of two enthusiastic, blundering young medical students. At the same time, some powerful things were sustaining the illness, something we were not appreciating. What were they in Ben's case—relationships, finances, sense of purpose, anger, helplessness? I just don't know.

Ben was a mystery, a challenge that I found irresistible. I kept thinking about the other patients too—Lisa, who found a way to live with the voices inside her; Emily, who showed courageous insight into her depression; and, of course, the young man who reminded me of my high-school classmate Bobby. These men and women, and their struggles, pulled me into psychiatry, a line of work that was at the time considered to be the outcast of the medical profession. They had changed me. I was no longer the boy who teased a socially awkward fellow student who had just come home from the hospital. Now, unlike some of my classmates at medical

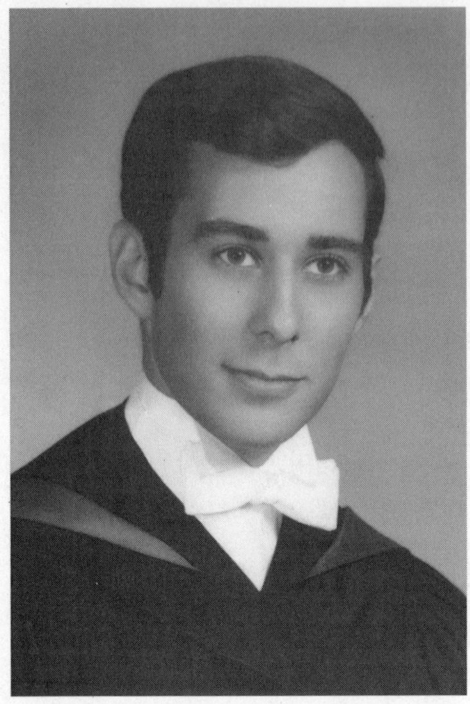

Medical graduation, University of Manitoba, in 1969.

school, I was starting to feel comfortable with people who had fully developed psychosis or serious depression.

Maybe it was the respect for the underdog instilled in me by my family. Psychiatric patients were underdogs; through no fault of their own, they were disadvantaged and did not belong. In many ways, though, they were worse off than the underdog, who sometimes triumphs in the end. Mentally ill patients at that time had little chance of ever being fully accepted again by their communities. They were defined by their illnesses—"He's schizophrenic" or "She's had a nervous breakdown"—and they were generally shunned. If their illnesses were chronic, family and friends had often long since deserted them.

I was intrigued by their cases and touched by their condition. Ben taught me that the field had real intellectual challenges. I could see a future for myself in this burgeoning but chaotic field. The patients were underserved by the medical world; there was a real need that perhaps I could fill. Nonetheless, as I considered my future, I felt ambivalent. Psychiatry was appealing because it was a multifaceted discipline: many factors—from genetics, hormones, and medical conditions to culture, relationships, family, and early experiences—played a role in the development of mental illnesses. One could take a broad view of health and illness that was not common in those days, even in general medicine. On the other hand, did I want to spend a lifetime tackling such complex puzzles as Ben's? I had been around long enough to realize that psychiatrists, like the patients they treat, were held in low esteem. I wanted to impress my hard-working parents, who had sacrificed so much of their own happiness to give their boys a chance to succeed. How could I do that in such a marginalized branch of medicine, scorned by doctors and even by medical students? I hesitated. But I had one advantage. I had graduated from medicine at age 23, so I figured that I could afford a trial year. I would try psychiatry. If I didn't like it, I could always transfer to internal medicine, which could lead to endocrinology.

Internship

Dorothy and I were both eager to leave Winnipeg and, like many young Canadian doctors just after Expo 67, I wanted to go to Montreal. I had applied to be a rotating intern to both Royal Victoria Hospital and Montreal General Hospital, but I didn't get accepted at either. I was extremely disappointed, but when a classmate recommended I apply to Toronto Western because it was a good community hospital, I did. I was accepted there, and within a few weeks, Dorothy and I had moved to the High Park area of Toronto; Dorothy got a position teaching in nearby Etobicoke, a borough just west of the Humber River.

The psychiatric patients at Toronto Western were fascinating. I remember one young woman, an attractive university graduate in her mid-20s, who had developed a habit of going to the seedier bars in Toronto, ordering a double Dewar's on the rocks, and waiting for someone to pick her up and take her home. It didn't make sense. She came from a loving family, and yet she ended up in hospital after overdosing one night, unable to deal with the breakup with her boyfriend, a responsible and caring young man. I was worried when the attending staff advised me to use medication sparingly and to encourage her to talk. I knew this was supposed to settle her, but deep in my heart I wondered how this could change such a repetitive and obviously harmful behaviour pattern. I felt woefully inadequate to help this young woman, but I was intrigued. Somewhere in psychiatry, clearly, there were pathways to understanding people that far surpassed my natural intuition about human behaviour.

Then there was a young man, a student of English literature, who was preoccupied with the number 27 because it represented the "trinity of trinities." He told me he was going to die in a car crash on Toronto's Highway 27 on his 27th birthday, which was approaching. Not knowing how to deal with this, and because he was all alone in the city, I had him come back to the hospital the night before his birthday. I admitted him for 36 hours—until the risk had passed. He may have had a crummy birthday, but at least he was alive. And I thought how great it would be to know how to really help these people.

Late in the fall of 1969, about five months after arriving in Toronto, I sent off an application to the University of Toronto's psychiatric residency program. I kept telling myself it was worth a try; I could switch to internal medicine after a year if I hated it. Weeks later I received a letter from Vivian Rakoff, the director of postgraduate education for the University of Toronto's Department of Psychiatry, in my mailbox.

"Congratulations," the letter read. "You've been accepted into the psychiatry residency at the University of Toronto." It seemed odd: I hadn't even gone for a personal interview. Nevertheless, I resolved to do the residency, though I was still so unsure of the wisdom of my decision that I didn't tell anyone at the Western until months later, after I had finished my pediatrics rotation at the Hospital for Sick Children. Then I grew a beard. I suppose I hoped it would make me and my decision look serious, but when I told colleagues that I was going to be a psychiatrist, they laughed, saying, "You? I never thought of you as crazy!" I took it in stride when a senior physician needled me: "Is that a Freudian or a rabbinical beard?" I was able to reply with some confidence, "Both."

CHAPTER 3
A Profession Split

In 1969, in my last year of medical school in Winnipeg, I had a little taste of the tumult that was engulfing my future profession. The head of the Psychiatry Department was Dr. George Sisler, an old-school psychiatrist who wore a white coat and carried a stethoscope in his pocket, as if to align himself with the other medical practitioners. Sisler ran a biologically oriented department that valued careful observation and description of mental illnesses before selecting medication or ECT and supportive therapy.

In the late 1960s, a group of young psychiatrists came home from academic centres in the United States, where they had picked up the ideas and practices of dynamic psychiatry. These brash young psychiatrists wore sports jackets and ties, not white coats. They had studied Freud's theoretical model, and now they spoke an entirely different language from the one the white coats understood.

The psychodynamic psychiatrists would talk about the "mechanisms of defence," the unconscious ways we keep conflict and anxiety out of our awareness. For example, "projection" refers to attributing to another person thoughts and feelings that are our own, as when a patient says one thing ("He really hates me") but means another ("I really hate him"). Psychoanalysts referred to "splitting" as an unconscious defensive strategy that aims to keep us ignorant of feelings in ourselves that we're unable to tolerate. They'd use terms like "isolation of affect" to describe how patients carve off feelings from the thoughts accompanying them, or "displacement" to describe how people redirect feelings from their intended target to a more neutral one, such as kicking the cat instead of the neighbour.

The surgeons and internists didn't know what to make of it. To be honest, neither did I.[1] During my internship at the Toronto Western I had spent one month in the Psychiatric Department, and a second month in the Emergency Department, where day and night we saw patients with all kinds of mental problems—severe depression, suicide attempts, delirium associated with medical illness, LSD overdoses. When the psychiatrists sat down at the lunch table, other medical doctors gave them a cool reception. I felt a little bit deflated; after all, I was still ambivalent about my career choice, and I suspected that the other doctors were uneasy around psychiatrists because of their association with the mentally ill.

Little did I know that their derision was rooted in the contempt many physicians had for psychodynamic thinking, which they deemed not only nonscientific but fraudulent. As an intern working day and night, I had no time to keep up with the bitter debates ripping apart my chosen profession. All I knew was that psychiatrists, no matter their approach, were clearly outsiders in the medical world. We were not like the other medical doctors.

And within the field of psychiatry itself the divisions were percolating. There were the descriptive organic psychiatrists, like Sisler, who depended on careful observation to describe what they saw, and looked to medicines or ECT to provide help. Then came Freud's followers, the psychodynamic/analytic psychiatrists who probed unconscious drives, usually sexual or aggressive ones. But this was by no means the only divide among those in the profession. The proliferation of therapies cropping up in the late 1960s was nearly overwhelming, and it was certainly confusing.

From the world of psychology emerged several approaches, sometimes at war with one another. In client-centred therapy, launched by Carl Rogers in the 1940s, a therapist who is nonjudgmental, empathic, and genuine permits patients to explore feelings and behaviours in a nondirective manner.[2] William Glasser

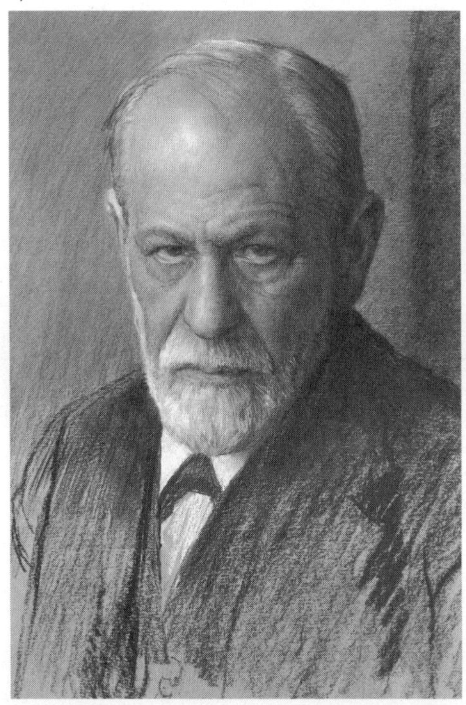

Sigmund Freud, a neurologist by training, became the founder of psychoanalysis. Courtesy Freud Archives.

developed reality therapy in the mid-1960s, promoting his view that mental health is mostly a matter of personal choice. Gestalt therapy emphasized the role of emotion and perception, and the relationship of the self to another, in the moment. Fritz Perls, a German-born psychiatrist, and his wife, Laura, developed many of the techniques involved and even a "prayer" (I do my thing and you do your thing; I am not in this world to live up to your expectations; and so on). In the early 1970s, Gestalt therapy was gaining ground in Toronto. It was all about you, the individual, and your goals and desires relative to your group.

Group psychotherapies were gaining popularity too.[3] Family therapy was supposed to relieve emotional distress and promote the mental health of family members.[4] If you read psychologist Rollo May's 1969 book *Love and Will*, you could look at anxiety from an

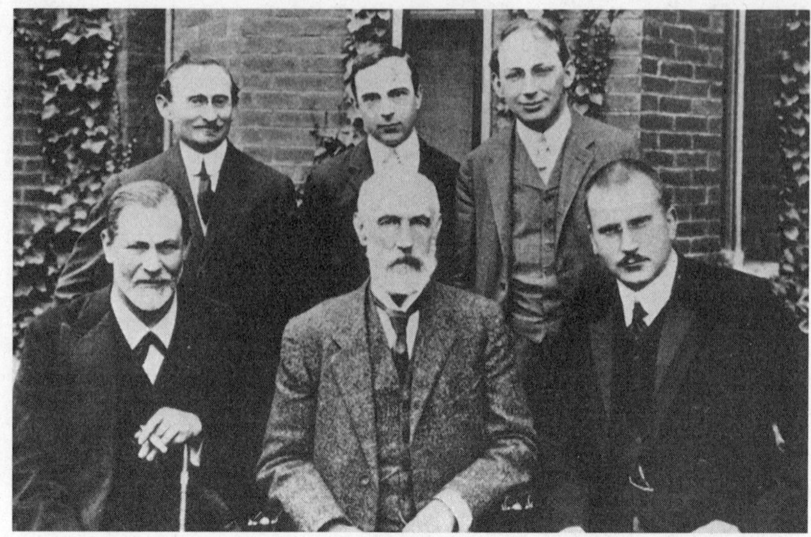

Freud's trip to North America. He visited Clark University in 1909. Front row: Sigmund Freud (left) and Carl Jung (right), and between them the president of the university. Back row: A.A. Brill, Ernest Jones, and Sandor Ferenczi. Courtesy Freud Museum, London.

existential point of view. Adlerians emphasized significance, security, and inferiority. Hypnosis was supposed to change behaviour. Psychedelic drugs could open up the psyche. Behaviour therapies could stop you from repetitive unwanted behaviours. And cognitive behaviour therapy, which was being developed by American psychiatrist Aaron Beck, would soon prove to be a success.

Beneath all this was an uncertainty about whether talk therapy worked at all. Hans Eysenck, an influential German-born, British-based behavioural psychologist, had published a highly discussed paper in the 1950s that asked the critical question, does psychotherapy work?[5] He studied the literature published to the time and demonstrated that the effects of dynamic therapies for "neurosis" were less favourable than for general practitioner–administered care, hospital-based treatments, or eclectic psychological support.

As Eysenck put it, his data "fail to prove that psychotherapy, Freudian or otherwise, facilitates the recovery of neurotic patients." His book spurred controversy, but he would go on to publish another paper nine years later showing essentially the same results. He felt that dynamically oriented therapists were administering ineffective treatments. This work prompted much research on treatment effectiveness and patient selection, but in 1969, I believed that Eysenck had a point: all this emphasis on talking about one's problems could just be a waste of time. Yet teachers who I respected said otherwise.

I was in no position to know from direct observation because as interns we were rotating to other medical departments and were not with any patient long enough to really see the impact of dynamic therapy. I was confused. The late 1960s were about "going your own way," especially if it defied authority. But there was so little science, and what there was was of such poor quality (the psychotherapy researcher Hans Strupp blasted Esyenck for his reliance on poor science). Who knew what was right for our patients?

If it was confusing for psychiatrists, it had to have been confusing for patients or families looking for help. The practitioners of various forms of talk therapy didn't feel they had to prove its effectiveness. Evidence apparently didn't matter. There was no way of knowing what worked and what didn't, and so many different types of treatments were heralded as the next major cure. People were being treated by ineffective means, or hurt by the treatments they received.

The crux of the problem was a huge gap between traditional methods of psychiatric care and the application of scientific inquiry into the treatment of mental disorders. This gap has existed since the beginning of modern psychiatry, when two very different models of care dominated the treatment of mental illness: the asylum, and Freud's theories of the unconscious. As different as these approaches were from each other, they had one thing in common: neither submitted itself to the rigours of the scientific method, which would transform most other parts of medicine. It would take almost 100 years for psychiatry to catch up. And the result, as I could see when I entered the field, was a chaotic proliferation of competing theories and methods for treating mental disorders.

In looking back at the birth of modern psychiatry in the asylum and particularly in psychoanalytic theory, one can discern a similarly fertile theoretical period, much of it born of disputes between competing ideas.

The Birth of Modern Psychiatry

Asylums emerged in the late 18th century as a humane approach to treating problems like depression and schizophrenia—as illnesses.[6] Vincenzo Chiarugi, as director of the Santa Dorotea hospital in Florence, outlawed chains of restraint in the 1780s. Jean-Baptiste Pussin and Philippe Pinel in France famously unchained the patients in the Bicêtre and Saltpêtrière in the early 1790s.[7] In the United Kingdom, William Tuke, a coffee and tea merchant, opened the York Retreat in 1796. Although he was known among fellow Quakers for stern self-discipline and high moral standards, Tuke treated the mentally ill with respect and kindness. York Retreat emphasized personal relationships as a healing influence, as well as the importance of useful occupation, the quality of the physical environment, and self-discipline. It was a revolution in mental health, termed "moral therapy."

By the mid-19th century, asylums were booming as a place to house, clothe, and feed the insane. Toronto's own Provincial Lunatic Asylum opened in 1850, with great expectations. The architect, John George Howard, was a social progressive who believed patients with depression and schizophrenia would improve in an idyllic environment that included fresh air and healthy work in the gardens. The early advocates of the asylum were so optimistic, they thought they could cure mental illness. In the mid-1800s in the United States, it was common to claim 70 to 90% cure rates. Dorothea Dix, a leading American proponent of asylum care, claimed that severe mental illness, when treated early, was as easily cured as the common cold.

However, asylums served another, less noble goal: patients were separated from society, in an institution, out of sight of the public, who feared and misunderstood them. The inmates (they considered themselves more prisoners than patients) could be housed, clothed, and fed, and the population as a whole could be spared regular encounters with members of this group, who were both not understood and feared. Politicians and bureaucrats, mindful of the public purse, jammed mentally ill patients into rooms designed for far fewer people.

In these crowded conditions, administering moral treatment wasn't feasible, so asylums resigned themselves to simply housing chronically ill patients. Fewer and fewer people were sent home. The conditions at these institutions became increasingly deplorable. Medical treatments such as bloodletting, cold baths, laxatives, and morphine were introduced. Sedatives such as chloral hydrate (by the 1870s) and barbiturates (just after 1900) were administered for sedation, even though they did nothing to relieve the florid symptoms of psychosis.

By 1900, the asylum doctors' early optimism had vanished. Psychiatrists had begun to view the seriously ill as having hereditary degenerative diseases. They started to look for outward deformities to indicate the inner degeneration that was to follow. This was particularly significant when a young man was to choose a spouse, because heredity meant the condition was irreversible and would be apparent in future offspring. This fear of mental illness in future generations helped spur the eugenics movement of the early 20th century, which initially isolated mentally ill people, and then sterilized them.

A History of Schism: Freud and Psychoanalytic Theory

Just when the asylums were seen as hopeless for mentally ill patients, Sigmund Freud revolutionized the practice of psychiatry. Freud, a neurologist and not from the asylum tradition, invented an entirely new approach, talk therapy, to probe the unconscious part of the mind, where feelings and ideas were silently guiding everyday behaviour.

Freud had been greatly influenced by neurologists who set up offices to treat people, mainly women, with "nervous disorders," including "hysteria." One such neurologist was Jean-Martin Charcot, in France. Charcot thought "hysteria," manifested as episodes of paralysis, blindness, muteness, and other somatic symptoms, was an inherited nerve disease. To diagnose hysteria, Charcot tested the patient to see if she was hypnotizable. Freud studied with Charcot in Paris in 1895, and when he returned to Vienna he hypnotized his early patients and applied electric currents. Later, Freud came up with a different theory about hysteria: he proposed that it was rooted in unconscious conflicts rather than in weak nerves. He believed hysterical symptoms developed when painful memories were converted into bodily symptoms.

Freud thought that symptoms and illnesses could be the result of highly significant and traumatic events that had been actively pushed into the unconscious. This was not normal forgetting but an active repression. Freud claimed that by using free association, which meant the patient was to say whatever came to mind with as little self-censorship as possible, or through the interpretation of dreams, in lengthy sessions conducted with the patient lying on the couch, he could raise the noxious ideas to the surface and, by having the patients incorporate and then accept these thoughts and feelings in a safe setting, cure them of mental disease.

Freud's early work borrowed heavily from others, as you would expect. Charcot's student Pierre Janet wrote about unconscious processes, as had many others. However, Freud made it acceptable to examine the mechanisms of the mind. He rejected the religious-based mind cures that were popular at the time as an affront to science and reason. He infused the field and its practitioners with an optimism for psychological treatments, and he hoped to develop his theories into a science.

Many of Freud's theories have become staples of our popular culture—the unconscious, repression, the Oedipus complex, and the reformulation of our basic selves into the id, the ego, and the superego. However, his impact would be far greater than these popular theories. He made us appreciate that we, as human beings, are far more complex than we know; it is the parts of us we do not know that can cause the most trouble in our lives and our relationships.

Freud's ideas were controversial from the outset. Both the neurologists and the asylum doctors in Vienna were so offended by his unorthodox approach to mental illness that they wouldn't let him speak at their conferences; some of his earliest lectures were addressed to the B'nai Brith instead. Gradually, the psychoanalytic movement became identified and bound up in Freud's Jewishness. It was seen as a Jewish science and was later banned in Germany in 1933 as a "Jewish science."

Freud surrounded himself with a group of loyal psychoanalysts. This inner circle had been formed just after 1910 to help promote psychoanalysis. Freud gave each member a golden ring symbolizing a new force, psychoanalysis, and securing their loyalty to Freud.[8] Even within Freud's inner group, it didn't take long for the fighting to begin. The most serious and infamous split occurred between the Swiss psychiatrist Carl Jung and Freud. Between 1906 and 1912, they had an intense personal and professional relationship, and Freud had high hopes for Jung to succeed him as the movement's leader. Since Jung was the only Gentile in the group, Freud felt that his leadership might ensure the longevity of psychoanalysis—it wouldn't continue to be seen as a Jewish treatment. They quarrelled initially over theory; Jung felt that the unconscious was not only a personal repository of drives and emotions but also a collective unconscious. Jung also differed in his views of religion and myths. Later the dispute became personal: Jung spread false rumours about Freud and his relationship with Freud's sister-in-law.

Alfred Adler, a Viennese physician, was part of Freud's early inner group. He emphasized the role of birth order and of inferiority. He had rickets as a child and did not walk until age four. Having been infirm, Adler was preoccupied with equality and self-esteem in theory and therapy, and he emphasized treating the "whole person." In this regard he was the first to emphasize the social element in therapy, and he split with Freud over this in 1911, becoming the first of the inner circle to form his own competing institute. When Adler left, Freud demanded loyalty from the remaining members: either avoid Adler or leave the group.

The various splits had an advantage: they generated some helpful new thinking. Following Adler, Erich Fromm emphasized the effect of culture and society on the individual and personality development. In fact, he stressed that one's "social character" was modified by the external world. He was sharply criticized for undercutting the importance of inner drives or instincts, but after writing a series of wildly successful books between the 1940s and the 1970s, Fromm became a highly read public intellectual and social critic. He was also a lifelong Marxist who attempted to unite Freudian and Marxist theory.[9] A lay analyst (he was a sociologist), Fromm maintained an analytic practice throughout his career, modelling it after that of Georg Groddeck, a colleague of Freud's; that is, the role of the analyst was to feel the patient's emotions within himself in order to feel the totality of the person. Groddeck emphasized kindness, truth, and courage, and placed less importance on theory.

The psychoanalytic movement divided itself into different streams of thought and practice, often related to power, dominance, and incestuous relationships. Analysts formed their own institutes, separate from the universities, and because of the infighting, most cities had at least two. Since these institutes evolved outside universities, they lacked checks and balances, and this lack of oversight only fomented further rivalries and divisions.

The infighting would become a key feature of the culture of psychoanalysis, according to T.M. Luhrmann, an anthropologist at the University of Southern California who studied psychiatrists and residents in psychiatry. "The history of psychoanalysis is a history of schism," she wrote in her 2003 book *Of Two Minds,* on the fragmentation of the psychiatric field. "Analytic institutes are famous for their tribalism, the smallness and ferocity of their quarrels."[10]

Complicating matters was the fact that there was no reliable way to test psychoanalytic theories. Freud considered psychoanalysis to be a science of the mind, one that explained phenomena of our worlds based on his observations. He believed that others would replicate these observations over time. But it was a closed loop: disagreement with some or all of it was considered a form of resistance, part of your pathology, or, worse, a betrayal.

Psychoanalysis, then, was never a scientific proposition. It couldn't be tested (though some of its tenets are testable today), or disproved, so its practitioners could make up their ideas without the necessity to test their hypotheses, or to see whether their results could be replicated by other scientists. They could say whatever they wanted without being constrained by the discipline of science.

The psychoanalysts were, in this respect, similar to the asylum doctors. Asylums were located away from the large cities, where the science and teaching were conducted, and the people who worked in the asylums often had little or no background in science. At times, they were more concerned about the population as a whole than about the individual: they wanted to prevent "hereditary degeneration." What's more, the asylums were starved of cash; the best scientific minds stayed away.

Neither the psychoanalysts nor the asylum doctors paid much heed to the emerging science that was about to transform modern medicine.

Science and Psychiatry: Uneasy Bedfellows

The main body of medicine had been developing science as a base over this same time. The scientific revolution had been building since the Renaissance. Galileo, the 16th-century engineer and astronomer who was educated in the liberal arts, transferred the spirit of the Italian Renaissance to mathematics and to observational science. Using a telescope, he evaluated Copernicus and Kepler's idea that our earth was spinning around the sun—and proved that they were right. This was the power of the scientific method, a disciplined way to study the natural world, with observation, explanation, and prediction. It would transform medicine in the 19th century and produce us all kinds of innovations, from the science of genetics, evolution, new vaccines, and anesthesia to handwashing.[11]

Universities had been teaching medicine in some parts of the world for hundreds of years—in Bologna and Padua since the 1200s, and in Oxford since the 1300s. By the late 1700s, the First Vienna School of Medicine aimed to put medicine on new scientific foundations, "promoting unprejudiced clinical observation, botanical and chemical research."[12] By the 19th century, the scientific approach to medicine was being developed in medical schools. The University of Toronto, for instance, started teaching medical students in the 1840s, then passed the task onto proprietary schools for four decades before resuming it. These proprietary schools did not have the financial means to conduct scientific research properly, and they could not grant university degrees. It was hard for the proprietary schools to obtain philanthropic gifts, and some students began going elsewhere—for example, William Osler, later a preeminent physician and educator, went to McGill—because they wanted a stronger base in science. One of the leaders of the Toronto proprietary schools, William Aikins, had close ties to the university and he wanted his school, the Toronto School of Medicine, to become the foundation for the new university-based Faculty of Medicine. When the university took over the medical training in 1887, Aikins became the first dean, and he emphasized the new scientific base to medicine.

But the medical profession did not know how to treat people with mental illness, or how to empirically measure a therapy's effectiveness. So when physicians interested in improving treatment for mental disorders were confronted with these serious, puzzling problems, they did what they could. The results varied widely, from partial success to abject failure. Along the way, experimental treatments and surgeries were conducted on thousands of unsuspecting mental patients.

In the early part of the 20th century, people with mental illness were given malaria parasites, with the belief that the fever it induced might cure insanity. The theory proved to be correct for those suffering from psychosis brought on by neurosyphilis. The disease was spread by an organism, and if you injected a patient with malaria parasites, the patient would get a fever, and the patient would improve. This discovery earned Julius Wagner-Jauregg the Nobel Prize in Medicine in 1927. However, creating a fever didn't help other patients with mental illness.

Other theories led to bizarre treatments with poor results. By the 1920s, Henry Cotton in the United States linked mental illness to bacterial illness, calling it "focal sepsis," and also to auto-intoxication from the toxins derived from different areas of the body, but especially the bowels. He felt that if one removed the area of sepsis, 80% of people could be cured. The result was that tens of thousands of patients had all their teeth removed, and that then led to an epidemic of tonsillectomy and sinus surgery, and eventually removal of abdominal organs in people in the mental hospitals. The surgery persisted for years in spite of a mortality rate of about 45% and no benefit.

The late 1930s brought in a new wave of shock therapies. The first of these, insulin coma therapy, like many medical discoveries, was an accident. A Viennese physician, Manfred Sakel, began treating drug addicts in Berlin. In 1930, Sakel inadvertently gave an overdose of insulin to a morphine addict with diabetes. This resulted in a mild coma, but when the patient recovered, her desire for morphine had abated. Soon, Sakel gave insulin to other drug addicts and claimed spectacular successes. Another accidental overdose of insulin produced a coma in a psychotic addict. Upon recovery, his psychotic symptoms had improved. After some initial animal experiments to establish a safe method of administering an insulin coma, Sakel began treating people with schizophrenia. In 1933, he published a short paper reporting the success of his method.

Joseph Wortis, an American psychiatrist who was being analyzed by Freud, brought the technique back to the United States in 1935, and the following year, Sakel came to the United States and began instructing psychiatrists from New York State hospitals in the new treatment. In early 1937, Norman Easton, a Toronto psychiatrist, was sent to Bellevue Hospital in New York for two months to learn how to administer insulin coma therapy, and work and study in this area began over the next two years in Toronto. Canada's Nobel laureate Sir Frederick Banting was part of the research applications for this work, though he was quite removed from any of the actual research.

Soon after insulin coma therapy was introduced, Ladislaus von Meduna of Budapest started giving metrazol to produce epileptic seizures in schizophrenic patients. The therapy was based on the erroneous assumption that there was an antagonism between the convulsive state and the schizophrenic process. It was abandoned after doctors discovered significant side effects, such as difficulty in controlling the number of seizures. Insulin was more reliable. In the mid-1950s, however, controlled studies found insulin coma therapy to be useless, and it gradually faded out over the next 15 years.

Electroshock or electroconvulsive therapy (ECT) was the next new thing for mental illness. It was first used in 1938 by the Italian neuropsychiatrist Ugo Cerletti, in Rome. Like insulin and metrazol, electroshock rapidly spread to the United States, where it was in extensive use by 1941 because it was easier on the patient (less fear, nausea, vomiting, and fewer severe headaches). The inherent simplicity of electroshock, its significantly lower cost than that of drugs, and its relative lack of apparent side effects led to its widespread use. It turned out to be highly effective for severe depression, but it was used far more widely for conditions that did not benefit from ECT, and it came with problems such as memory loss. Of significance, it didn't prevent recurrence of a depression.

The experimentation continued over the first half of the 20th century. The most extreme example came from Egas Moniz of

Portugal, who invented the lobotomy and shared a Nobel Prize in 1935 for his work. Moniz's theory was based on the assumption that all serious mental disorders were the result of fixed thoughts maintained by nerve pathways in the frontal lobes of the brain. Destruction of these abnormal pathways was the only effective cure. Two years later, neurologist Walter Freeman and his partner James Watts, a neurosurgeon, introduced it to the United States. Despite the tenuousness of the theory and inadequacy of evidence supporting it, doctors performed lobotomies on approximately 40,000 people in the United States and on 17,000 in Great Britain.

In January 1938, the Ontario Health Department sent psychiatrist Clarence B. Farrar and neurosurgeon Kenneth McKenzie to Washington to visit Freeman and Watts and learn about lobotomies. While they expressed concerns about the selection of patients, they felt that the procedure had promise, especially since it was supported by the father of neurosurgery, Harvey Cushing. Lobotomies began in Ontario in 1941, but surgeons were more cautious than were those in the United States. By the mid-1960s, just over 1,400 patients in Ontario had had this surgery. When Toronto psychiatrist Abe Miller later reviewed the results, he found that 55% of the patients improved enough to leave the hospital. Only a small percentage did not improve at all. In 1967, when he checked the patients again, Miller conceded that the value of the lobotomy "is clearly limited" but still thought it could be a "useful therapeutic technique" in "certain chronic, intractable, distressing psychiatric conditions."[13]

Looking back, these theories and treatments seem primitive, and it would be easy to conclude that they were prime examples of the blatant lack of scientific rigour in the treatment of mental illness. We need to qualify this view. These physicians were desperate to find something to help. Not all of them were bad either: ECT has saved many, many lives. Used appropriately, it is

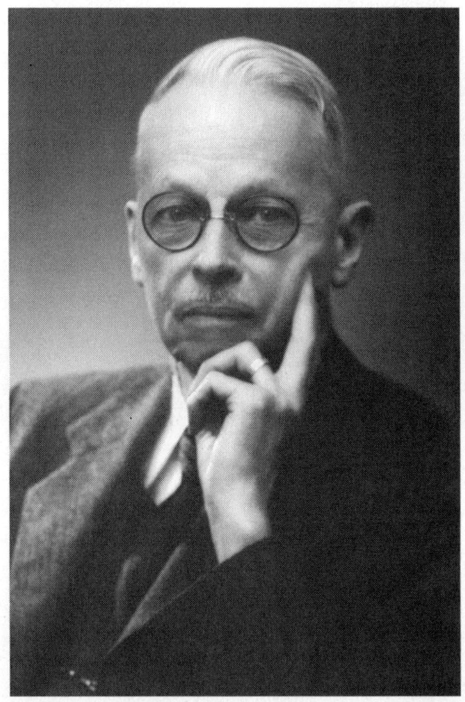

C.B. Farrar, Clarke's chosen successor, was the second professor of psychiatry at the University of Toronto. He was editor of the American Journal of Psychiatry *for over 30 years.* Courtesy CAMH Archives.

an effective treatment. It's also important to put these experiments into historical context. First, scientists at that time didn't have sophisticated means to study the effectiveness of treatments. It was not until the late 1940s that a randomized control trial was used to study a medicine, in that case, streptomycin to treat tuberculosis. (This kind of trial randomly allocates patients into two groups, one to receive the experimental therapy and the other to receive a placebo or a standard existing treatment.) This methodology was then applied for many forms of treatment, including psychiatric medicines that would revolutionize the field in the 1950s.

There was also no real regard for the ethics of experimenting on the mentally ill. But mentally ill patients were not the only ones to suffer from medical experimentation. For every example of this type of research on the mentally ill there are as many experiments conducted on prisoners, people captured in wars, or on poor people in the United States or in the developing world. Between 1932 and 1972, for instance, researchers from the US Public Health Service enlisted several hundred poor black sharecroppers in various stages of syphilis with promises of free medical care and free burial insurance. Then they watched to see how the untreated syphilis in the men developed. They gave them a "treatment" (that wasn't a treatment) and never told them they had the disease. They never gave these men treatment, even after 1947, when penicillin could have cured them. Disgraceful experiments such as these have been repeated numerous times in medical history.[14]

Just as science must be coupled with compassion in the clinic, it must be coupled with ethical behaviour in research. Unethical treatment of human subjects in research experiments is more likely to occur when groups of people are dehumanized (from "these people are different from us" right up to "they are not really people at all") and when ambitious scientists put their own careers and the needs of the broad public ahead of the individual's rights. Such research is generally conducted on disadvantaged people who can't protest, and often when there is a lack of oversight. Mentally ill people, then, have been vulnerable. Their families may be embarrassed or put their trust in "important" authorities; the public can be apathetic; and they, the patients, have been out of sight.

These days, scientists have to abide by ethical rules that put the rights of the individual human subject before the benefits of the study for the broader good. The people participating must provide fully informed consent, and they must be informed about the purpose of the research, the procedures to be used, the benefits to the participant, if any, and the potential risks of participating. These rules have helped protect human subjects, although they have been violated numerous times.

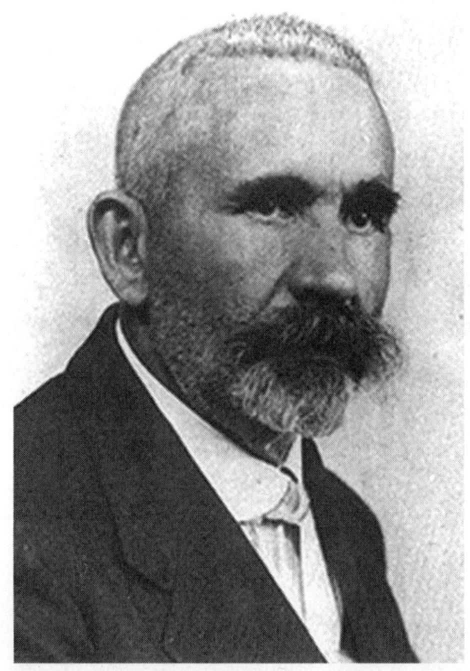

Emil Kraepelin (circa 1900). Kraepelin was a leading German professor of psychiatry who developed a clinic that integrated clinical care with research and education. CAMH Archives; photo courtesy Professor C.B. Farrar.

The Next Wave: Emil Kraepelin, Science, and Psychiatry

During the tumultuous period of the late 19th century, there was a German psychiatrist who rejected Freud's theories of the unconscious and insisted that the scientific method ought to be deployed in the study of mental illness. His name was Emil Kraepelin, and he would become a hero for the biologically minded psychiatrists of my time.

The nature of German universities played a huge role in how Kraepelin developed. The German universities in the 1800s were largely state supported. They developed teaching and research side by side and had a tradition of the doctoral dissertation for all medical students.[15] Students were therefore oriented to science through research and publication. By 1865 internist and psychiatrist

Wilhelm Griesinger had become professor of psychiatry in Berlin, moving psychiatry away from the custodial asylum to the university stance of enquiry and education for the first time.

Emil Kraepelin, born in the late 19th century, founded modern scientific psychiatry and psychiatric genetics. Kraepelin believed that psychiatric disease was related to genetic and biological mechanisms. Although he did consider stress and traumatic early development in his theories of illness, Kraepelin rejected Freud's hypotheses regarding sexuality. To him, this was unscientific speculation. Kraepelin also spoke out against the then barbaric treatment of mentally ill people in psychiatric asylums.

His biggest contributions, though, related to diagnosis. Kraepelin noticed that symptoms found in a person with schizophrenia, for example, may also appear in a person with bipolar illness. As a result, he identified disease not by its dominant symptoms but by the patterns of symptoms, or syndromes. We follow this today in our modern psychiatric diagnoses. Kraepelin also demonstrated the role genetics play in psychiatric disease. He observed that relatives of schizophrenic patients have a higher rate of schizophrenia than the general population, while manic depression is more frequent in the relatives of manic-depressives than it is in the general population.

Kraepelin's key observation was that schizophrenia has a chronic deteriorating course while the course of manic depression is intermittent—patients could be relatively symptom-free and then experience acute episodes.

Kraepelin's emphasis on empiricism and diagnosis took hold not only in Germany, but at the Maudsley Hospital and its Institute of Psychiatry in London, and at Johns Hopkins School of Medicine in the United States. Through these influential institutions, Kraepelin would play a profound role in shaping the history of the Clarke Institute and psychiatry at the University of Toronto.

Johns Hopkins was the first American medical school to emphasize the German approach to integration of science, education, and clinical care, under the leadership of the preeminent physician William Osler. In this great institution, Swiss psychiatrist Adolf Meyer would have a tremendous impact on North American psychiatry. Meyer was about a decade younger than Freud and trained in neuropathology. As professor of psychiatry at Johns Hopkins from 1910 to 1941, he tried to strike a balance between science and psychoanalysis. He introduced Emil Kraepelin's classificatory system, but he also introduced Americans to Freud's ideas, especially those about the importance of sexuality and of the formative influence of early experiences on the adult personality. He insisted that patients could best be understood through consideration of their life experiences and situations. Careful interviewing as well as detailed case histories and records were vital. Meyer was at first intrigued by Freud's theories but over time became more antagonistic to them. He strongly encouraged an empirical base and scientific inquiry for psychiatry.

Meyer's writings were an inspiration for me, as he thought that both science and caring deserved a place in the practice of psychiatry. But he was way off in believing that mental disorders were not diseases but reactions to stress. We know now that many psychiatric disorders—autism, schizophrenia, and bipolar illness, for example—can be called disease, whereas other conditions, like some depressions, can be products of life experience and stress in the vulnerable person.

The Maudsley Hospital began in its academic form in the 1890s when Dr. Frederick Mott, a leading neurologist, proposed university-level training courses in subjects related to psychiatry. It was named after Dr. Henry Maudsley, a prominent British psychiatrist who wrote extensively about mental illnesses in the 1860s; he also provided funds to establish the hospital in Denmark Hill, in southeast London. The academic arm of the institution changed its name in 1948 to the Institute of Psychiatry when it amalgamated with the Bethlem Royal to form a joint teaching hospital. Its first leader, Aubrey Lewis, kept alive the Kraepelinian tradition. Lewis, an Australian, studied with Meyer in Baltimore. His interest was in empiricism; he was a skeptic and had little regard for analysis. Many Toronto academics went to the Maudsley after residency in the 1960s and 1970s.

Meyer's insistence on care and science was unusual because, in the years after World War II, psychiatry was polarized between two main camps: psychoanalysis and observational science. You had to choose a side, and it became more difficult to appreciate the value of both.

By the time I got into medical school, psychoanalysis was the winner in the United States. Freud's intellectual heirs, who had emigrated from Nazi-occupied Europe, were so powerful that you had to be a psychoanalyst to get ahead in the field, at least in the United States. In the 1960s, psychoanalysts accounted for less than 10% of psychiatrists but well over 50% of the academic chairs, according to Leon Eisenberg, a leading American academic psychiatrist at Johns Hopkins and Harvard. By the 1960s, there was a two-class system of psychiatric care in the United States, with the yearly cost of an analysis more than 80% of the median income of an American worker.[16]

In the 1950s and 1960s, analysts controlled the development of the psychiatric system of classification (the DSM, or *Diagnostic and Statistical Manual of Mental Disorders*) of the American Psychiatric Association. As a result, most diagnoses were written in the psychoanalytic language of reactions and neuroses. They were based on the presumed unconscious conflict and the means to keep it unconscious, or the breakthrough of symptoms when defences failed.

Some of Freud's theories were wrong. Freud believed that women had a moral inferiority, relative to men, an inferiority of reasoning and conscience, for example. Later study has shown women and men do reason differently when coming to moral judgments, the difference lying in women's more nuanced approach relative to men's more black and white stance, a difference that cannot be considered inferior. Or take Freud's theory of penis envy. This was based on his conviction that women are anatomically inferior, so they must therefore envy men's penises. In the 1960s, when I was a medical student, many psychodynamic psychiatrists still considered penis envy to be a serious problem for women. But this idea was culture-bound, based on women in Vienna in 1900 when the theory was first formulated, not those in Winnipeg in 1965, and certainly not in Toronto in 2014. With the societal changes over the next generations and new opportunities for women, and their successes, we see this theory's limitations; it's no longer of use. But although penis envy may be an outdated concept, its derivative, competitive envy, is important for some people of either sex.

Another problem was that psychoanalysts routinely confused cause and effect. They would observe that an autistic baby didn't mould to the mother and conclude that it was because the mother was a "refrigerator mother." In fact, the baby's inability to mould was the result of being autistic. It had nothing to do with the mother's psychology. Leo Kanner, who developed the term "refrigerator mother," later wrote a book recanting his earlier work.

In science, it's perfectly normal to have theories that are proven incorrect. That's how science progresses, as scholars try new approaches in order to add to the foundation of knowledge. Yet, perhaps for lack of empirical evidence of its effectiveness, psychoanalysts adhered so rigidly to their approach that they oversold its value. By the 1940s and 1950s, people began to analyze even young children in order to prevent mental illness later in life. A few even thought that psychoanalysis could channel human aggression and prevent war.

By the late 1960s, Freudians were stuck in a time warp. They adhered strictly to the orthodoxy of Freud's original ideas and practices, right down to the insistence on the one-hour sessions on the couch and the silent therapist as mirror. Their focus on repressed drives, sex, and aggression seemed anachronistic, or at least in need of some serious reconsideration. Ironically, Freud himself was far more flexible in his own approach than his adherents proved to be. For example, he believed in short analyses, he took patients on holiday to continue the work, and he favoured lay analysts (those without a medical degree). He felt that psychoses were not helped by analyses—something his followers had to painfully relearn. Some of the traditions that the Freudians clung to came from simple expediency. Abram Kardiner, an American-born physician who was studying psychiatry, went to Freud for an analysis in 1921.[17] Freud accepted five Americans and one European to Vienna that fall to begin analysis with him. He had earlier let them all know that he would see patients six times a week for six months. All six candidates turned up, a surprise to Freud because he expected one to drop out. His schedule was clearly overloaded, so he reduced the frequency of sessions for the new candidates to five times a week. It became the tradition.

By the time I entered the field, psychoanalysis was being attacked for its lack of scientific rigour. Was it even a science? Karl Popper, the exceptional philosopher of science, wrote that the basic criteria for science involve the testing and discarding of conjecture and hypotheses. Freud's ideas didn't pass the test as far as his critics were concerned. Peter Medawar, a Nobel Prize–winning immunologist, put it this way. Psychoanalysis, he said, is the "most stupendous intellectual confidence trick of the 20th century."[18] But Freud didn't think his method could be tested in an empirical way, and many analysts who followed him claimed that the emphasis on evidence somehow undermined the humane and caring side of psychiatry.

Whether or not psychoanalysis is a science or an effective treatment, it provided explanations for strange symptoms. It taught doctors to listen to people and to try to understand their distress rather than classifying them and then putting them in the asylum. The concept of unconscious forces and the primacy of internal conflict in personality development and relationship patterns has remained valuable particularly for psychodynamic therapy, an offshoot of psychoanalysis.

While psychiatrists were waging war against one another in the United States, those in Toronto and Winnipeg were still largely following the path forged by Kraepelin. This wasn't inspiring work, though. Most of the psychiatrists in Winnipeg, as in the rest of Canada, spent their time trying to get an accurate and detailed picture of the patient and his or her symptoms and past, in order to come up with the right diagnosis. These psychiatrists, donning white lab coats, focused on caring for severely ill people with psychosis such as schizophrenia or bipolar illness. They did offer therapy, generally of a supportive nature based on common sense, reality, and encouragement, not on repressed drives. They reinforced patients' ability to cope, and their strengths. They treated many people with ECT or medications. These psychiatrists often had to be content with small gains over lengthy periods.

But the scientific approach fell short. For one thing, there was no objective way to diagnose mental illness. To be really useful, a diagnosis should say which signs and symptoms cluster, what this means for treatment and outcome, and hopefully something about the mechanisms involved in producing the illness. For many medical diseases, such as diabetes, we have biological markers—for instance, blood sugar levels (for heart disease, they're the cardiogram, enzymes measured in the blood, and, now, imaging the vessels.) For mental diseases, however, there are no such markers for diagnosis. There is no blood test for depression or schizophrenia. Psychiatric diagnosis can't describe the mechanisms of illness. If you have two doctors disagreeing about the presence of prostate cancer, there is an objective marker for the illness—a biopsy. Psychiatry has no such tool (this is also true for some other areas of medicine such as many forms of headache, for example).

Psychiatry's inability to accurately diagnose led to embarrassing disclosures. In one famous 1972 study published in *Science*, David Rosenhan showed healthy volunteers how to simulate hearing voices that were threatening harm, and sent them to emergency wards of hospitals. They were all admitted to hospitals with a diagnosis of schizophrenia. While in hospital they returned to their normal behaviour and took detailed notes. To some staff, this was a sign they were ill, suspicious, or paranoid. The volunteers were all discharged with a diagnosis of "schizophrenia in remission." The psychiatrists and hospital staff were easily fooled. One group, however, wasn't fooled: the fellow patients. The people who suffered from genuine mental illness all knew that the simulated patients were phonies.

In the late 1960s, one often heard people say that mental illness wasn't real. But people who were sick knew they were ill (except when psychosis eroded insight). They knew these were not romantic disorders any more than tuberculosis was in the 1800s.

In another study, clinicians in several countries were shown videotapes of physician interviews with patients. They were asked to diagnose patients on the basis of what they saw on the screen. Clinicians in the United States diagnosed many more people with schizophrenia, while clinicians in Great Britain were more likely to diagnose patients with bipolar illness. We in Canada, as expected, were in between, if somewhat closer to the British.

As psychoanalysis came under attack, so too did psychiatry itself. French philosopher Michel Foucault argued that mental illness is not an illness at all but a scheme to contain poor people who don't fit into the new industrialized order. Other critics railed against coercion by the state and by psychiatrists.[19] Scottish psychiatrist R.D. Laing had been a physician in the Royal Army Medical Corps in the early 1950s; there he became enraged at the inhumane treatments that dominated care—insulin-induced comas, physical restraints such as straightjackets, and seclusion. He advocated for more and better communication between doctor and patient. He spent lengthy periods with psychotic people listening and being with them. Biological therapies that ignored social, intellectual, cultural, and existential concerns were, in his view, harmful.

As for the asylum, conceived as a humane way to protect mentally ill people from the street, it too was crumbling in esteem. Canadian sociologist Erving Goffman saw it as a "total" institution, which cuts patients off from the rest of the world, so that they are completely dependent on staff and have no say in how decisions are made. The result is a loss of identity, interest, and drive, which can be mistaken for symptoms of mental illness.

The answer to institutionalization was supposed to be community health clinics, recommended in 1960 by the American Joint Commission on Mental Illness and Health. While there was early optimism, it became apparent over time that the community mental health program had also been greatly oversold. Deinstitutionalization without passing on the funding to the community had poor results. It became a way to cut costs. When people left the state mental institutions, they needed help with housing, jobs, and income support, but community psychiatry was not up to the task. When the approach of community psychiatry could not provide solutions to all mental illness, it too fell from grace, and a new model took hold: the re-medicalization of psychiatric care.

Amid all this controversy, science was planning a comeback, and it would soon deliver a new model to transform the treatment of mental health disorders. This was the re-medicalization of mental illness. Starting in the 1950s, a combination of happy accident and clinical research would create new drugs that would transform our understanding of mental illness, and the lives of people with problems like schizophrenia and depression. It started in places like the Rhône-Poulenc Laboratories in 1950, when the surgeon Henri Laborit was looking for a better antihistamine to prevent surgical shock. He tried the antihistamine chlorpromazine and discovered it had artificial hibernation effects; that is, people could be sedated without narcosis (a state of deep stupor). Psychiatric clinical trials were conducted in 1952 in Paris, and in 1954, Heinz Lehmann of the Douglas Hospital in Verdun, just outside Montreal, and later of McGill conducted the first North American work on chlorpromazine. When it was introduced throughout Europe and in America over the next decade, chlorpromazine transformed the treatment of schizophrenia. People no longer had to cope with hallucinations and delusions, although they did suffer severe neurological side effects such as a Parkinson-like state. (A second generation of antipsychotics, the atypicals, emerged in the 1990s, but they come with a new set of problems, such as severe weight gain that could lead to a metabolic syndrome and diabetes.)

There is a great, almost unknown story that deserves to be told. While Lehmann was doing his research, an Ontario-based psychiatry resident, Dr. Ruth Koeppe (later Kajander), independently conducted chlorpromazine clinical trials at the Ontario Hospital, London. Koeppe was European-trained and was able to read the preliminary European journal findings. She delivered her report a few months ahead of Lehmann, but unfortunately for her, she reported to a professional meeting of the Ontario Psychiatric

Association rather than in a peer-reviewed journal. Therefore, Lehmann got the lion's share of the Canadian glory.

The antidepressants were developed in a similar mix of research and serendipity. In the early 1950s, scientists at the pharmaceutical company Geigy, in Switzerland, were working with the chlorpromazine molecule. They modified it slightly and came up with imipramine. It did not help control delusions and hallucinations, but when the Swiss psychiatrist Roland Kuhn tried it, he found it did elevate mood. These tricyclic medications were introduced to clinical practice in the early 1960s. The monoamine oxidase inhibitors (MAOIs) had been discovered a few years earlier when scientists were looking for new antitubercular agents and noted the improved mood and activity of people treated with the drug iproniazid, chemically related to a drug used to treat tuberculosis. MAOIs came to market in 1958 and were popular for a while, but they quickly lost ground to the tricyclics because of their serious interactions with foods containing tyramine (the so-called cheese syndrome).

In 1954, in the New Jersey–based laboratories of Hoffmann-La Roche, Dr. Leo Sternbach began to study a class of unexplored compounds he had previously worked with as a postdoctoral student in Poland. When the lab was being moved, an assistant found a sample of one particular chemical and asked whether it should be thrown out. Sternbach sent the sample to Roche's research lab for study. It was the first benzodiazepine, a class of drugs that enhance the effect of the neurotransmitter gamma-aminobutyric acid (GABA) and induce sleep, soothe anxiety, prevent convulsions, and relax muscles. The benzodiazepines became the most widely prescribed drugs worldwide. Librium was introduced in 1960 by Hoffmann-La Roche. Three years later came a more potent tranquilizer from the same family, Valium.

John Cade, an Australian psychiatrist, discovered lithium in 1949. Cade was interested in mania and used lithium in animal experiments, noting how apathetic the subjects became. He then tried lithium for his manic patients. Pleased with the result, he published a paper on this. Lithium worked, and yet it was not used in Canada for another 15 years or so. Since lithium is a naturally occurring salt, it can't be patented, so the drug companies were not interested in funding research or talks to spread the news. The slow acceptance of lithium was also in part because some psychiatric leaders wouldn't believe it worked. Then a Danish psychiatrist, Mogens Schou, entered the picture. The son of a psychiatrist, Schou was fascinated by bipolar illness. His research confirmed lithium's ability to relieve mania, and he showed in the early 1960s that it could prevent recurrences of bipolar disorder. He campaigned hard for lithium—even wearing cufflinks made of lithium—and eventually he won over the world's psychiatrists.

The drug revolution that began in these labs in the 1950s would soon transform the lives of mentally ill patients. Science had finally entered the world of psychiatry, permitting us to not only prescribe drugs but to also test psychotherapies to see whether they work, and for whom. By now, 70 to 80% of the patients who suffer from bipolar disorder live gratifying and independent lives, especially when drugs are combined with therapy. Patients with even the most severe forms of schizophrenia may now be greatly helped by advances in pharmacotherapy, as well as by tailored therapy, social-skills training, family education, and outreach. Major depression and the anxiety disorders, including obsessive-compulsive disorders, may all respond to a combination of drugs and specific, tailored psychotherapy. Science has helped alter the course of mental illness and of clinical care, replacing ice wraps with lithium, insulin shock with olanzapine, and psychoanalytic regression with cognitive behaviour therapy.

In 1970 we were on the cusp of the great swing from psychoanalysis and its fascination with the unconscious to the scientific model of mental illness, with its heavy emphasis on drugs and detailed diagnostic rules. But even with new drugs already on the market, our profession hadn't begun to change in a meaningful way. Psychoanalysts were still entrenched in their powerful seats in US academia. They were still influencing the diagnosis and treatment of mental illness. The critics were still biting from all sides. The war was still on.

This was the world I was about to enter when I accepted the invitation to do my psychiatric residency at the Clarke. It was an institution with a new name, a new building, and a complicated past.

CHAPTER 4

The Clarke Institute

The Clarke Institute of Psychiatry was established in 1966 as a research and teaching setting for the University of Toronto's Department of Psychiatry. As a clinical research institute with hospital beds, the Clarke was to take the lead in the university's psychiatric system. It had just moved into a Stalinesque new concrete tower on the edge of the vine-covered University of Toronto campus, which reflected the Clarke's position in Toronto's mental health system at the time: it was powerful, but remote from the world around it—from both the chronic psychiatric patients who lingered in the asylum or wandered from street to jail, and from the medical establishment in the general hospitals who felt that psychiatrists had veered way too far from the beaten path of medicine and science.

Culturally, the Clarke was one of the most cautious research institutions on the continent. The men who shaped the Clarke's culture had embraced the scientific, evidence-based approach that Kraepelin had pioneered in the late 19th century. They did not join their American colleagues in converting to psychoanalysis; some of them fiercely opposed psychoanalysis as a travesty of science.

In 1966, just as the Clarke set up in its new building on the edge of campus, everything was about to change. The institute had a new leader: Robin Hunter, a psychoanalyst. This appointment was a real departure for the world of psychiatry as practised in Canada. To appreciate this, we need to look back at the roots of the Clarke and how it was formed.

The Clarke was named for Dr. Charles K. Clarke, the first professor of psychiatry at the University of Toronto. He was a 19th-century alienist—as the asylum doctors were called—who felt that mentally ill people suffered from an alienation of their reason and spirit from their bodies. He had good reason to want to keep psychiatry in the asylum. Clarke had been lured to the Rockwood Asylum in Kingston by its superintendent, his brother-in-law Dr. William Metcalf, who shared Clarke's convictions about the treatment of the mentally ill. Working together, the two were able to achieve a great deal, but in August 1885, as the two doctors were making their rounds, they were attacked by a knife-wielding patient. Clarke was able to subdue the patient physically, but not before the patient fatally stabbed Metcalf. Clarke experienced another attack some years later when he was inspecting a boat dock at the lake. A patient seized Clarke by the throat and the two plunged into Lake Ontario. A passing blacksmith dragged Clarke to safety.

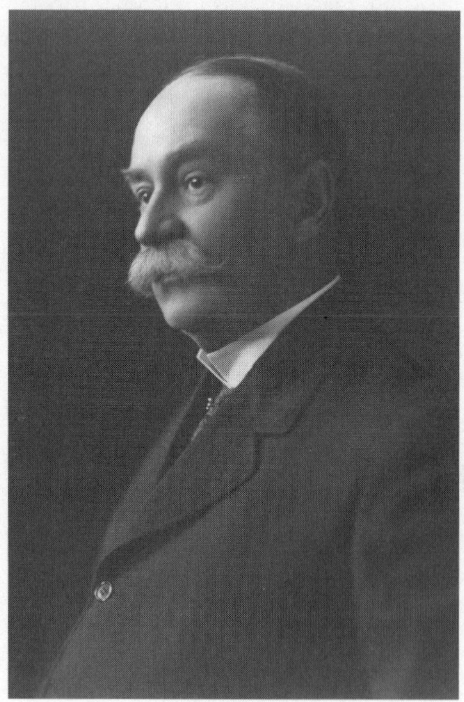

Ontario-born C.K Clarke was the first professor of psychiatry at the University of Toronto. He was a strong advocate of treating the mentally ill in the asylum and also for developing a Kraepelin-style university clinic. Courtesy CAMH Archives.

When Clarke took charge of the Kingston asylum in 1885, the so-called lunatics were locked up alongside the criminally insane. He immediately removed all traces of the jail era. He introduced formal training for nurses and attendants in managing the mentally ill so they would treat inmates as patients, not prisoners. He also tried to find useful occupations for his patients, in the belief that regular and steady work and habits, along with good food, would speed their recovery. In this precursor of occupational therapy, Clarke enlisted the aid of a patient who was a skilful brushmaker to teach other patients brushmaking. In spring 1886, Clarke noted in his diary that some 20 patients were occupied in the "brush factory" and demand for its brushes was outstripping supply. But the brush factory was short-lived; after complaints from competing brush manufacturers and politicians, the Inspector of Asylums forced Clarke to shut it down.

A man of indomitable spirit, Clarke was chagrined but not deterred. An accomplished musician himself, he formed an orchestra and brass band for patients, as well as a dramatic society. A photography club was added, as was a birdwatching club (Clarke was also an avid birdwatcher) and various sports. In 1893, when the Kingston asylum needed an additional building, Clarke once again gave the patients useful employment. As he wrote in the 1893 annual report on the asylums for the insane of Ontario: "All the stone for the hospital has been quarried by our people; they have also made the excavation, dug the sand, dressed a certain portion of the stone, and supplied most of the unskilled labour in connection with the building operations. In this way, the cost of the structure has been greatly reduced and pleasant occupation furnished for many of the inmates."[1]

Today we might take a more cynical view of these money-saving work projects, considering these practices an infringement on patients' rights. But at the turn of the 19th century, engaging the minds and hands of mentally ill patients in a hospitable environment was a revolutionary concept. Health professionals from Europe and the United States converged on Kingston to see how things were done.

Clarke came to Toronto in 1905, eager to introduce a scientific approach to psychiatric practice. Although he was an alienist at heart, he still wanted to bring science into psychiatry. His model was the Psychiatric University Clinic in Munich, where Kraepelin had championed the concept of a clinic associated with a university, where treatment would be based on "science" and research would be conducted to expand the knowledge of psychiatric disorders. All this would be integrated into the teaching of students.

As Clarke was making his plans for the Toronto Psychiatric Hospital to offer credible research and humane care for mental illness, he encountered another challenge, this time from the heart of medicine.

Toronto General Hospital, which began in a small building in 1812 to care for the wounded in the war against the United States, had launched a program in psychiatry. It threatened Clarke's plans because it could greatly diminish the importance of both the asylum and the psychiatric institute that Clarke was longing to build.

The new venture was the product of neurologist D. Campbell Meyers's determination. Meyers was a follower of the American neurologist Silas Weir Mitchell, professor of neurology at the University of Pennsylvania. Weir Mitchell was antagonistic to the asylum doctors for their lack of science—as the 19th century was ending, Weir Mitchell delivered a talk to the asylum doctors at their 1894 annual convention and criticized them for their isolation: "Want of competent original work is to my mind the worst symptom of torpor the asylums now present … [Where are] your careful scientific reports[?] … You live alone, uncriticized, unquestioned, out of

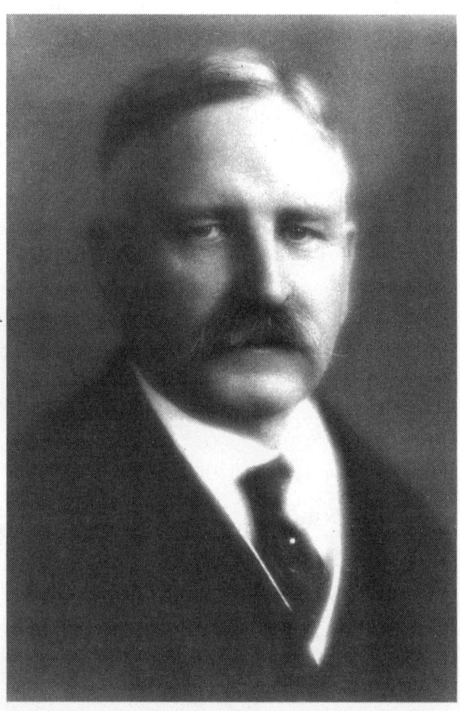

D. Campbell Meyers was Ontario's first neurologist. Working at Toronto General Hospital, he clashed with C.K. Clarke over the role of psychiatry in the general hospitals. He set up a private clinic at 72 Heath Street, and an outpatient clinic at Toronto General Hospital. Courtesy CAMH Archives.

the healthy conflicts and honest rivalries which keep us [neurologists] up to the mark of the fullest competence."[2]

At the time, the insane were kept in the old asylum on Queen Street, separate from people with other illnesses. But Meyers believed that if you treated the mentally ill early, in close collaboration with other branches of medicine, you could prevent the chronic psychotic state. He thought asylums should be reserved for the incurable cases. In 1894 he established a neurological hospital on Heath Street for his private patients. A decade later, in 1906, he persuaded Toronto General's board of trustees to open the first public unit in Canada for nervous diseases in a general hospital. Like other physicians on staff at the General in the late 1800s, Meyers was very familiar with treating some types of short-lived psychoses, such as deliria from infections, epilepsy, strokes, Huntington's disease, and those that were alcohol-related. Hysteria, hypochondriasis, and neurasthenia were also being seen by neurologists in the United Kingdom and the United States in general hospitals.

When Meyers proposed to set up a psychiatric department at the General, Clarke was running the Toronto Hospital (formerly Asylum) for the Insane and held the post of "extramural professor of mental diseases" at the university. Over the next few years, Clarke would be on the defensive as Meyers showed that his treatments were keeping people out of the asylums. But Clarke proved to be an able politician. When the Ontario government established a commission to examine policies on care of the mentally ill, Clarke and other alienists were named to the commission, but neither Meyers nor his younger colleague Francis Hyland, the only two neurologists in Ontario at that time, were included. Predictably, the commission did not support Meyers's model. It was this commission that established the pursuit of a university-based, Munich-style clinic for Toronto, rather than Meyers's proposed hospital-based psychiatric department.

Meyers fought back, claiming that the alienists should not be teaching medical students, since they saw only people who had been chronically ill, so couldn't possibly teach about the preexisting condition. But Clarke prevailed. He was elevated to dean of the medical school, and from that powerful post he campaigned against admission of psychiatric patients to Toronto General. He became chief of its psychiatric service in 1909, and brought Ernest Jones from Britain to run the outpatient program at Toronto General.[3] Once in Toronto, Jones set up an ambulatory "prevention" program, which at the same time was to facilitate transfers to the asylum when admission was required.

Meyers continued to present his results: several hundred people had been treated by then, and no one needed to go to the asylum.

Meyers desperately wanted a psychiatry inpatient unit to be part of the new general hospital when it opened on College Street in 1913. This wasn't to happen. In 1911, Clarke resigned his position as head of the asylum to become superintendent of Toronto General. Meyers retired to his Heath Street hospital and died in 1927.

Meyers, correctly, had seen the need for and efficacy of providing care to people with medical and surgical conditions (postpartum psychosis, depression after a heart attack, or an infectious or intoxicated delirium) in a general hospital. But he erred in thinking that, without clinical intervention, such patients would inevitably go on to chronic schizophrenia. Still, when it came to the politics of making his case, he was just no match for Clarke.

It was Clarke who gave psychiatry special status within the university system. In the first decade of the century, when Clarke was dean of medicine and soon-to-be superintendent of the new Toronto General, he wanted psychiatry to be separate from other medical teaching and remain based at Queen Street, with himself as professor of psychiatry at the university. He got his way. Under the 1911 Toronto General Hospital Act, the head of each service at Toronto General also got to be the head of the department at the university. There was one exception: psychiatry. It was not represented at Toronto General, so the Department of Medicine's Division of Neurology was in charge of general hospital psychiatry, while Queen Street and the Toronto Psychiatric Hospital (after the mid-1920s) were the centres of psychiatry. This political game had a big impact, because the Toronto Psychiatric Hospital inherited from Queen Street an asylum tradition of psychiatry, which separated it from the general hospitals.

Despite considerable obstacles, including public apathy and a government long on promises but short of funds, Clarke helped give Canada a standardized, professional treatment of mental illness. As founding medical director of the Canadian National Committee for Mental Hygiene (now the Canadian Mental Health Association), he established rehabilitation centres for soldiers returning home from World War I, and training programs for nurses and social workers.

Psychiatry and the Eugenics Movement

Clarke was in many ways a visionary, ahead of his times. Ironically, he also played to public fears and suspicions about people who were mentally unstable. Clarke was concerned about the overcrowding of Canadian mental facilities; asylum populations were growing, in part because of returning shell-shocked soldiers in need of treatment. It presented a huge cost for a young country. Clarke put the blame squarely on immigration policies that allowed insane and "defective" immigrants into the country to become a burden on the state.

He had plenty of allies in the growing eugenics movement. It encouraged the "right kind of people" to breed and tried to stop the "defective" kind from reproducing. Clarke and his allies in the eugenics movement persuaded the Canadian government to amend the Immigration Act in 1919 to exclude people of "psychopathic inferiority" and mental "defectives," as well as alcoholics, illiterates, people from countries that had fought against Canada during the war, those guilty of espionage, and those who believed in the forcible overthrow of the government or who "disbelieved" in government at all. To put this new law into practice, Clarke even spent a month in 1920 instructing immigration inspectors on how to assess the mental stability of immigrants.[4]

It's not a huge step to go from charging the public to gawk at the insane (as was common at the turn of the 19th century) to the eugenics movement. The thoughts behind them are similar: *These people are not like us, they are not really people like we are at all—by distancing ourselves, we are protected from ending up like that.* Although

Clarke may have had the welfare of Canadian asylums and their patients in mind when he aligned himself with the movement, the effect on that patient population could only be a negative one, stigmatizing an already marginalized group even further. It was a sad, even tragic irony that many early Canadian leaders in psychiatry were active proponents of eugenics. They readily adopted the theories of the day, partly because it was easy to dehumanize the mentally ill. The dangers of such theories are apparent. As Robert Jay Lifton has described, this psychic numbing made it possible for Nazi doctors, many of whom were psychiatrists trained to do no harm, to participate in the death and torture of an entire population of European Jews.[5]

Clarke died in 1924 of a heart attack, only one year before the founding of the Toronto Psychiatric Hospital, which would realize his vision of combining scientific research, education, and care for the mentally ill. But before he died, he made sure, through key appointments, that the leaders and many of the staff of the Toronto Psychiatric Hospital would bring scientific rigour to the practice of psychiatry by following the Maudsley, Johns Hopkins, and Kraepelinian approaches to mental illness. These men were careful observers of the behaviours of their patients and tried to be focused on evidence. Unlike the psychoanalysts, they were trained to observe the evidence, based on what patients said and how they appeared.

Clarke's hand-chosen successor as the second professor of psychiatry at the University of Toronto was Clarence B. Farrar. Farrar was an American from New York who came up to Toronto during World War I to advise the Canadian Army on shellshock. After receiving his medical training at Johns Hopkins, Farrar had gone to Germany to study with Nissl, Kraepelin, and Alzheimer, who were then professors of psychiatry in Heidelberg. He immersed himself in the Heidelberg school, later bringing back to North

America the need for careful description before generalizing about a phenomenon.[6]

Although psychoanalysis was stronger in the United States than it was in Canada, Toronto did have a key connection to the psychoanalysts and Freud's inner circle. British neurologist Ernest Jones, a close personal and professional friend of Freud's, had come to Toronto for five years, tapped by Clarke to run the outpatient clinic at Toronto General. He'd also taught psychiatry at the University of Toronto and worked as pathologist for the Toronto Hospital for the Insane, all the while conducting a private psychoanalytic practice. While he was in Toronto, Jones helped build support for the psychoanalytic movement in the United States, and he joined Freud's inner circle after returning to Britain. He even rushed to Vienna in 1938 to negotiate the exit of Freud and his inner circle, when Freud's escape from Nazi Germany became imperative.

Clarence Farrar, however, viewed psychoanalysis with contempt. In fact, he once told his wife that the Four Horsemen of the Apocalypse were "Communism, Catholicism, unionism, and psychoanalysis."[7] He refused to jump on the bandwagon as psychoanalysis gained popularity, even in the late 1940s when psychoanalysts were beginning to run most major facilities in America. It doomed him professionally. By 1947 Farrar's enemies had lined up against him and ousted him.

Farrar had the odds stacked against him in another way as well. During the World War I years, when he was based in Ottawa and travelling often to the military hospital in Cobourg, Ontario, his wife left him and returned to Virginia. When, in 1923, he became superintendent of the Homewood Sanatorium in Guelph, Ontario, he began an affair with the wife of an alcoholic patient. When he moved to Toronto, the two "lived in sin," much to the shock and dismay of virtuous Toronto society. Life was difficult for the couple socially and may have also had an impact on

Farrar's professional credibility. (They finally married in 1964, on the death of Farrar's first wife.)

Among his principal detractors was Brock Chisholm. Chisholm, who had graduated in medicine from the University of Toronto in 1924, had been in general practice before going, in the early 1930s, to London for a training analysis. When he returned, he opened a psychotherapy practice in Toronto. During World War II, Chisholm became the director of medical services of the Canadian Army and had considerable influence. He brought well-known New York analyst Lawrence Kubie for a group of weekend seminars, held at various military medical establishments and intended to reorient army psychiatrists toward psychoanalysis. In 1944 Chisholm became Canadian deputy minister of health. Thus, when in May 1945 Chisholm wrote to Sidney Smith (the new president of the University of Toronto) on the subject of Farrar's replacement in the chair of psychiatry, the letter came truly from a position of influence. Chisholm wanted Aubrey Lewis from London or an analyst. Fortunately for Farrar, the dean in charge of the search didn't listen.

Probably the greatest contribution Farrar made was his advocacy among family physicians of informal psychotherapy, a treatment based not upon rigid doctrinal systems but upon the intrinsic healing power of the doctor-patient relationship. Of course, Farrar had learned from Osler that the physician possesses the power to do great good just by talking with the patient and through the laying-on of hands.

The Stokes Era

Farrar was succeeded by Aldwyn Stokes as professor of psychiatry and director of the Toronto Psychiatric Hospital. Stokes, the former medical director of the Maudsley, came to Toronto in 1947. Stokes was an erudite, gentlemanly psychiatrist. Although not enthusiastic toward Freud and the psychoanalytic movement, he was far more diplomatic about it than Farrar. Stokes was from Newport, Wales, but became very much the Oxford scholar.[8] He was curious about everything. He was not above jumping up from the evening meal and racing to his study to look up the exact meaning of a word. His qualifications were diverse and included a physiology degree, a diploma in psychology, and extensive research work. Stokes entrenched the Kraepelin approach by instituting a kind of exchange program with London. For the next quarter century, he would recruit colleagues from London, and send academically oriented Toronto psychiatrists to spend a year or two at the Institute of Psychiatry in London as a kind of finishing school. I was proud that when the institute was looking for a dean in 2008,

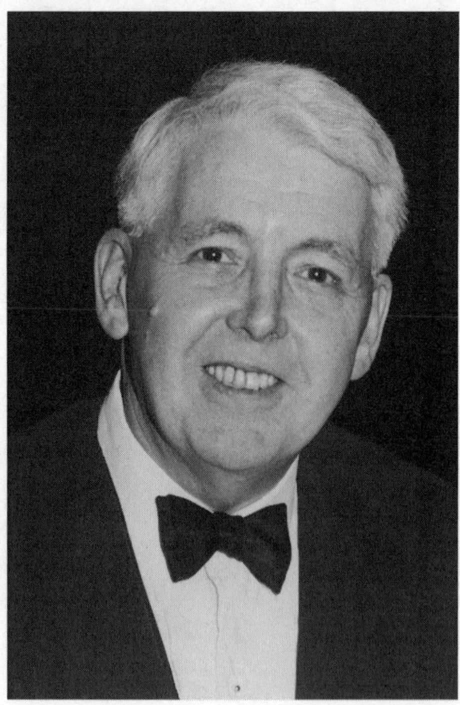

Aldwyn Stokes, a Welsh psychiatrist who studied at Oxford before coming to Toronto as the third professor of psychiatry. He oversaw the expansion of psychiatry in the general hospitals and planned the Clarke Institute. Courtesy CAMH Archives.

it recruited one of our top people, Shitij Kapur, in a reversal of the old process.

Although Toronto was not an international centre of psychiatric research, it did make some contributions to the understanding of mental illness. Stokes was interested in periodic illnesses—those that had abrupt onset and endings. He brought Rolf Gjessing from Norway to set up a metabolic clinic and laboratory at the Toronto Psychiatric Hospital. The two meticulously studied patients over time and found changes in nitrogen metabolism in different phases of an illness, periodic catatonia. This led to their successful use of thyroid hormone to treat this disorder. We no longer see periodic catatonia, likely because antipsychotic drugs prevent the illness progressing that far.[9] Stokes also brought John Lovett-Doust, an expert in physiological psychiatry, from London to do research that would connect low oxyhaemoglobin levels to disturbances in schizophrenia.

Stokes stimulated research in the mental health of schoolchildren. The famous Crestwood Heights study, the first major psychological research project undertaken in a Canadian community, focused on the emotional adjustment of schoolchildren by examining all aspects of their life in a community. He also encouraged Elvin "Bunky" Jellinek, a scholar of alcohol abuse, who did more than anyone at the time to make acceptable the concept of alcohol abuse as a disease.

One of Stokes's priorities was the development of psychiatric wards in the general hospitals, first at the Wellesley Hospital (from 1949 to 1960 that hospital was administratively part of Toronto General. It was merged with St. Michael's in 1998). This model was soon extended to other teaching hospitals: Toronto Western Hospital in 1953, St. Michael's Hospital in 1954, and Women's College Hospital in 1956. Throughout the 1950s, this slow integration of psychiatric services into the general hospitals proceeded. By the

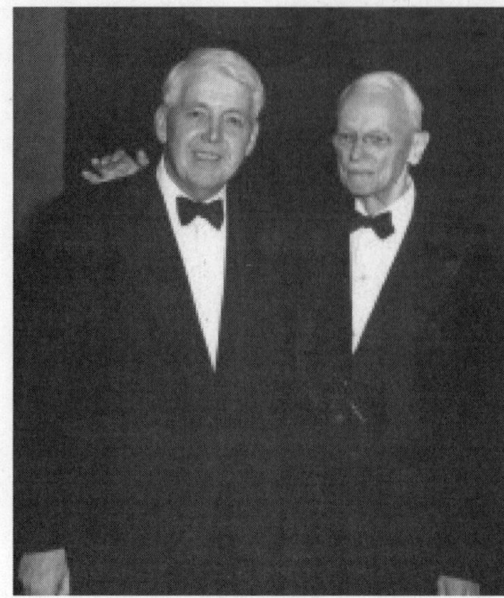

Professors Aldwyn Stokes and Clarence Farrar at the Canadian Psychiatric Association annual meeting in 1965. Courtesy CAMH Archives.

end of the decade, 11 hospitals and institutes were affiliated with the Department of Psychiatry for clinical teaching, bringing psychiatry toward the mainstream of medicine.

Stokes built up psychiatry wherever he could. He wanted the 72-bed Toronto Psychiatric Hospital to expand, both physically and intellectually. Over the course of the next 20 years, he added outpatient and forensics clinics, brought in specialists who contributed to the hospital's multidisciplinary approach, and added more classes in psychiatry at the university. Stokes worked tirelessly for the establishment of a larger university facility; like Clarke, he struggled to find the support he needed, and like Clarke, he succeeded. His greatest contribution in this regard was the establishment of the Clarke Institute of Psychiatry. He had started in the mid-1950s with task forces to build momentum for a new building. He also started lobbying the minister of health, Matthew Dymond, with whom he had a personal rapport.

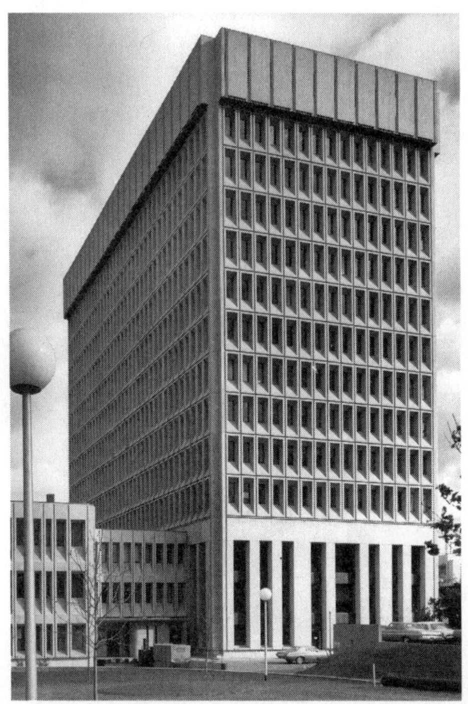

The Clarke Institute of Psychiatry opened in 1966 as a clinical research facility for the province and for the University of Toronto. Courtesy CAMH Archives.

The Clarke was chartered in legislation as the "Ontario Psychiatric Research Institute." However, as word of this name spread to the province's other medical schools, they registered their alarm with Minister Dymond—the new "Ontario Institute" would appear to represent psychiatry for the province as a whole and would thereby eclipse the others in attracting faculty, students, grants, and fundraising. What to do? Dymond asked for advice from his ministry staff. Their social work advisor, history buff Cyril Greenland, had acquired an admiration for the long-deceased C.K. Clarke, who was now otherwise largely forgotten. Greenland pitched this name, gently sheltering Dymond and Stokes from the worry of Clarke's eugenics advocacy, anti-Semitism, and other less-admirable traits. Dymond and his bureaucrats shrugged—why not? And so the legislation was hastily amended in time for the 1966 official opening ceremonies.[10]

The Clarke Institute opened in June 1966, established under the Ontario Mental Health Foundation Act, which made it a public hospital with a clinical research institute dedicated to mental illness. Research, education, and treatment were to be intertwined, just as Clarke envisaged. An independent board of directors was to govern the new facility, as occurred in general hospitals in order to minimize direct government interference.

The psychiatrist-in-chief of the Clarke would continue to be chair of the entire Department of Psychiatry at the University of Toronto. That would include the psychiatry departments at general hospitals such as the Hospital for Sick Children and Mount Sinai, and at Toronto General, which would set up a department one year later, in 1967. As chair of psychiatry, the head of the Clarke would also be directly involved in the appointment of the head psychiatrist at the province's largest mental health institution, the old asylum on Queen Street now known simply as 999.[11]

By the late 1960s, Queen Street had only a few hundred inhabitants. Asylums in Ontario and all over the Western world were in the process of emptying, dispatching their patients into the community, where they were supposed to be able to live comfortably with new drugs and on-the-ground care. The reality was completely different: people often ended up on the streets or in jail because community programs to help mentally ill people live outside the hospital weren't actually developed until the late 1970s. The result was that, at the very moment when the Clarke opened its tower to be a beacon of scientific research into mental illness, the people with the most serious chronic sickness had no place to live, just as hundreds of years before.

In 1966, when the Clarke opened in the brutalist tower on College Street, everything changed. A new leader was selected: Dr.

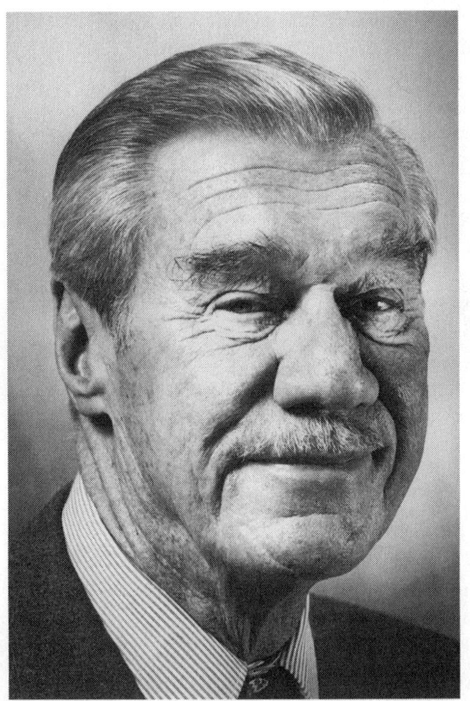

Robin Hunter changed psychiatry in Toronto during the 7 years he led the University Department and the Clarke Institute. His clinical skills spanned the breadth of psychiatric practice, and he was an outstanding teacher. Courtesy CAMH Archives.

Robin Hunter, a psychoanalyst, would attract a new breed of creative and optimistic psychoanalysts, some of whom thought the old-style generalists, the psychiatrists who depended on observable behaviour, were stuck in the past.

It's not clear why Hunter was selected, but Toronto wanted what McGill had. And McGill had Dr. Ewen Cameron, a man of particular prominence, having served as president of the Canadian, American, and World Psychiatric Associations. Cameron was not an analyst but was considered to have breadth and an ability to bridge the gap between the neurologically oriented psychiatrists and those in the asylum. Hunter was an analyst but also had breadth. I believe that Toronto also envied the United States and its analytic leaders.[12]

Hunter, the former chair of psychiatry at Queen's University in Kingston, was a handsome, tall, aristocratic-looking gentleman from an old, Caucasian Jamaican family. He had joined the Royal Canadian Air Force in 1940 and was shot down over Europe during the war. He spent four years in a prisoner-of-war camp. It left its mark. Before flying, Hunter always had to have a Scotch or two at the airport. At the end of the war, Hunter went to medical school at McGill, returning to London to complete his psychiatric residency. In 1955 he began his decade-long association with Montreal's Royal Victoria Hospital.

Hunter was an analyst who immersed himself in the thinking of Melanie Klein, the Viennese-born British psychoanalyst who was the first to psychoanalyze children. He would bring up Klein's metaphors about the good breast and the bad breast, and how a child needs to understand both can exist in the same person; the mother who nurtures is also the one who withholds nourishment at times. Hunter was never dogmatic, however. He could think as an analyst and as an eclectic clinician. He had even run a clinic in Montreal that put psychotic patients into insulin comas. Hunter did not shun drugs or other therapies that most psychoanalysts spurned. He appreciated the breadth of therapeutics that could be of value in various clinical circumstances. When patients were not responding, he pushed for greater use of medication and convulsive therapies. Always patient-centred, he made a point of going to the inpatient units, reviewing the charts of patients, and interviewing some to ensure they were getting the best care possible.

Hunter had a deep sense of ethics. At university he refused to join an anti-Semitic fraternity, and at the Clarke he was blind to colour and race. He was never prepared to pursue groundbreaking research at any cost. He often spoke about his teacher at McGill, Ewen Cameron, chair of the university's Department of Psychiatry and director of the Allen Memorial Institute in Montreal. He spoke about Cameron's expansive views that could leave science in the background. The Scottish-born Cameron was interested in memory and in schizophrenia, and he thought that mentally ill people could recover if they experienced a radical brain repatterning. To do this, Cameron administered a bizarre treatment involving three kinds of barbiturates and chlorpromazine to put his patients into a prolonged sleep. They'd be woken up several times a day for feeding, elimination, and repetitive electroconvulsive therapy.

Cameron's idea was to blot out psychotic behaviour and reeducate the patient. The theoretical basis for this was not only slim but dubious, and it led to severe memory problems with little upside. It turned out that Cameron's research was funded through an indirect route by the CIA, and after Cameron died in a mountaineering accident in the late 1960s, numerous lawsuits were launched against the Allen. Cameron is reviled today for his experiments on patients, many of whom had only relatively minor mental problems before the sleep treatment, but back then, in the 1960s, he was considered to be a bright star. He didn't hide his experiments; on the contrary, he reported the results in detail at a 1962 lecture at the Maudsley and later in a publication in the respected journal *Comprehensive Psychiatry*. Still, Hunter as his student never bought into that form of experimentation on humans. He wanted to hit a home run, just as Cameron did, but his moral compass was strong.

This was the world I entered when I accepted the invitation to do my psychiatric residency at the Clarke. The Clarke had successfully navigated its way through the stormy waters of 20th-century psychiatry, and now here it was, a tower of research on the edge of campus, a place where the men and women from competing psychiatric factions were on the brink of a great new revolution in psychiatry, one that would change the nature of psychiatric research and our understanding of mental illness.

CHAPTER 5
My Early Years

The Clarke Institute of Psychiatry was designed in the 1960s by the well-known Toronto architect John Parkin. When I first saw the building, in the fall of 1969, three years after it was opened by Ontario premier John Robarts, I wondered what Parkin could possibly have been thinking. This building was not designed for comfort or for healing. It was a forbidding 13-storey concrete tower that loomed over the University of Toronto's genteel, ivy-covered campus. The 1960s-style fortress made no effort to blend in with the jumble of little shops on the street below. The windows were so small you couldn't see in, and the steps leading up to the entrance were oddly spaced, so you'd have to take a step and a half to go up each stair. It was a classic example of brutalist architecture that looked as though it belonged in a totalitarian state, not in the heart of Canada's mental health care system. Perhaps it is appropriate that the creator of this ugly building would be immortalized in Timothy Findley's 1994 book *Headhunter*. Findlay named his asylum the Parkin Institute of Psychiatric Research. I never knew whether he was referring to the architect or to Alan Parkin, one of the fathers of Canadian psychoanalysis, who was later found to be sexually abusing his female patients.

I was really nervous that day I first went to the Clarke, and the unwelcoming building didn't make me feel any better. I was about to meet the man who had invited me there, Dr. Vivian Rakoff, the University of Toronto's director of postgraduate education and one of the legends of Canadian psychiatry, and I still wasn't sure how I, a 23-year-old intern with a meagre background in the field, could ever develop the skills to help the patients inside.

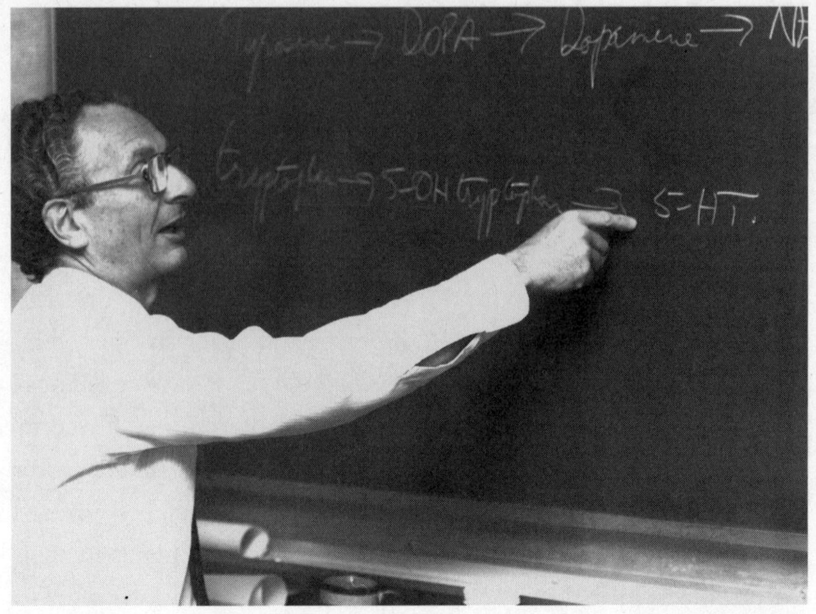

Harvey Stancer leading a discussion on the neurotransmitters in the 1970s.
Courtesy CAMH Archives.

I stepped into the elevator, and when I got out, I knew I had stepped into a different world.

Patients were shuffling stiffly down the hall, past institutional paint and pictures bolted to the wall. Most of them were smoking and grossly overweight. Many clearly hadn't brushed their hair or tidied their clothes. Some were drooling and gazing blankly into the distance as they slumped into stained furniture. I could tell right away that many of them were suffering from psychosis and were on drugs to suppress hallucinations and delusions. Chlorpromazine, the first antipsychotic drug, introduced to North America in 1954 by McGill University's Heinz Lehmann, relieved the terror of the hallucinations and delusions, but it was a dirty drug that caused nasty side effects. So did the new antidepressant drugs, such as Tofranil, Elavil, and Parnate. Although they relieved the depression, they caused blurred vision, constipation, sleepiness, and significant weight gain, which distressed many of the women. Nearly everyone had a parched mouth. You could hear the smacking of lips and gums as they spoke.

In my state of nervous preoccupation, I had clearly gone to the wrong floor. This was General Psychiatry, one floor above Rakoff's office. At the giant nursing station just opposite the elevator, I saw what must have been nurses, orderlies, and doctors milling around, drinking coffee and smoking cigarettes, though they didn't look like any hospital staff I'd seen in the general hospitals. The psychiatrists wore natty sports jackets and ties, not white coats; the rest of the staff wore jeans and tie-died shirts and beads, the style of the 1960s counterculture. I wondered how you could tell patients from the staff. The senior resident would later give me the answer: slippers. I would eventually come up with my own clue. It was the key rings. The staff always made sure they were visible; they wouldn't want to be confused with a patient.

I sheepishly headed down to the eighth floor, where Rakoff awaited me in his handsome office, just off the elevator. Rakoff was smallish at five foot eight and beautifully dressed and groomed, with a small, greying goatee. He was worldly, articulate, and charming, with a lovely and distinctive South African accent. I'd heard his voice before, as he was frequently on radio, speaking about the gift of adolescence, which was, in his view, an extended period of self-discovery. (My mother-in-law thought he was the most eloquent man she had ever heard.)

Born in Cape Town, he had studied psychology and then medicine at the University of London before coming to Canada in 1961 to join the Psychiatry Department at McGill. While at McGill, Rakoff had distinguished himself in family therapy and adolescence; there he also examined the effects of the Holocaust on children of concentration camp survivors.

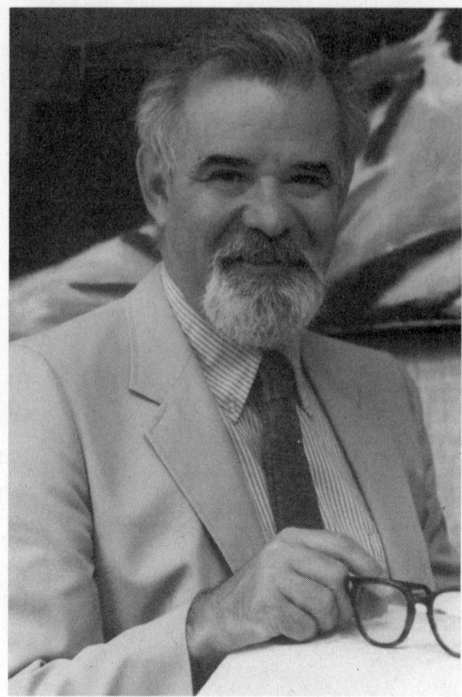

South African Vivian Rakoff trained in London before studying psychiatry at McGill. He was recruited to Toronto by Robin Hunter in 1968 and became a leading educator and later the chair of the University of Toronto's psychiatry department and director of the Clarke Institute of Psychiatry from 1980 to 1990. Courtesy CAMH Archives.

Like many other English-speaking Quebecers caught up in the turmoil of the time, he joined the exodus from Montreal in the late 1960s. He came to Toronto to be chief of psychiatry at St. Michael's, one of the large downtown teaching hospitals in the Toronto system, but he soon felt the sting of anti-Semitism in Canada's largest city. After he had accepted, the St. Michael's offer was mysteriously withdrawn. Rakoff learned why from Robin Hunter: it was because Rakoff is Jewish.

In our first meeting, he described the role of psychiatry so beautifully. Like all of medicine, it involves a social interaction, he said. It is an art but based on science. In conventional thinking, art and science are separate worlds—one creative, passionate, and romantic; the other cold, rigorous, and objective—but both are driven by a passion for understanding and explanation, both work from imagination and informed intuition. Rakoff would often say how much of medical practice was an art until the end of the 19th century. By the end of World War II, medicine aimed for science, but much of medicine was still in the realms of the creative and the humanistic.

I was deeply impressed, but if I was going to practice psychiatry, I asked him, then why should I start out in Toronto instead of in Montreal? Montreal's McGill had built a strong international reputation in the field over the past 20 years and in the late 1960s was still the most exciting place for psychiatry in Canada. And Montreal was a delightful city, still enjoying the afterglow of Expo '67. True, separatist radicals had planted bombs in mailboxes in Westmount, where many English-speaking executives and doctors lived. But the terrorists were denounced by everyone, including René Lévesque, the sovereignist leader. So wouldn't this be a great place for a Winnipeg boy to study psychiatry, and enjoy the city's wonderful restaurants and joie de vivre?

Rakoff shook his head. He still had an extremely dark view of Quebec. Even in 1969, it was clear that Quebec nationalism made his blood boil. "Going to Montreal now," he warned me, "would be like a Jew moving to Germany in 1933."

That was Rakoff: brilliant, sharp, and provocative. Many of his colleagues were uneasy around him—he took up so much energy in a room, and his tongue was like a sword, to the extent that people were often hesitant to confront or disagree with him. Instead, they'd makes jibes about him behind his back, such as at an alcohol-fuelled dinner when a fellow psychiatrist would get up to make a speech and reassure his audience that he was going to be brief, not like Rakoff.

Still, Rakoff's view of psychiatry was thrilling to me. He could envision where the science could take the field but would never lose sight of the fundamental role of the healer. This was a model that could encourage my growth as a professional, a framework of science in the service of caring for others. Of course, I said yes to his offer.

When I arrived at the Clarke in June 1970, Rakoff assigned me to the Clarke's Clinical Investigation Unit, where some of the most puzzling cases in psychiatry were sent to be studied in a comprehensive manner. These patients were the mysteries that couldn't be helped by conventional psychiatric techniques. The aim of the unit, as its name suggested, was not only to treat patients but to study them in a controlled environment in order to contribute to the scientific understanding of these mysterious mental illnesses and also to see if there could be alternatives to the standard treatments. The patients had been handpicked by the scientist who created the Clinical Investigation Unit, Harvey Stancer, and his colleague Harvey Moldofsky, for special treatment.

Stancer was a slight, intense man with prominent glasses and short curly hair. A chemist by training, he spoke in short, clipped sentences. He came from a business family; his parents had been milliners and then owned a movie theatre in Toronto. After getting a PhD in chemistry and a medical degree in Toronto, he had lived in New York, where he did his psychiatry residency at Columbia University, and then in London, England, where he had worked as a fellow in the chemistry of psychiatry.

Stancer was a pioneer in the early days of the drug revolution. Doctors were just beginning to use the first antidepressant and antianxiety drugs to relieve the dark pit of depression, and Stancer thought the answers to the problems of illnesses like depression lay in the chemistry of the brain. He was well positioned to play a leading role in this revolutionary approach, and he had several offers to work in the United States, but he wanted to make his mark in his hometown.

When Stancer returned to Toronto in 1963, he intended to apply his scientific principles and rigour to the practice of

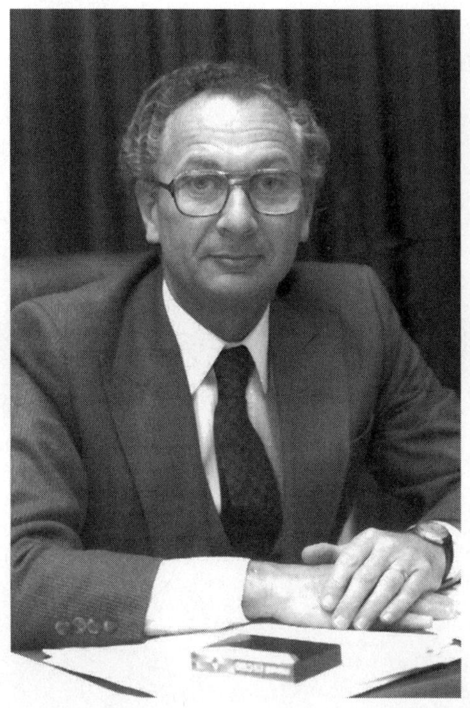

Toronto-born Harvey Stancer was originally an organic chemist who studied medicine and psychiatry. He returned to Toronto in the early 1960s and later became professor of psychiatric research, before moving to California in the late 1980s. He played a leading role in developing science in Canadian psychiatry and was a major influence in the career development of several academic psychiatrists, including that of Paul Garfinkel. Courtesy CAMH Archives.

psychiatry. Unfortunately, what he saw in Toronto did not inspire him. Toronto, as far Stancer was concerned, was a psychiatric backwater where the modus operandi was "anything goes." In those days, psychiatrists might have had a background in neurology or in psychiatry, but lacking training in science, they didn't use the scientific method. From his perspective, they weren't objective—they relied far too often on their impression or experiences, rather than on scientific principles or statistical study data. Random assignment, blind or double-blind studies were standard practice in medicine but only beginning to be so in psychiatry, which infuriated Stancer. He was even more bothered than most psychiatrists of that time, who didn't care about the application of science to the field. He thought that most psychiatrists relied on personal impression far more than did physicians in other branches of medicine. This

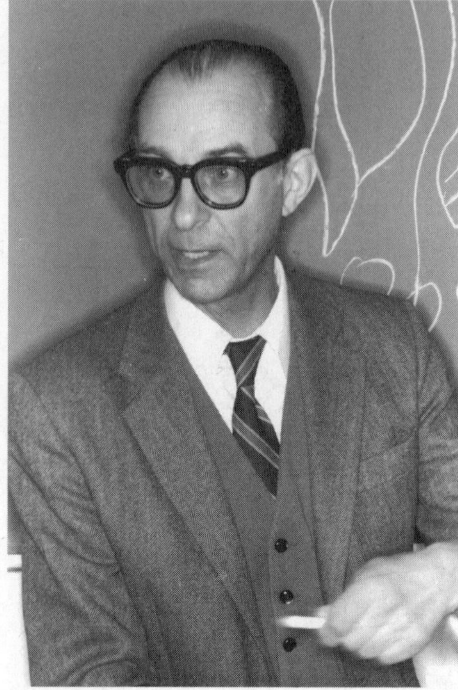

Oleh Hornykiewicz, an outstanding neuroscientist, made fundamental discoveries that led to new treatments for Parkinson's disease. He moved back to Vienna in 1987 to lead the Institute of Biochemical Pharmacology at the University of Vienna's Faculty of Medicine. Courtesy CAMH Archives.

meant that treatments were being determined by physician bias rather than evidence.

Stancer came from a world where the scientific method ruled. This included careful observation and rigorous testing of a hypothesis. He didn't see any reason this shouldn't apply to psychiatry too. He reserved particular contempt for psychoanalysis, which aimed to bring to the surface the repressed from the unconscious. The unconscious, by its very nature, couldn't be observed or measured directly. The treatment, talk therapy, wasn't being submitted to rigorous testing to see if it worked. Stancer didn't believe it was scientific: "Imagine grown-up people doing this!" he'd say.

He wanted to bring scientific rigour to psychiatry in Toronto, and especially to the diagnosis and treatment of mental illness. He felt that this would make the field more effective, more respected, and also more accountable to a broad public. Accountability was important to Stancer, long before others became concerned with it.

Harvey Moldofsky, then about 35, was second-in-command to Stancer in the Clarke's Clinical Investigative Unit. He couldn't have been more different from the intense and opinionated Stancer. He was quiet and so absent-minded that he once arrived at an early morning meeting with his comb still in his hair. A Torontonian, he had been an intern in Vancouver and then studied psychiatry in Toronto before going on to do part of his postgraduate training at St. George's Hospital in London with Arthur Crisp, one of the world experts on eating disorders. Moldofsky was interested in mind-body problems and would see the occasional person with anorexia nervosa, as well as people with other unusual problems, such as Tourette's syndrome, obsessive-compulsive disorder, or pain syndromes. In 1970, when I was the junior resident on the unit, he took a six-month sabbatical to work with William Dement at Stanford, coming back to establish Toronto's first sleep clinic. He subsequently made important contributions to the relationship between sleep and pain.

Stancer and Moldofsky liked to tease naive young residents like me. That summer of 1970, six weeks after my arrival, I hoped to drive in my '67 Mustang to visit relatives in New York, so I asked for time off. Moldofsky turned to Stancer. "We don't usually let people go until they've cured one patient," he said; "should we make an exception this time?" Stancer shook his head. "I think not."

The Clinical Investigation Unit was on the fifth floor. As you came off the elevators, you turned right down a long corridor. In the centre was a large common room, a dining room, and a kitchen designed for the supervision of a diet if a study required it. On either side of this large common area were a set of rooms; one group of single and double rooms housed the 11 inpatients. At the other end of the corridor were a series of offices for the residents,

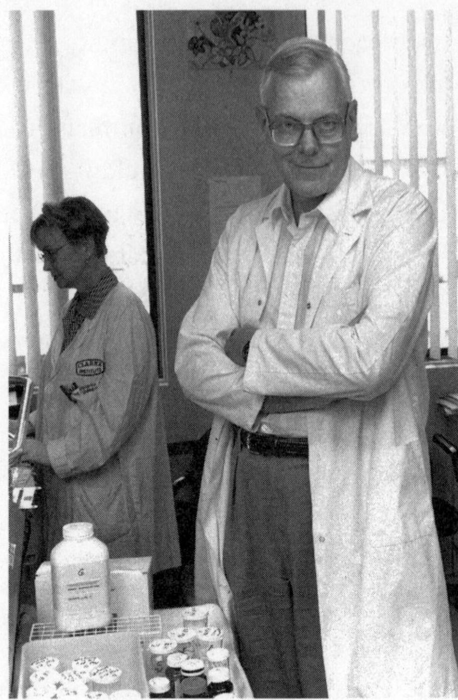

Greg Brown, a psychiatrist and neurendocrinologist who studied the role of a variety of hormones in psychiatric disorders. He became chair of Neuroscience at McMaster University and, later, vice president of research at the Clarke Institute. Courtesy CAMH Archives.

social worker, and psychologist. In contrast to the other inpatient units at the Clarke, the heads—Stancer and Moldofsky—didn't have offices on the floor of their unit; they wanted the residents to feel they were in charge of their own patients.

The patients were fascinating. There was a former teacher in her 50s, living with a benign pituitary tumour and a severe depression, and almost immobilized by headaches and apathy. A well-dressed racing groom was an impeccable conversationalist, until he burst out with a string of "Fuck, fuck fucks!"—a sign of a then little-known syndrome called Tourette's. An emaciated young woman paced up and down the halls all day. Their conditions were mysterious and captivating. But the patient who most stands out in my memory, the one who marked my commitment to this messy field, was a woman in her 50s called Margaret.

Margaret had been transferred to the Clarke from Kingston Psychiatric Hospital with a long-standing catatonic illness. She would sit frozen, immobilized. She had what was termed a "waxy flexibility." If you lifted her arm, it would remain in place until it was moved again, as if it were made of wax. Margaret always wore a simple, printed housedress, and her grey hair in a pageboy. She had to be assisted in all activities of daily living, and a dedicated and empathic nurse, Carolyn Smale, endlessly comforted and supported her. As did I. I was both fascinated and saddened. I pored over her history and the relevant literature. We tried everything, but to no avail. After several months, however, one of our experimental medicines, L-dopa, a drug newly introduced for Parkinson's disease, seemed to make a huge difference. Margaret recovered; she was animated and described her life experiences in detail. She told us about being a single schoolteacher in the area around Kingston, about her life with her family. I was exhilarated. It was an extraordinary awakening. But several months later, after being switched to placebo (as called for by the research trial), she woke up in her old catatonic form. We tried the same medicine a second time, but with no results. Nothing worked, and there was nothing more we could do for her. This was a research facility, so she had to go back to Kingston. The morning she left, I went down to the Spadina Avenue doors, where the ambulance came to get her. I could barely watch as it pulled away from the Clarke. But at that very moment, I knew I was fully committed to finding answers for patients like Margaret, or if that wasn't possible, at least helping them live better lives.

Under Robin Hunter's leadership, the Clarke as an institution was changing dramatically. Hunter himself used drugs and several forms of talk therapy, whatever worked for the patient. Now, after taking over the leadership of the Clarke in 1966, he expanded the institute's mainstay, the careful scientific branch of psychiatry. But he also brought in psychoanalysts and good general psychotherapists. In keeping with Hunter's high standards and with Stancer's urging on the science side, he insisted on recruiting top people.

The range of intellects at the Clarke was astonishing. From Vienna and Oxford came Oleh Hornykiewicz, who had revolutionized the way Parkinson's is treated with his discovery of altered levels of the neurotransmitter dopamine in the basal ganglia, clusters of tightly interconnected nerve cells deep in the brain that have a role in initiating and regulating motor commands. This research led to the development of L-dopa and other pioneering medicines.

A distinguished, slight, sophisticated European man with flip-up glasses, Hornykiewicz was also an excellent mentor. Although he returned to Vienna in 1987 to head up the Institute of Biochemical Pharmacology at the University of Vienna's Faculty of Medicine, newly created for him by the Austrian government, for the next 10 years and more he commuted between Vienna and Toronto so that he could head the Clarke's new Human Brain Laboratory (later the Human Neurochemical Pathology Laboratory). He was a force at the Clarke for more than 20 years. Many of us thought he deserved the 2000 Nobel Prize, awarded to three researchers who had determined how nerve cells exchange their signals.

Gregory Brown, then a young psychiatrist who had been a student of Stancer, got his PhD in the relatively new field of neuroendocrinology, working with the pioneering Dr. Seymour Reichlin at the University of Rochester School of Medicine and Dentistry in Rochester, New York. He returned to Toronto in 1968 and was working on developing measurements for a number of hormones that might be implicated in mental illness.

From Hong Kong came the distinguished transcultural psychiatrist P.M. Yap, who studied the manifestations of psychiatric disorders in different cultures. He was fascinated by Koro, a belief

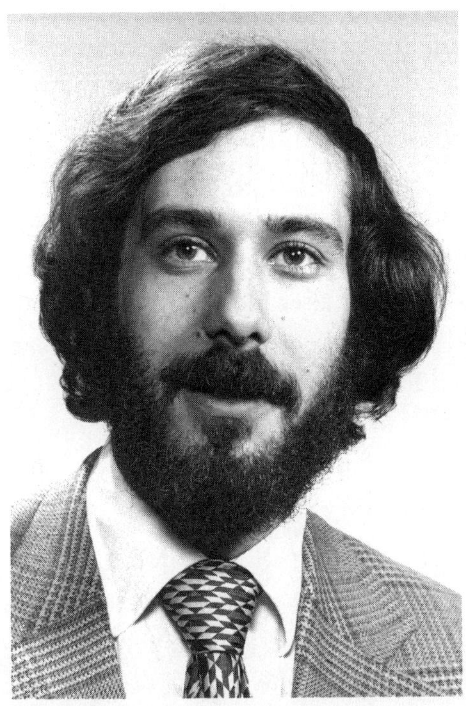

Paul Garfinkel when he was working with Robin Hunter as chief resident of the Clarke Institute in 1972. Courtesy CAMH Archives.

that one's penis is shrinking into the abdomen. It had occurred in epidemic form in southern China, but sporadic cases have been reported in many parts of the world. (One day this interesting problem caused Dr. Yap some grief: he was stopped at Canadian customs, and his slides showing a man with weights attached to his penis, to prevent its disappearance, were examined at length.)

From Britain came Dr. Betty Steiner and her work on gender, including transsexuals, now transgendered, men (usually) who felt they were women. This was a new field for medicine and psychiatry. At the Clarke, neuroendocrinologist Greg Brown assessed and measured hormone levels, while Dr. Kurt Freund, a Czechoslovakian physician/researcher, measured sexual arousal with a phallometer, which measures blood flow to the penis. As an index of sexual arousal, it is a very effective instrument that is still in use today.

This was a new frontier in gender, and the team drew up an elaborate protocol to learn more about the physiological, hormonal, and psychiatric implications of a man who wanted to turn into a woman. As the junior resident, I did the physical examinations. These could be startling because, although these patients were on hormones, they were still biologically male. Starting from the head, I checked the patient's breasts and then later moved on to examine the penis. It took a little adjustment in perspective for me to see both on one individual.

Stan Freeman, a firebrand Torontonian, believed in community-based care. He and his team occupied the other half of the fifth floor, opposite the Clinical Investigation Unit. They were studying stress in air traffic controllers, and the mental condition of meteorologists in isolated, harsh environments such as remote Arctic mining and oil-drilling installations. His team also studied the borough of East York, a part of metropolitan Toronto, to determine how to prevent and identify mental illnesses and how to link services from an academic centre to a community.

The forensic group had been strong since Ken Gray, both a lawyer and a psychiatrist, built a team in the 1950s and early 1960s. Ed Turner, and a younger man, Ken McKnight, were the leaders when I arrived. Turner, a kind Hamiltonian who studied in Bristol, England, was a true organization man and would go on to be the medical director, really, Hunter's right-hand man.[1]

The Clarke had good clinician-teachers. Emmanuel Persad had just completed his psychiatric residency in 1969 and was brought on staff. He was a Trinidadian, educated in England before coming to Canada. A gentle, thoughtful clinician, Emmanuel was an excellent teacher; later he became chair of psychiatry at the University of Western Ontario. Gerry Shugar, a Torontonian who became a Canadian squash champion, was also a leading teacher. One of the first manic patients I ever saw, a hypertalkative Jewish woman, kept describing him as "Sugar-meshuga" ("meshuga" being Yiddish for "crazy").

From Ireland via Kingston, clinician-teacher Joel Jeffries worked with people with schizophrenia and wrote successful and practical books on the pharmacology of treating the illness. Hunter recruited from Scotland Jim Davie, an analyst who could read you so clearly that you'd feel your skin was transparent. The son of a prison guard in Kingston, Doug Frayn led the Outpatient Department and went on to become an excellent analyst and supervisor. The arrival of so many outsiders—analysts and clinician researchers—shook up the Toronto establishment.

As a young resident, I was studying both descriptive psychiatry and psychodynamics. The descriptive side readily fit with all the training I had received in medical school: What are patients' symptoms, what contributes from their current, past, and family history? And what objective signs do I observe? I found psychodynamics as an area of study intriguing but not easy. Analytic language was obscure, much of it metaphor. I liked the psychoanalytic concepts but became increasingly frustrated with the terminology. Ideas like "regression in the service of the ego," "the good and bad breast," and "object relationships" were difficult for me to grasp. Why couldn't these ideas be put into sensible language? But over time I found there was real value in this approach to understanding patients and especially to being with people who were seriously ill or hopeless. Exploring past experiences, the meanings of illness, recurring patterns in relationships, and patients' fantasy life could have real bearing on current circumstances. The techniques helped develop relationships with patients and permitted patients to explore their world. These psychodynamic psychotherapists focused on feelings and the expression of emotions. They explored why patients were avoiding distressing thoughts and feelings, and the issue of recurring themes or patterns. They focused on interpersonal relationships, the fantasy life, and the relationship patients form with the therapist rather than on just the observable phenomena and practical recommendations. I learned that being understood is hugely important to people and in itself offers hope.

This type of thinking is important to psychiatrists. Of course, if patients are acutely suicidal or psychotic, getting on top of the practical issues is critical. But so is being able to sit with patients and absorb what it means to be in their world. What did this hopelessness feel like? How did patients understand their feelings in relation to their past history and the people in their world? Although I'm not a psychoanalyst and I was never psychoanalyzed myself, this dynamic thinking helped me to be with people. This was a means of understanding people, one of several, that could be useful in some circumstances, and less so in others.

It helped me to be more patient, a virtue that I had seen in great clinicians in other fields of medicine. As an intern, I had worked with an excellent cardiologist Susan Lenke at Toronto Western. She could see how I urgently wanted to fix things, and when a man came in with acute pulmonary edema, she asked what I would do. We'll administer morphine, oxygen, a diuretic, and rotating tourniquets (common in those days), I replied. What next? she asked. I began to consider every possible drug in the ER. She would have none of it. "No," she said. "Now we go for coffee."

What I particularly liked about psychodynamic thinking was that it pushed you to explore and enquire, beyond the superficial level. I have always kept a notepad and pen by my office chair. I take notes, especially upon first meeting the patient. I let the person know I'll be taking notes while we talk, and may not always be looking at him or her. People have different responses to note taking. They might ask, "What are you going to do with these, who will be seeing them?" Or think, *I am so grateful that you are going to be listening, my last therapist was not invested in understanding me—I was neglected.* Or, *I must be so important to have you write down what I say—I'll have to make sure you get it right.* Three people responding to the same thing in very different ways.

In the seven years that Hunter ran the Clarke and the university's Psychiatric Department, he changed Toronto psychiatry. It became much more diverse, but with an often uneasy truce between the disparate groups. There seemed something fixed and inflexible, almost fetishized about the psychoanalytic approach as well, which didn't quite jibe with all the other new ideas and therapies cropping up. This was really brought home to me when Harold Searles, a prominent American analyst, visited the Clarke to review his lengthy experience using intensive psychotherapy to treat a handful of people with psychosis. Freud himself didn't think that psychotherapy worked for psychosis, but psychoanalysis was so appealing in the 1950s and 1960s in the United States that many analysts, like Searles, tried it anyway. Some, like Searles, had clung to the idea even when good controlled studies showed how important the medicines were for psychosis. The case for drugs was made in a landmark 1964 study by Philip May, a Californian psychiatrist. He demonstrated that the new phenothiazine medicines (such as chlorpromazine) relieved psychosis better than did traditional care, psychotherapy, or a placebo. He also found that the combination of medicine with the psychotherapy did not prove more effective than the medicine alone. In other words, the drug was the critical ingredient for treating psychosis. These medicines became the cornerstone of treatment for schizophrenia.[2]

When Searles visited, he described his intensive work with a handful of psychotic people over many years. I felt sad for him, and even sadder for his patients. They had done so much work, and yet they had so little to show for it and at a time when new drugs could have relieved the psychotic symptoms. I knew that I wasn't alone in thinking that, as important as analytic thought was, it was by no means a treatment option for most patients, especially those most critically ill.

Sometimes the debate between the scientific types and the psychoanalysts interfered with basic patient care. I saw it in my second year of residency while I was working with children and adolescents at the Hincks Treatment Centre in Toronto.[3] One day I presented the case of a late adolescent suffering from a serious depression. I used analytic concepts to make sense of the story, but the treatment I recommended was an antidepressant drug, along with psychotherapy and career counselling. The first question came from a senior member of staff: Was I worried that the use of the antidepressant drug might kill the motivation of the patient for therapy? At that time, rather than accept that seriously ill people could be helped by medications, the analytic community often felt threatened by the use of medications.

These debates seemed theoretical on night call, though. Most admissions to the Clarke came through the ER, as they do for the Centre for Addiction and Mental Health (CAMH) today. Patients were in traumatic circumstances; they may have attempted suicide, or were having a severe reaction to street drugs. (Recreational drugs had become the "in" thing in the 1970s, and reactions to them were common; with music clubs the Silver Dollar Room and the Comfort Zone just across the street, the Clarke was unhappily close to the action.) People came in on their own, were dragged in by family members or friends, or were brought in by the police. As well, our own outpatients might come in during off-hours if they were having side effects to their medicines or were experiencing a recurrence of symptoms or disturbing events.

The ER in those days was quite simple: a tiny interview room on the first floor behind the switchboard operator. There wasn't any security, but in those days we weren't particularly security-conscious. Then one Friday night, my colleague Steve Kline was on duty. A man pulled a handgun on him and discharged it, only to have the gun misfire. That incident certainly made us all more than a little nervous. The next night, I was on call dealing with a man reeking of alcohol who was demanding admission. I repeatedly refused, suggesting instead we find him a hostel. He became exasperated with me, paused, and reached into the inside pocket of his short leather jacket. My heart was in my mouth, anticipating a rerun of the previous night's events. But he brought out a bottle of cheap sherry, saying, "Let's talk about this over a drink."[4]

As a resident, I felt anxious and insecure a lot of the time, and not just when working nights in ER. Although I loved the idea of understanding and treating people with complex mental illness, and I felt a real compassion and caring for the seriously ill, I worried that I didn't have the competency I needed to make a difference to my patients, and confronted with complicated and mysterious problems, I felt helpless. I wasn't sure I would ever master some of the more abstract psychodynamic views that could be of use in understanding people.

CHAPTER 6
Training Takes Its Toll

The profession of psychiatry didn't pay enough attention to the mental health of its own members, especially residents. That was obvious to me from the very beginning of my training just by listening to conversations with my colleagues. So I dealt with my anxieties in my typical fashion: by learning about them. Young physicians are clearly capable, ambitious, motivated, and extremely bright. They can grow at a phenomenal pace in the right circumstances. At the same time, too many of them suffer. I found an article, published just a couple of years earlier, in 1967, that described what I saw around me. As authors Lewis Merklin and Ralph Little, who worked at a private hospital in Pennsylvania, said, the first year of residency training is "that most difficult year." Students, feeling anxious and helpless, search for strategies to cope. They simultaneously feel the need to control and the fear of being controlled. They can even develop what Merklin and Little described as the "beginning psychiatry training syndrome," characterized by temporary neurotic symptoms such as anxiety and worry with depressive features, sleep loss, and often with bodily aches and pains.

Residency is hard for all specialists: between 25 and 30% become depressed or develop an anxiety disorder during their residency, far more than in the same age group in the general population.[1] (In the general population, 8 to 12% experience these symptoms at any one time.) Rates as high as 40% have been documented for impaired performance due to anxiety or depression lasting for four weeks or longer.[2] When my colleague Ted Waring did studies of medical and psychiatric residents, he found that between 15 and 20% scored as cases with a high likelihood of psychiatric disturbance during their first year.[3] It seems to be worse for psychiatry residents. Although they make up 5 to 8% of the residency population, in some reviews from the 1970s, they account for up to 30% of the suicides.

What's more, psychiatry residents faced a high risk of failure: in the early 1970s, about 50% of residents who started in the training program either failed their specialist exams (35%), often after four years of hard work, or dropped out of training (15%).[4] This was a higher percentage than the failure and dropout rates in other branches of medicine. Why was this happening? Was it the people who chose psychiatry, or was it the pressures of the profession?

Residency requires learning new skills just after you've received a hard-earned medical degree—in many ways it feels like starting over. This is true for all specialists. Residents often move to a new city, work long hours, do thankless tasks, miss their partner, and try to handle their looming debt at a time when they feel they are novice students again. They often have to make difficult decisions while being at risk for errors due to fatigue and inexperience. Residents are faced with human tragedies and have to learn to deal with some of life's most sensitive issues, such as death, dying and loss. It is hard, especially when residents in all specialties face intense competition for post-residency jobs while experiencing constant demands, criticism, and, perhaps, harassment from teachers and supervisors. They do all this while frequently separated from supportive networks, such as family and friends, adding to the stress. Sometimes just moving to a new hospital every six months or year adds to the feeling of not belonging.

Residency for most physicians occurs at a particular time or phase in life—in their 20s. Forming a personal identity is a continual, never-ending process, but it is a critical function at this time in life, when young physicians are so devoted to becoming professionally competent. For some, personal growth is stunted, their identity becoming merged with work. For others, autonomy and performance are emphasized at the expense of intimacy and friendships; loneliness can ensue.

Psychiatric residents have to live with the demands of all medical residents, but they also face the prospect of violence, often for the first time—as did my colleague. Between 40 and 50% of psychiatry residents will be physically attacked by a patient during their four-year training program, according to a study from Wayne State University.[5] Psychiatrists are far more likely to be assaulted than other professionals. According to the US Department of Justice's National Crime Victimization Survey conducted from 1993 to 1999, the annual rate of non-fatal, job-related violent crime was 12.6 per 1,000 workers in all occupations. Among physicians, the rate was 16.2 per 1,000, and among nurses, 21.9 per 1,000. However, for psychiatrists and mental health care professionals, the rate was 68.2 per 1,000, and for mental health custodial workers, 69 per 1,000.[6]

Psychiatric residents also have to live with cutting comments from other medical colleagues about their chosen specialty. Then, while colleagues are ridiculing the profession, psychiatric residents get their first taste of the burden: the emotional pressure of dealing with patients who might harm themselves after they leave the office. One psychiatrist who trained in both internal medicine and psychiatry put it this way: "Being a medicine resident and being a psychiatric resident were both really hard for different reasons. As a medicine resident you were just so goddamned exhausted. You were on call one night in three. After your night on call you would go home the next morning at seven o'clock; you did your laundry and tried to get your life going, and the next night you're there until eleven o'clock and the next day up all night again. You were exhausted. In psychiatry, this demand was less, but there was a different kind of stress. You know, I still remember discharging patients from emerg and going home and thinking, *"Did I do the right thing? What if they kill themselves? Am I going to be there?"*[7] Constant worry is draining.

Anthropologist T.M. Luhrmann described the early residency period well.[8] Most residents feel an inadequacy to some degree through this part of their training, often seeing themselves as a fake or imposter. Because they find it so difficult to master psychodynamic thought, many turn to descriptive psychiatry and psychopharmacology, as it is easier to learn and feel a sense of efficacy. Luhrmann was also right, in my view, in saying that residents turn to this because it helps to avoid awkward intimacy with patients.

Nevertheless, it's shocking to see the high rate of suicide among psychiatric residents. Why were so many killing themselves? In 1975, Robert Pasnau and his colleague in California studied five psychiatric residents who committed suicide.[9] Although Pasnau found no single cause, he did see some striking similarities between the five residents. They all were having trouble with their marriages. They didn't have close friends. They all abused either drugs or alcohol. Residency was considered very difficult and stressful. In other words, they succumbed to a deadly mixture of personal, peer, and institutional factors.

Still, it was a mystery. Why do so many psychiatric residents suffer depression or even consider suicide? Is it the job? Or is it the personality of the people who choose psychiatry as a profession?

I started studying this problem of residents at the Clarke in the early 1970s, with Betty Steiner, one of the senior psychiatrists I was working with, and Robin Hunter. Later a colleague, Ted Waring, and I did tests of residents using several psychological instruments. In the first studies we found that the high failure rate on fellowship exams was partly due to the type of people who entered the field. The psychiatrists who had trouble tended to be older physicians entering psychiatry later in their careers, or were people who were not familiar with the culture or language. But more important, some of the psychiatric residents who failed their exams were identified by their supervisors as being not suited to the field, or were troubled. The residents who developed signs of emotional disturbance in their first six months of training scored more like bankers or accountants on aptitude tests. They scored high on tests of depression, neuroticism, isolation, and introversion. The problem, in other words, did not lie in their intellectual ability to do the job. It wasn't even the volume of work; the on-call hours were less frequent for a psychiatrist than for many other medical residents. Instead, they were hindered by personality factors coupled with the stress and emotional upheaval that occurred during residency.

Our profession can help residents who are having emotional problems become useful members of the profession. A 1976 study in the United States by Floyd Garetz, Otto Rath, and Richard Morse reviewed 200 psychiatric residents who had trained at one university over a 25-year period.[10] Some 13% of them were considered disturbed (psychotic, addictive, severely neurotic, or with serious character problems). Of these, 80% were considered disturbed enough for faculty to consider asking them to leave the program. However, many of these residents benefited from psychotherapy and, after follow-up, only 10% could be considered "failures" in their careers. The answer from this study, then, was that, with therapy, psychiatric residents with emotional troubles can heal and go on to successful careers helping others.

I dealt with my own anxiety by studying fellow residents, and it gave me a lifelong interest in the mental health of my own profession. I suppose it helped. I passed my professional exams, and I would be a fully licensed psychiatrist by November 1974.

Even as I dealt with the professional challenges of my psychiatric residency, I faced deep personal trials. In November 1971 my brother Marvin called to say my mother might have an aortic aneurysm that could be rupturing. I rushed back to Winnipeg, but when I got to her bedside, my mother was sitting up, cheerful and relaxed. I shouldn't have come out, she assured us; it wasn't necessary. Her physicians thought she would be fine. It wasn't a ruptured aneurysm, they said, just an infection around the heart.

It turned out she had metastatic cancer, but it was not recognized for another month or two. In the third week of February, Barry called me. "You have to come quickly," he said. I got on the next plane and, upon landing, raced to the hospital. But my mother had just died. I didn't get to say goodbye.

I was in shock. I took three weeks off, and then went back to work at the Hincks. But my sleep was poor, and for the first time in my life I felt lonely. It seemed as though everything, myself included, was unreal. Moldofsky, who had recently lost a parent; Barry, my brother; and I would go together to the morning prayers at the Anshei Minsk congregation in Kensington Market. In late afternoon we would go to the Beth Tzedek synagogue, near our homes. One of the people at the Minsk, clearly at one time a psychiatric patient, would announce our arrival: "Here come the psychiatrists. They feed *chazer* [pig] to the patients at Queen Street."

Grief did not feel like anything I had read about. It was so intense, so painful and full of guilt. I hadn't been there to say goodbye to my mother. But I also felt that Mother, who died at age 58, had been cheated out of the fruits of life. She would never meet her grandchildren, never have the pleasure of our accomplishments. My wife, Dorothy, had been very close to my mother, and she shared the sense of grief and loss. Being connected to her was a comfort and extraordinarily helpful to me in surviving this period and moving forward.

Three years later, in June 1975, my father died of a stroke. He was 68. It wasn't so surprising—he had been hypertensive for years and had once smoked heavily. But it was jarring.

I again felt guilty. Had I thanked him properly? He had lived a hard life, coming to Canada at age 20, uneducated, with no one giving him a break. He had worked so hard for the family, only to lose his wife before he could start to really enjoy life. I again felt lonely, the existential loneliness that we experience at the loss of the second parent.

I grieved for my parents for a long time. I thought about them every day. Life, as it turned out, wasn't fair after all.

On some level I was still grieving when my own children were approaching the age I was when my mother died. I am not certain why I held on to this for so long. I had always felt that I would be likely to die as my mother did, in my late 50s, but when I actually arrived there, I realized I didn't have to die, and in fact could reinvest in living fully.

Grieving is a process that helps us deal with mortality. There is also a social element in that it demonstrates the bonds between people. There is an experience to the grief—a sense of permanent loss, sadness, preoccupation with the lost person, an adoption of some of his or her mannerisms, and sleep loss. But there is also a meaning to this grieving process, a part of letting go as well as paying one's respects. The intense pain involves recognizing the loss of something truly vital in one's life and the beginning of the remaking of life. The manifestations and duration of grief have a cultural component too (in some cultures, it is a lifetime phenomenon). No one who has experienced grief can doubt the complexity and mystery of human emotions. My own enduring experience of grief would inform, even drive, my work as a psychiatrist in a positive direction.

CHAPTER 7

Depression: Beginning in Research

In the difficult period following the loss of my parents, Robin Hunter, now the vice-dean for postgraduate education in the Faculty of Medicine, and a mentor, provided great comfort and insight. Particularly after my father died in 1975, Hunter and I had several significant conversations. He helped me channel my grief and guilt into anger about the misfortune of my parents' premature deaths. The anger fuelled a drive to make a difference, to work even harder to fulfill the gifts my parents had given me.

Fortunately, I didn't slide into a depression. In those years, while I was grieving my parents' deaths, I was fully engaged in both my family life and my professional life. Dorothy had given birth to our first child, Jonathan, on August 8, 1973. Jonathan was a delight from the beginning and still is; he has my drive, a type of focused preoccupation that he has channelled to writing. A month after my father died, our son Stephen was born. He would turn his capacity for empathy into a thriving career as a therapist, focusing on people with anorexia nervosa. Four years later, on December 31, 1979, Joshua was born and, like his brothers, he too has lived a life true to his temperament. He has made environmental causes and concern for people his career. It was a joyful time for us. Dorothy was an outstanding and devoted mother, and as our family grew we moved to a small house in the Forest Hill neighbourhood, where we would stay for two decades.

Meanwhile, my career as a psychiatrist was progressing. In July 1972, while I was going into just my third residency year, Hunter asked me to be chief resident at the Clarke. It was an honour and a responsibility. This was my first taste of management, overseeing a group of about 30 residents, at various stages of training, assigned to the institute for 6 or 12 months.

In addition to arranging the call schedule and the rounds, I would help individual residents deal with their worries and life changes. We held a few social events and gathered together for the Canada-Russia hockey games. Most residents were capable and responsible physicians. But my first taste of "administration" occurred when Hunter called me into his office early in the summer. I thought he wanted me to help him consider some important issue facing the institute, but what he really wanted was to get one of the residents to stop sleeping with the nighttime switchboard operator while he was on call. I remember thinking that administration was way out of my depth and experience.

Then Stancer, my mentor at the Clinical Investigation Unit, insisted I do a master's degree at the university's Institute of Medical Science, a graduate department at the university that had been set up a few years earlier to provide physicians with an opportunity to learn science. Here I would acquire knowledge in statistics, pharmacology, and radiotracers. Studying statistics and radiotracers was taxing for a clinician like me, whose satisfaction comes from understanding the complexities of patients, but this work, Stancer promised, would prepare me for a research career in an exciting new field, the chemistry of depression.

Stancer could be very persuasive. After I received my certification to practise as a psychiatrist, in the late fall of 1974, he took me under his wing, making room for me on the 5th floor of the Clarke to conduct my research. He moved to the 11th floor's new Mood Disorders Unit, to work with Emmanuel Persad.[1]

I was enormously grateful to him, but like many sons, I faced a real dilemma. Should I follow in his footsteps and plunge into this promising new field that was attracting large research grants and scientific interest? Or should I chart another course entirely, into a lesser-known field that interested me deeply?

Sitting quietly on the sidelines of scientific inquiry was an illness called anorexia nervosa. It was a fascinating puzzle, waiting for new ideas, perhaps from someone like me. I was intrigued by the people we saw with anorexia nervosa, which typically afflicted young women. Between 8 and 10% of those who sought treatment died from the affliction. I had seen quite a few disturbing cases, since the local expert on the illness, Harvey Moldofsky, had gone to Stanford to study sleep disorders. Somehow, I couldn't get these patients out of my mind.

I decided to do research on both anorexia and depression at the same time. To make this possible, Stancer displayed extraordinary generosity. He gave up some of his Clarke salary so I could afford to research two big topics without having to scramble to make money by seeing as many patients as other clinical psychiatrists did.

Depression was undoubtedly a big field. A complex, diverse illness that affects 15% of us at some point in our lives, it had fascinated psychiatrists for decades. When I immersed myself in the field, the symptoms were well-known: affective changes such as sadness, despair, anxiety, irritability, a feeling of reduced self-worth, relative lack of pleasures; behavioural changes such as withdrawal, weepiness or wanting to cry but being unable to, self-medicating with alcohol or drugs; vegetative changes such as poor sleep or increased sleep, poor appetite or increased appetite, lack of energy, lack of interest in sex, dry mouth, and constipation; and cognitive changes such as poor concentration, reduced memory, preoccupation with the self, loss of social interests, and at times delusions, including believing oneself to be worthless. Not surprisingly, there were a variety of intriguing insights into the source of this grim malady.

For Freudians, grief and mourning are instances of sadness caused by the permanent loss of someone we have loved. But loss may also trigger rage and hostile responses. They postulated that if that rage, or hatred, is turned on the self, depression is the result.[2] Depression, from this point of view, can then be seen as a maladaptive expression of loss or mourning.

The outstanding British psychoanalyst John Bowlby thought the roots of sadness began in infancy, particularly through disruption of attachment processes.[3] Bowlby believed that attachment in infants is primarily a process of seeking closeness to the mother in situations of upset to ensure emotional survival. Infants become attached to adults who are sensitive and responsive in interactions and who remain as consistent caregivers during the first two years of age. These responses lead to the development of patterns of attachment. Those infants whose mothers are rejecting, unresponsive, or too smothering will experience different patterns of relationships later in life, such as anxious, ambivalent, or avoidant attachment styles. Such individuals are prone to react to life stresses with anxiety, sadness, and depression. Bowlby stressed that the earliest bonds formed by children with their caregivers have an impact that continues throughout life—from "cradle to grave," as he put it. Bowlby's work is supported by an empirical research base and has fostered newer psychodynamic thinking and treatments focusing on interpersonal relationships.

Cognitive psychologists see depression from a different point of view. Since the 1970s they have found that depressed people have distorted views of themselves characterized by negative thoughts of themselves, their relationships, and their surroundings, as well as negative perceptions of their past, present, and future. Often they brood (women more than men, and this may partially account for the gender differences in frequency of depression) or see minor events as catastrophes, and they end up deriving generalizations about themselves and their world that further reduce their sense of self-worth. These dysfunctional thoughts can lead to low mood states and into a depressive syndrome. Childhood adversity, including the death of a parent, physical and sexual abuse, parental drug abuse, parental psychopathology, and severe illness, may be the initial triggers of a negative and pessimistic cognitive style, which predicts a vulnerability to depression. An adult mood disorder may then be precipitated by losses such as divorce or the death of a parent, or by financial adversity.

The evolutionary biologists tell us that psychic pain may have evolved as a warning signal. Most evolutionary theories of major depressive disorder see the psychic pain as a motivator to conserve the self, to save resources. If this is so, it is a brutal way to warn a person. The pain of depression can be more exquisite than physical pain, and it's not just the individual who suffers. The entire family can be affected. Depression traps people who have it. They tend to look inward, which makes them look selfish to the outsider. Depression causes great misery and early death.

The world has known about this illness since ancient times, but until a few years before I entered medical school, we didn't have an effective way to release people from the grips of deep depression other than through electroconvulsive therapy, and otherwise providing support, while waiting and hoping for a spontaneous remission. That changed just before I started my psychiatric training.

The world of mood had just been rocked by groundbreaking articles that pointed to a new cause of depression: the chemistry of the brain. If this were so, it would make a profound change in the way depression was treated. It was a thrilling moment in psychiatric history because it offered new, tangible hope of reasonably quick recovery to patients who suffered from severe depression. For a young researcher like me, it was an exciting moment to follow Stancer into the lab, even if it meant less time with the patients whom I found so intriguing.

The idea that depression is a chemical problem goes back to the time of the ancient Greeks, when it was thought that humans had four humours, or basic bodily liquids. Personality types were determined by the dominant humour in a particular person, and an imbalance in one or other of the four humours would cause disease. Hippocrates thought that melancholia was caused by an excess of black bile. Even Freud thought that brain chemistry must somehow correspond to the more abstract psychological issues he was considering.

The modern era of neurochemistry of mood was ushered in at the National Institute of Mental Health in the 1950s when Julius Axelrod began working on the mechanisms of effect of caffeine. He turned his attention to the chemicals that transmit messages between the neurons, or brain cells. The brain sends messages electrically within brain cells. But there is a tiny gap between the brain cells (a synapse). To get one cell to communicate with another, the cell releases a chemical messenger and then takes that messenger back in; it returns home, like a diplomat having sent its vital information. One of these messengers, or neurotransmitters, was norepinephrine. It was a stimulant that promoted alertness and a sense of well-being, but if it's overproduced, it can cause fear and anxiety. In the late 1950s, Axelrod discovered that norepinephrine went out with a message to another cell and then returned to the cell where it came from. This research later won him a Nobel Prize and eventually lay the groundwork for a whole new class of antidepressants.

The first antidepressants, the monoamine oxidase inhibitors were actually serendipitously discovered in 1951 when doctors at a Staten Island hospital began treating tubercular patients with a new drug, isoniazid. These chronically ill patients were also severely depressed, and, surprisingly, they had a significant mood response to the drug. The second group, the tricyclics, evolved after Roland

Kuhn recognized the antidepressant effects of imipramine while the pharmaceutical company Geigy was looking for a chlorpromazine-like (antipsychotic) drug. The current generation of antidepressants, the SSRIs, or selective serotonin reuptake inhibitors, such as Prozac, were developed a bit later, in the mid-1970s, and introduced clinically in the 1980s. These drugs were based on the work that followed Axelrod and were designed to target the neurotransmitter serotonin. Later refinements of these drugs also increased the levels of norepinephrine.

The theory was that if you could prevent the norepinephrine (or serotonin) from returning to home base, there would be more of this neurotransmitter circulating in the brain, and more available for transmission of the next message at the synapse as a result. This is how the tricyclics and SSRIs and SNRIs function in the brain.

In 1965 Dr. Joe Schildkraut, a Boston psychiatrist who spent four years at the National Institute of Mental Health, in the United States, published a speculative but intriguing paper titled "The Catecholamine Hypothesis of Affective Disorders." What Schildkraut did was link brain messengers (especially norepinephrine, but also epinephrine, dopamine, and serotonin) to depression through indirect evidence. He reviewed how these substances naturally occur in our brains and their importance in transmitting nervous impulses from cell to cell. Using earlier research in people and rodents, Schildkraut pieced together the evidence. He noticed that people treated with an antihypertensive agent, reserpine, often became depressed. Reserpine lowered monoamines in the brain. From this type of evidence, he created a hypothesis: lowered levels of these chemicals might be linked to depression.[4] This paper set the agenda for biological research on depression for the next 25 years. The article was recognized in 1997 as the most cited of all articles ever published in the *American Journal of Psychiatry* and as one of the most-cited papers in the entire history of psychiatry.

When I entered the field of depression, we knew we were onto something significant, but we had to overcome some serious technical barriers. In the early 1970s, Stancer was troubled by a critical question: How exactly does one measure these important neurotransmitters in the living human brain? This was long before modern brain imaging, so we had to rely on measurements from urine, blood, and cerebrospinal fluid. The problem was that these measurements would not just be an index of brain levels of these chemicals but would be contaminated by the presence of large amounts of these very same substances that occur elsewhere in the body. We could measure chemicals at autopsy, but this may not tell us anything about the living brain. We could infer what is happening in the brain from the actions of drugs, but this was too indirect to be accurate. The brain was, at that time, like a black box.

Stancer and his postdoctoral fellow, Jerry Warsh, were examining a unique way to approach this issue by using what is called the blood-brain barrier. This is a protective, semipermeable membrane that permits some substances to enter the brain, while others are kept out. It protects the brain from foreign substances in the blood that may injure the brain and helps maintain a constant physiological environment for the brain. Warsh became aware of a new compound, then called MK-486 (now carbidopa). This compound blocked an enzyme (dopa decarboxylase) required for the synthesis of the brain amines we were interested in. But it could not get into the brain because of the blood-brain barrier. As a result, theoretically, it would block production only in the rest of the body, not the brain. So what was measured in the blood and urine would then be an index of what was present in the brain.

Warsh was working on an animal model for this, and I set out to design a clinical study. We wanted to see whether there were differences between people with depression and healthy controls when they took MK-486. If so, could this help us predict who would respond to an antidepressant? Since the antidepressants took from four to six weeks to work and were administered by trial and error, an ability to predict treatment responses would be a major advance.

My task was first to develop a research study for humans that would permit us to assess the model, and second to develop a means to measure the end product of serotonin in the lab (the end product was 5-hydroxyindoleacetic acid). But I had a problem. I hated working in the lab. I had always been clumsy, and I kept breaking the glass test tubes. I just couldn't wait to get out of there.

Then I did what business guru Marcus Buckingham recommends. I played to my strengths and wrote a grant to hire someone who could do the lab work. Thanks to the Ontario Mental Health Foundation, I hired Ahmed Naqvi, a talented young scientist, so that I could concentrate on the clinical side of the research.

The clinical side wasn't any easier. People had to be in the study for 10 days and submit to various restrictions, among which was eating the exact same foods every day for a three-day baseline and seven days of the active study. Stancer and I were the first controls. We ate most of our meals on the unit, but if we had to go somewhere, we'd take with us a little box of the food for each day. I couldn't drink coffee, or enjoy my daily morning swims. We had to collect all our urine and have repeated blood tests over the 10 days. But we did produce results. We were able to show that the use of carbidopa for seven days produced a substantial decrease of some of the urinary end products, including neurotransmitters like tryptamine. In people with bipolar depression, the end product of norepinephrine metabolism was much lower than in controls. Although we were able to show differences in people with depression in the production of these chemicals, in the end, it didn't make a difference for patients. We still couldn't tell which antidepressant people should receive, and four decades later, even with sophisticated brain-imaging techniques, we still can't predict accurately.[5]

No one would do a study like this now—brain imaging makes it feel ancient. Also, we have moved on from Schildkraut's original hypothesis. Whereas the original work on neurotransmitters focused on monoamines, more recently the field has expanded greatly to look at other neurotransmitters (e.g., those that relate to acetylcholine or nicotine). Even more exciting are two very different other areas, that of neurogenesis or how antidepressants stimulate nerve cell growth in specific brain regions, and that of the fascinating relationship between depression and chronic inflammation.[6,7]

Stancer was a demanding mentor. He could be extremely critical of himself and others, and he insisted on honesty and accountability. He also helped me navigate my way through a complex institution and university, get grant funding, and publish my findings. He was a perfectionist. To ensure there were no spelling errors, he even insisted that a couple of my papers be read out loud word for word, backwards. At the same time, Stancer was kind. He supported our body-image studies in anorexia nervosa, even though the money for them came from his neurochemistry laboratory, and he showed genuine concern for my wife and family too. We grew close over these years.

On the other hand, he would unfailingly comment on the wasteful expense of the Cuban cigars I smoked. Whenever we travelled to a conference, he would reluctantly agree to stay in the conference hotel, even though it could cost $40 or $50 more than one down the street, but he would then insist on breakfasting at the other hotel because the orange juice might save us 50 cents. Then he'd brood all day, in Larry David style, if the diner didn't have just the right fries.

Stancer railed against the foolish side of clinical care and how easily people can delude themselves into believing that whatever they're doing is right. Harvey knew that science was the way to guard against this kind of self-delusion. He was years ahead of others in insisting a rigorous scientific training accompany good clinical knowledge and experience. Nevertheless, I felt that his clinical psychiatric views were too one-sided, too much on the biological end. He could easily dismiss or not notice psychosocial problems or even personal details that were evident to me. Perhaps it was because he was so committed to the biological research model, particularly on the study of brain chemistry and these neurotransmitters. This has been a useful area of research, but the model is limiting in clinical practice if applied exclusively, at the expense of understanding the patient as a whole person.

Stancer's lab was booming; patients were plenty and money was flowing in. The chemistry of depression was a hot topic for researchers; therein lay a problem for me. I was just one player in a crowded field. Lots of researchers in North America and Europe were studying and chasing monoamines, chemicals that are important when people become depressed or addicted. I was, and still am, interested in whether one can predict responses to antidepressant drugs based on these chemical changes, but again, it seemed less original in its scope. Even my thesis work, on blocking the peripheral effects of decarboxylase, was largely based on my colleague Jerry Warsh's more basic research. Although all research develops from the work of others, in the affective disorders area, I felt more like a cog in a machine than a scientist getting ready to be independent.

Some of the work we did had a more practical side. One study, of the drugs for mania, helped clarify an important concern: an earlier report had suggested that combining lithium with one of the popular neuroleptic drugs, haloperidol, could prove toxic to the brain and cause serious side effects (a type of encephalopathy). When we studied the combination—with patient safety being carefully monitored—we found that lithium and haloperidol could be given together safely. Also, as others had found, we saw that haloperidol alone was an effective antimanic agent, and that lithium was useful in the prevention of further episodes. Lithium was interesting from another perspective too. It was a naturally occurring substance, discovered by an Australian, John Cade, in 1949 to have mood-stabilizing qualities. But, as mentioned earlier, because it was a natural substance and cheap, drug companies were not interested in it and it was slow to catch on. When I was a medical student, lithium was not yet used in Winnipeg; I believe it was first used in Canada by Eddie Kingstone, then in Montreal, in the mid-1960s. Lithium has transformed the care of people with bipolar illness and has led to the use of other mood stabilizers for this condition.

But again, the chemistry side wasn't exciting to me. I was more intrigued by the patients themselves. I remember one young man in his mid-20s who turned up in my class on psychopathology in the Faculty of Social Work. As it was the first day of the course, I asked the students how they wanted to be graded—by an essay or a multiple-choice exam? Classes usually preferred multiple choice, but this time the exuberant young man in the front row convinced his fellow students of the great merits of an essay. After the class, when I went up to the 11th floor to meet a new patient who was coming in for mania, I was startled to find he was the same front-row "student" who had convinced the entire group on the merits of an essay exam.

The manic-depressive patients could be entertaining in their manic phase but also could be quite dangerous to their own or their family's well-being because of impaired judgment. It is in these phases that people can spend a fortune, become promiscuous, or have difficulty with drugs and alcohol or the law. Mania can feel exciting: many patients love the feeling of specialness and strength, but dread the depression that so often follows.

One patient, Ron, experienced depression in his late 20s. He had a strong family history of this, including the suicide of a close relative; there was a great deal of alcohol abuse in the family, and in at least one relative, periods of mania in which huge fortunes were made and then lost. His depressive illness first began when he worked in the stressful financial sector. After treatment he wisely moved to a quieter environment and married a supportive, caring woman. Still, over the last 30 years, he has had at least three more depressive episodes and at least one manic episode that landed him in conflict with the law.

A second depressed patient, Susan, a woman of close to 50, came from a professional family on her father's side, and a business family on her mother's. Susan studied business at university, entered the male-dominated field of stock trading, and in her late 20s married a lawyer. When I saw her 20 years later, she had three children, to whom she was devoted, and had given up all hopes of reentering the business world. She was passionate about art but had not been supported in pursuing this passion. She felt helpless in her marriage and helpless to leave. After treatment she was able to pursue her passion for art as her children went off to university. Her husband's inability to tolerate any independence in his wife precipitated the end of the marriage. Several years later, Susan connected with a supportive man with similar interests to hers. Despite this, she has had two depressive episodes in the 10 years since. (Most depressions after the first episode require less and less stress to provoke an episode.)

Jessie, a 50-year-old physician when she came to see me, had been molested by her older brother, their mother's favourite son, over many years while she was a child and then an adolescent. There was a clear family history of depression in one of the brothers and likely the mother too. Her abuse could never be discussed within the family. Years later, Jessie, now married and a mother of two, became severely depressed as her eldest daughter was approaching the age at which the incest had begun. She was haunted by memories and became enraged with her mother and brother. Jessie could not recover until the story of her abuse was revealed to her family as part of the treatment. Subsequently, she has done very well and has had no further depressive episodes.

These cases show that there is no single route to the final common pathway to depression. Two of my patients had a clear family history of depression leading to a biological vulnerability that resulted in depression in the face of severe life events. Depression can also be part of other medical illnesses, such as hypothyroidism (when the thyroid gland is underactive), cancer, or chronic infection. It can accompany disorders such as schizophrenia and anorexia nervosa. It's a common side effect of steroids, antihypertensive agents, and hallucinogenic drugs. Depression can be part of brain diseases, such as Parkinson's disease or stroke. Previous personal or familial history of depression creates a vulnerability to the syndrome. Depression can be affected by a person's temperament, personality, intimate relationships, and self-worth. Personality features such as self-criticism, high levels of perfectionism, extreme shyness, and a high degree of sensitivity to the judgments of others can put people at risk. Genetics have a significant role in producing a vulnerability to depression, or to manic depression (bipolar disorder). Earlier experiences with physical or sexual abuse can predispose people, as it did Jessie to depression, along with addictions and eating disorders. But it's even more complicated than that: the emergence of depression in a single person depends on all kinds of factors; however, the mere presence of known vulnerabilities does not reliably predict the development of depression. Some people who have experienced abuse as a child end up with depression; others do not.

No single model could explain depression—not the thrilling new findings in brain chemistry or the psychoanalysts' deep insights on attachment theory. What most appealed to me about my work with depression was, in fact, our incomplete knowledge of the disorder. It was a mystery, one that would require an intense, single-minded, scientific pursuit of neurobiology to lead to new and more specific treatments for this terribly painful state. With my disinterest in lab work, I knew that I was not the person to pursue this.

Meanwhile, the equally compelling mystery of anorexia nervosa—the mystery of why girls (primarily) would starve themselves in a time of plenty—still drew me powerfully. Some of the deep appeal was that even less was known about it; the syndrome was just emerging from a brief paragraph in psychiatric texts in the rare disorders section. It was also appealing because it was so serious: there was a high mortality rate, and real endocrine changes were apparent. I just had to study it.

Stancer was very kind and generous regarding my decision. In many ways, our circumstance reminded me of a young man whose father has a prosperous *shmatte* (clothing) business and is desperate to have him join the business. Initially, the son gives it a try but eventually finds he has to go his own way. My decision marked the end of our father-son working relationship, but not our close friendship.

The field of neuroscience was exploding with results both endlessly fascinating and holding promise for new treatment. I felt privileged to be part of this exciting endeavour, but I couldn't get the patients with anorexia nervosa out of my mind. I knew I wouldn't be satisfied until I tried to work on solving the perplexing problems of eating disorders.

CHAPTER 8

Changing Fields: Anorexia Nervosa

Just over a year after I started my residency at the Clarke, I met a 19-year-old woman called Marcia at Toronto General, where I was assigned to a six-month rotation. Marcia had anorexia nervosa. Her story would haunt me for years.

Hers was a complicated case. In addition to anorexia, she had an autonomic nervous system problem that made regulating her blood pressure problematic. When she stood up, she'd get weak and dizzy because of her low blood pressure, so unlike many people with anorexia, she mostly stayed in bed or in her room. She had many of the classic signs of anorexia: dry skin, hair loss, and fine, downy lanugo on her back. She looked terribly ill but put on makeup when we filmed a session for training purposes. With makeup on, she looked like a Barbie doll.

Her family life was chaotic. She had an abusive father, who disappeared from time to time and did not support the family, while her mother worked menial jobs. Her brother had died of a drug overdose around the time that she developed anorexia nervosa. Her mother was all she had. Marcia had dropped out of high school. Her friends had deserted her. She could not work, and she spent her time at home with her mother or at Toronto General, where she was seen first by the endocrinologists who diagnosed her with anorexia nervosa.

Marcia was admitted to the psychiatry ward on at least two occasions. She weighed only 70 pounds (she was about five foot two), but she strongly resisted eating and getting heavier. She hid food and had hidden laxatives in a Kleenex box, presumably to induce diarrhea. (Many patients with anorexia mistakenly think diarrhea will stop their bodies from absorbing calories, when in fact most food is absorbed before it reaches the colon.) It was all to keep her only measure of identity and self-worth, being thinner than anyone else. We were able to stabilize her, particularly after the second admission. At that point, she weighed 90 pounds, and although no one would have thought this was a decent weight, at least it was safe. Over the next three years, I saw her regularly at whichever hospital I was assigned to, and she maintained her weight and even enrolled in a cosmetician course.

But then her mother died of a massive coronary at just age 55. Marcia was bereft. About one month later, she drowned in a hot bath after suffering hypotension. She knew all about her illnesses' effects on her blood pressure, and yet the death was ruled an accident. I was so sad for weeks. What more could we have done? We couldn't keep her on a ward for life. But she had had such a meagre existence, alone.

Anorexia is so puzzling. Why would someone wilfully and defiantly starve, sometimes to the point of death, in a world of fast-food outlets, microwave meals, and supermarkets as large as city blocks? It makes no logical sense, but our brains can take us to strange places. We can all understand that if a blood clot lodges itself in a particular area of the brain, speech or movement are affected. But a brain that says "Starve yourself" seems unfathomable.

Anorexia in the early 1970s was still unknown territory for most psychiatric researchers. It didn't draw the money or the scientific interest that depression did. Many of my colleagues seemed to trivialize those who suffered from it as stubborn "spoiled girls." This field was outside the mainstream of psychiatry, but this was where my heart was. This was where I could make a difference.

There was a risk involved in pursuing this area. Anorexia nervosa was thought to be rare in the 1970s: Would there be referrals in sufficient numbers, and would granting agencies support research on such a "peripheral" topic? I soon discovered that this could be a more busy and interesting practice than I had imagined at the outset. Fellow clinicians were all too happy to send their anorexic patients to me. And research money was no problem. I was very pleasantly surprised when my first grant applications on both depression and anorexia were funded through Canadian agencies. And, shortly after, I was able to secure funding for the anorexia work from the US National Institute of Mental Health. This was not an easy task at that time for a non-American; the institute had to be convinced that the work was unique.

As I started to read about the history of the disease, I discovered that, as misunderstood as it was, and as little research as there had been, reports of anorexia nervosa in the medical and historical literature go back many centuries. In the Middle Ages, many women were inspired to starve themselves by the story of Saint Catherine of Siena. Born in the mid-1300s, Catherine turned inward at age 15 after her mother died in childbirth. She began to eat less and spend more of her time praying, especially when her father wanted her to marry. Devoting her life to God, she cut off her hair, began to meditate, and flagellated herself in imitation of Christ and his Passion. She ate almost nothing, or forced herself to vomit after she had eaten. She lived an austere, ascetic existence, devoting herself to helping other people, until she died of starvation at age 33. Catherine's story led countless women to fast to the point of death, all in the name of devotion to God. The Church approved, at least at first, and some of these "holy anorexics" were elevated to sainthood.

Were these women anorexics as we know them today? I don't know, but probably not. It appears they were motivated by religion, or even by their desire to avoid an unwanted husband and children. The illness we know today was first described in the medical literature in 1689 by Richard Morton, a clergyman educated at Oxford who became chaplain to New College before turning to medicine.

His main interest was tuberculosis, but his 1694 *Phthisiologia: Or, a Treatise of Consumptions* noted a separate condition of body wasting, or "nervous consumption," caused by sadness and anxious "cares." One of the patients Morton described was a young woman who had been losing weight for two years. She "fell into the total suppression of her monthly courses from a multitude of cares and passions of her mind but without any symptoms of the green sickness following upon it," Morton reported. "I don't remember that I ever did see one that was conversant with the living so much wasted with the greatest degree of consumption (like a skeleton only clad with skin) ... A nervous atrophy or consumption, is a wasting of the body without any remarkable fever, cough, or shortness of breath; but it is attended with a want of appetite, and a bad digestion, upon which there follows a languishing weakness of nature, and a falling away of the flesh everyday more and more." Only a few months later, the young woman was "taken with a Fainting Fit and died."[1]

For the next 200 years, anorexia disappeared from the medical literature, only to be rediscovered by French and English physicians Ernest Charles Lasègue and Sir William Gull, within a few months of each other and acting apparently without each other's knowledge. Lasègue, trained as a teacher and philosopher in Paris, later became professor of clinical medicine at the University of Paris, where he made some astute observations about the syndrome that would be called anorexia nervosa: it was, he wrote, "a refusal of food that may be indefinitely prolonged. Woe to the physician who, misunderstanding the peril, treats as a fancy without object or duration, an obstinacy which he hopes to vanquish by medicine's friendly advice, or by the still more defective resource, intimidation." He clearly appreciated the tenacity of the disease, and the added frustration of dealing with a patient like this, who insists she is fine: "Not only does she not sigh for recovery, but she is not ill pleased with her condition."[2]

Sir William Gull didn't know Lasègue, but he described anorexia at about the same time. Born in Colchester, Gull entered Guy's Hospital at age 18 to study and won every prize and honour. He was even called in to help the Prince of Wales overcome typhoid fever. Gull published many papers, including several on hypothyroidism and myxedema in adult women. He presented a paper in 1868 to the Clinical Society of London on anorexia nervosa, the term he later coined. His mention was brief: "At present, our diagnosis is mostly one of inference from our knowledge of our liability of the several organs to particularly lesions, thus we avoid the error of supposing the presence of mesenteric disease in young women, emaciated to the last degree through hysteric apepsia, by our knowledge of the latter affliction and by the absence of tubercular disease elsewhere." In an 1873 address, Gull reminded the audience of his earlier comment, and added two case descriptions, including clinical findings of reduced heart rate, slowed respiration, lack of menses, sleep loss, and edema of the lower limbs. As to treatment, he wrote: "The treatment required is obviously that which is fitted for persons of unsound mind. The patients should be fed at regular intervals, and surrounded by persons who would have moral control over them, relations and friends being generally the worst attendants."[3]

At the beginning of the 20th century, anorexic girls and women faced outright hostility from the medical profession. Thomas Allbutt and Clifford Rolleston, for example, noted that "fasting girls from time to time become notorious"; their "exploits have been known to terminate in death." They had little sympathy for one patient, "a young maiden with small experience of the world," who "expects more from life than life can give. The sympathy desired is not forthcoming, hence dissatisfaction and discontent. In the extreme degree of melancholy, the patient suffers from first conceit and strange notions."[4]

It was in this setting of hostility and mistrust to starving young women that a twist was added. In 1914 the pathologist Morris Simmonds described a patient in whom extreme emaciation was associated with destruction of the pituitary gland. He amplified these observations in papers between 1916 and 1918 that described four more cases, and the condition began to be referred to as Simmonds' disease. Increasingly, it was understood that the hormonal deficiency of Simmonds' disease could be relieved with hormones or implants of the pituitary gland. Throughout the 1920s and 1930s, many articles were written on Simmonds' disease, though it seems in retrospect that many of the cases referred to were actually cases of anorexia nervosa. By 1939 it was estimated there were more than 80 such instances of this misreporting and consequent neglect of any psychological factors contributing to the clinical state.

When I learned that this puzzling mental illness might be somehow related to hormones, I was intrigued. Perhaps this could be the kind of mental puzzle that could be solved, and people cured. But I was also drawn by the patients themselves. Anorexics were outsiders, even in the psychiatric world. It was a dangerous disease too. In untreated situations, the mortality rate was a shocking 18%, the highest for any psychiatric condition.[5] What I didn't understand at first was just how frustrating anorexics could be.

When Cathy came to the Clarke in 1971, she was five foot seven and 73 pounds, with straggly blonde hair, pale skin, and pale blue eyes. She didn't seem to care about her emaciated state. Her problems started at 16, when she felt that she should lose a "few pounds" from her 125-pound frame to compete on her high-school running team. At first she just exercised more—getting up to two hours a day; but then she gradually restricted her food intake. This consisted of water or juice at breakfast, a large salad at lunch, and small portions of the family dinner, without starches whenever possible. Her diet was extremely rigid. Neither of her parents was overweight, but her mother, a homemaker in her 50s, had been chronically depressed and drank to relieve the pain. Cathy was an only child, and both her parents had aspirations for their only child's academic success.

Cathy's family doctor and an internist had had her admitted to a community hospital, where they thoroughly studied her physical and laboratory findings. There was not much to see here—a very mild anaemia, a high level of blood cholesterol, some carotene pigmentation of her palms, and some fine, downy lanugo on her back and neck. After losing a few pounds in that setting over eight weeks, she was referred to us.

Cathy settled in after a week or so. She was extremely quiet with staff and the other patients. We did not restrict her activities beyond the need to stay on the unit; only once she began exercising close to an hour a day did we decide to limit that to less than 20 minutes. Our nutritionist would confer with Cathy and go out daily to nearby Kensington Market, an old and vibrant neighbourhood of multicultural food shops. Cathy's long shopping list was mostly of greens, which were prepared for her individually. Cathy's weight stayed the same or was down a pound or two in the first month. I met with Cathy twice a week and tried to learn more about her. She was pleasant and polite, but not reflective about her circumstance; mostly she was just anxious and felt that her anxiety would increase if she gained weight. She liked the "safety" of a weight under 85 pounds but had no explanation as to why. She would appear to try to eat when a staff member sat with her, but she complained of very early fullness and anxiety during and after meals.

It was hard to understand, especially for me. I love eating; I relish a great Italian dinner with fine wine. So it was hard to comprehend why someone would starve in the midst of plenty. It was fascinating too: this was an extreme example of the split between mind and body. Anorexics like Cathy denied the obvious physical facts, that they were emaciated and needed nourishment. They thought they could live through their minds only.

My sessions with her were not fruitful. Her thoughts of her earlier experiences were bland, except for her needing to do well for the team and for her scholastics. Scholastics were difficult. She had worked extremely hard through high school to obtain an A average, and now in first-year university she was struggling, not so much with grades as with the sense that everyone else was so bright and could achieve with less effort.

Eventually, I did get angry with Cathy and insisted the next phase involve close nursing observation, and no further exercise. She was placed on total bedrest. In retrospect, my response was a classic for doctors who think they know best and that patients should follow the doctor's instructions. If patients don't obey, it's easy to get angry and frustrated. The result is that many punitive regimens have been imposed out of a sense of helplessness and frustration, rather than as part of a therapeutic plan.

It was hard to impose bedrest on Cathy, especially after she had free use of the ward for weeks and was not more ill than she was when she was first admitted. Some of the staff didn't agree with this new plan. They thought it was punitive. One of the older, motherly nurses even permitted Cathy time out of bed when she was alone with her. At other times Cathy exercised furiously in bed. Some people on the staff, however, thought we were still being too easy on her. The divided staff doomed the already frail treatment.

After many months, Cathy was discharged. She weighed 87 pounds, 14 pounds more than her weight when she was admitted to the Clarke. It was a healthier weight for her medically, but she hadn't broken the pattern of excessive dieting, and we still had not learned much about her inner world. We had run out of ideas, so when she left, we were quietly relieved.

Part of the problem was that we didn't have a framework to understand the illness, so we couldn't devise a coherent treatment. Without this, the staff started to criticize each other—and me. I couldn't have felt more frustrated and helpless.

Back then, there were a lot of theories about anorexia. Some thought it came from a family dynamic where there were no boundaries between members. Others blamed a passive father and a controlling mother, or a fear of sexuality, or of oral impregnation. Others saw it as a form of flight, running away from responsibility as a young girl moved into adolescence. Still others thought it represented a denial of pleasures, as food represents all pleasures of the flesh. Yet another theory was that anorexia is a form of manipulation to attain a sense of specialness. Some experts saw it as a biological problem, a disorder of the hypothalamus or a defect in genetic makeup. It was also described as a variant of normal dieting, or a different form of common illnesses such as schizophrenia or depression. The theories, in other words, were all over the map.

We knew almost nothing about the hormonal changes then, except for the lack of menstrual periods, as had been noted almost 300 years earlier, and some changes in adrenal steroid excretion, which could be measured. We didn't know much about the complications of starving, and we had just learned about the danger of rapid refeeding. A 1968 paper showed that one-third of the deaths from anorexia came from rapid refeeding. One-third were from starvation, and the remaining one-third were the result of suicide. There was risk on all sides.

When I started treating anorexia nervosa, a common method derived from physicians in the United Kingdom involved bedrest, insulin, and chlorpromazine, a drug used for psychosis. Insulin, however, makes hungry people even hungrier and comes with high risks of hypoglycaemia. And contrary to what many think, people with anorexia do not lose their appetite until late in the starvation

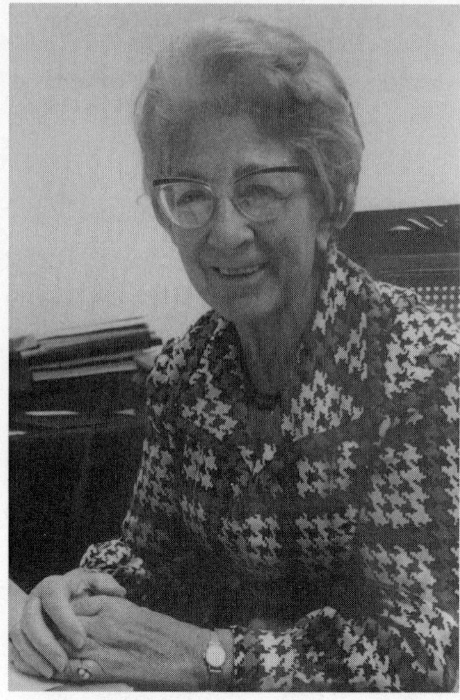

Dr. Hilde Bruch, a German-born psychiatrist and psychoanalyst, spent her career working on eating disorders at Columbia and Baylor. An independent-minded woman, she had a huge influence on our understanding of anorexia nervosa. Courtesy Dr. Stuart Yudofsky, Baylor College.

process. To make a hungry person hungrier and feel more out of control seems cruel. Chlorpromazine, associated with weight gain, has many severe side effects, such as a Parkinson's-like syndrome or other movement problems. These drugs were clearly inappropriate and didn't address the needs of the individual. Nonetheless, clinicians used them because they produced weight gain.

Into this vacuum came an independent and courageous psychiatrist, Hilde Bruch. Bruch, a Jew, had studied medicine and pediatrics in Freiberg, Germany, and was a practising physician until the rise of Nazism in 1933 curtailed her career. She begged her Jewish fiancé and parents to leave Germany, but when they refused, she went to London by herself, only to learn later of their deaths in concentration camps. She then went to America and worked in pediatrics—on childhood obesity—at Columbia University, but suffered a severe depression brought on by the losses of her loved ones. After treatment, she entered psychiatry and then did psychoanalysis, with Harry Stack Sullivan and Frieda Fromm-Reichman, two of America's leading analysts. She eventually moved to Houston to work at Baylor University; as a single elderly woman, she was concerned about crime in New York City. Before moving, however, she bought a Rolls-Royce because, as she put it, she didn't want to be "kow-towing to the Texas oilmen in their Cadillacs."[6]

I first encountered the powerful force of Bruch's thinking on anorexia when I read her 1969 paper "Hunger and Instinct." After seeing patients for many years in her analytic practice, she believed that, at their core, they felt helpless; their stance of tough defiance masked a sense of feeling useless. She saw them as tough little girls who felt ineffective in their worlds. Controlling the body was the only way they could feel effective.

Bruch criticized traditional Freudian psychodynamic approaches to the treatment of people with eating disorders as likely to backfire. To her mind, when clinicians explore the patient's sexual and aggressive drives by probing repressed ideas, the patient might feel as though she is once again being told what to feel and think. This would reconfirm her sense of inadequacy, and interfere with the development of self-awareness and trust in her own psychological abilities. Trust in oneself, and authenticity, became Bruch's key goals with these patients. She set out to treat patients in a way that encouraged the anorexic to seek out autonomy and an identity that did not depend on others' expectations.

Bruch believed that an essential characteristic of anorexia nervosa was a disturbance in the image of the body. She felt that the patient's inability to recognize her appearance as abnormal reaches "delusional proportions" and is manifest in the stubborn defence of an emaciated shape. She linked this to inner deficits in self-awareness—the ability to recognize internal feelings. Bruch believed that anorexics couldn't read cues about their bodies. They were unable to tell if they were hungry or full, but they also couldn't read other signals, like whether they were feeling happy or sad, aroused, enthusiastic, or bored. Bruch thought these distortions in body image and internal perception were closely tied to the sense of helplessness. Women, she thought, were searching for self-mastery and autonomy, but they were doing it in the wrong way, by trying to control their bodies.

I thought Bruch's approach made sense, so at the Clarke we began to adopt her approach. We focused on how a patient felt about her body, how she read signals regarding her mood states. We'd ask gentle questions: What does it feel like to have the wind in your face, or water around you when you swim? Or more direct ones such as: How does hunger make you feel? What does sadness feel like? What do you do when you are angry? Can you experience pleasure without guilt? I'd ask patients how it felt to be bored. Perhaps it was actually anxiety they were feeling and hence the urge to binge on alcohol. I would suggest they could find other things to do, like an hour of yoga or a walk outdoors. Or maybe they'd think about why they feel bored, anxious, and alone. Could they trust themselves enough to feel vulnerable? If they could, this would be a big step forward because, as Bruch observed, the inability to trust oneself and listen to the body's signals can lead a person to try to control themselves, sometimes by starving.

Bruch's basic frame for understanding people made sense, and we found that our patients would develop some awareness of their psychological states. But they didn't gain weight. They would remain in hospital for long periods, or go home and be readmitted the following year, as emaciated as before.

The experience with Bruch's methods taught me something important: you can have a good understanding of a condition, and yet, applying what we know based on this may have no beneficial effect on treatment in an acute situation.

Bruch faced strong opposition from all sides of psychiatry. Traditional analysts resented her criticism, whereas the more biologically oriented psychiatrists thought she was permitting patients to remain emaciated instead of getting on with life. Bruch held up against the withering criticism with her usual aplomb: "There is no more lonely feeling in the world than everyone is out of step but me."

Around this time, another new theory for treatment emerged: behaviour therapy. It came from a series of cases described by Bart Blinder in California and Mickey Stunkard in Philadelphia. They said a patient should be put on bedrest, and she should have to earn the right to get out of bed, use the phone, or watch TV. She could earn these privileges if she gained a certain amount of weight. This seemed to address the problem we were facing; our patients were in hospital for long periods and made what appeared to be psychological progress, but they still didn't gain weight.[7]

This approach had a number of advantages: it unified the staff, so the infighting subsided. Patients did gain weight. Sometimes they felt actively involved in their treatment, and other times not. But we did not yet understand how much weight patients needed to gain to be discharged safely. We tended to discharge people when their weight was still too low, which made relapse easier, since they were in a dieting mentality. Also, the details of the behaviour therapy became the focus of treatment. This meant we spent endless hours negotiating what we meant when we said that at 95 pounds the patient would be allowed three hours out of bed. It also detracted from getting to know the person behind the symptoms. This wasn't individualized treatment, and our follow-up treatments after hospital discharge were too brief. Not surprisingly, relapses were frequent.

Bruch strongly opposed the new method. In a *Journal of the American Medical Association* (JAMA) article, she warned that behaviour therapy could harm the patient if it didn't consider the individual and her particular psychological state and needs.[8] It might even push some of these anorexic women to become bulimic after discharge, or even to commit suicide. Her warnings unnerved us, so we conducted a follow-up study of more than 40 patients we had treated several years earlier.[9] Behaviour therapy, we found, did not lead to the problems Bruch had suggested, but it didn't improve the patient's health over the long term either. The results led us to put more emphasis on post-hospital treatment. Weight restoration, in other words, was a small but necessary part of treatment. Treatment after discharge was essential. Our treatment program slowly evolved to a multifaceted one.

It was at this point that I read a groundbreaking book that would give me a new way of looking at mental illness. It was *Psychobiology and Human Disease*, published in 1977 by Herb Weiner, who was a professor at the Albert Einstein College of Medicine, and later at UCLA.[10] Weiner, surveying both physical and mental illness, had posed an intriguing question: Why do some people get sick and not others, even when they are infected by a bacteria or have a well-known risk factor for a disease? Only a proportion of individuals at risk ever become ill—many smokers live until they're 90 without succumbing to heart attack, stroke, or lung disease. What's more, of those who do develop an illness, only a few risk factors will be present in any individual—some people who die of lung disease, for instance, never smoked. Also, if one has a predisposition to disease, it is not certain where it might lead. It could cause one of several health outcomes.

Weiner's book made a deep impact on my view of mental illness. The risk-factors model made sense and had many advantages. We wouldn't have to blame the individual or the family. We could create individualized treatment plans, and reject the one-size-fits-all approach that often leads to the "if there is a symptom, there must be a pill for it" mentality.

Weiner's work would be particularly important to me when I started thinking about how it applied to anorexia nervosa, an illness that is obviously physical and dangerous, but also very puzzling. Developing an illness like anorexia was not a simple story of a single cause and getting sick. Rather, my colleague David Garner and I argued that it is brought on by a symphony of factors—genetic, cultural, family, and others. When these factors converge at a certain time in a young woman's life, they lead her to starve herself.

The sequence of events is important. A young woman might be predisposed to developing anorexia by numerous factors. Then something happens that effectively places a demand on the person, and she stops eating. You could say that the onset of illness is determined by the individual's failure to adapt to the demands placed on her, but even that is not the whole story. There could be completely different circumstances that induce her to keep starving herself.

In this sense, anorexia is like agoraphobia, the fear of open spaces. Various events can lead to agoraphobia, but once it has developed, the course of the illness may be greatly influenced by the individual's attempts to deal with the severe panic on being alone in public places. The individual may avoid going outside, or insist that a spouse be present. This produces further problems, such as social isolation, marital disharmony, and depression.

For sufferers of anorexia nervosa, the illness may cause changes in personality and behaviour, which account for many of the later symptoms that perpetuate the disorder. The perpetuating factors are significant. Starvation can cause poor concentration, reduced memory, heightened rumination, and food preoccupation, as well as sadness, irritability, or heightened variability in moods. It can cause poor sleep, early morning awakening, and voracious eating because of intolerable hunger. These all work to make the anorexic person feel more out of control and helpless. A healthy response might be to nourish the body, but instead the anorexic increases her dieting and exercise in a vain attempt to reestablish control. On top of the starvation effects, the person is left behind socially and vocationally, and there may be changes in the family; all of these contribute to her getting "stuck." This perpetuation of the disorder has many similar qualities to addiction. Contrary to public perception, patients with eating disorders do not always come from wealthy families. They come from all social classes and types of occupation and background. Many families are dealing with other problems, such as depression or substance abuse, and by the time they seek help for the anorexic daughter they are feeling frustrated, angry, and helpless. At times, the parents are desperate and often they feel guilty—*If only we had done such and such earlier.* Frequently, the anorexic girl becomes dependent on her mother, but then, because she craves autonomy, she becomes hostile to the person she so needs.

During this period of developing treatment models, I was working with a young American psychologist, David Garner. Our perspective on the disease was a multidimensional one. We thought that it was necessary to understand people and illness from a complex point of view. Each person with an eating disorder, we argued, needs an individualized understanding and treatment. We also dispelled a variety of myths about eating disorders. They were not caused by a single traumatic event. It was not the patient's fault, or the family's fault. It was not caused by the cultural obsession for thinness either. Anorexia was caused by multiple factors, and each individual needed a careful examination by a multidisciplinary team.[11]

We have since learned of the many risk factors occurring within the individual, her family, and her culture. There is a definite hereditary component. Consider the findings of the studies of identical twins who share the same genetic makeup: if one identical twin has the illness, the other is five times more likely to be anorexic than a fraternal twin or another sibling. What is inherited is just not known. Is it something to do with perfectionism or regulation of self-esteem, or something we just don't understand yet?

Anorexia is a complicated and subtle illness, and some of the most important risk factors are not genetic. A strict diet may heighten the risk. Gary Rodin, Denis Daneman, and their colleagues have found that juvenile diabetics, who have been taught to follow a rigid diet in order to prevent later complications, have an increased rate of eating disorders.[12] So do people who have been obese: a high proportion of people with bulimia, which is marked by out-of-control eating followed by purging, have a prior history of obesity; they hate the stigma of obesity and will do whatever it takes to prevent it recurring. Bulimia is a known complication of anorexia also and may be predicted by particular predisposing factors. Sexual abuse can lead to both anorexia and bulimia. Some 35% of anorexics have been sexually abused, a rate that is far higher than it is for the rest of the population. But this data has to be interpreted carefully because abuse can also lead to drug addiction and depression. Abuse, in other words, can cause many kinds of problems, not just anorexia. Why it might manifest itself one way in one person and another way in someone else is not precisely known but relates to the nature of other risk factors.

Many people with anorexia nervosa have deficits in the sense of who they are and where they belong. How this arises is complicated. These deficits can be caused by the trauma and helplessness experienced after sexual abuse, or by neglect at an early age, which leads to relationship problems. Fragility in the sense of the self can emerge from competition with a parent, or excessive control by a husband. Bruch believed that an individual who has never had her internal sensations and feelings validated will grow up without inner signals to help her develop a sense of self-control and then will feel helpless in functioning separately from her parents. But similar difficulties may also be experienced by a child who grows up in a family with poor differentiation between members, or in a family with particular coalitions between parent and child, or in a family in which the parental conflict is expressed through a child. The biological phenomenon of an unusually early puberty may expose the individual to demands that she is not yet capable of meeting. This may cause difficulties in autonomous functioning. Struggles with autonomy may interact with other factors to trigger anorexia nervosa.

Hilde Bruch had observed that many anorexics have a distorted perception of their body. We began to work out the subtle manifestations of this feature. At first we studied the visual perception of self. Garner devised an ingenious way to assess how people saw their bodies. We would take a photo of the patient in a two-piece bathing suit, and then we'd have her view it through a lens donated by Stancer's chemistry lab. The lens distorted the photograph like a funhouse mirror, making the image of the person fatter or skinnier than she really was. In our assessment, the patient could adjust the lens to make the figure look up to 20% bigger or smaller. This would help us gauge how she saw herself or would ideally like to look. When anorexic patients looked at photos of other people, they usually had a pretty accurate view. But when they looked at themselves, they thought they were bigger than they actually were. Soon we realized that how you saw your body and how you felt about it were two different things. Three-quarters of women in general surveys think they are too fat, but only about half of these women are extremely unhappy with their bodies. For some women the degree of loathing of the body is striking, and we found body loathing to be especially high in people with bulimia nervosa.

I was deeply immersed in anorexia by the time an American magazine suggested an entirely different type of risk factor. Could it be that anorexia was caused by the media? The question came up after the *New York Times* Sunday magazine did a piece on anorexia in 1973. The big question was this: Did the media obsession with Twiggy-style thinness cause women in the real world to starve themselves in greater numbers? If so, how did this happen? Then, we had no way to answer the question. We now know, from community surveys in North America and throughout the Western world, that about 5% of women are impaired psychologically, socially, or physically by an eating disorder during their lifetime; of these, 0.6% of the female population suffer from the full-blown illness, anorexia nervosa (males represent about an extra 10% of cases). But back then we could only speculate.[13]

We were intrigued by the question, but we had no way to assess the prevalence of the disease, especially in a large population. So Garner and I developed a scale (the Eating Attitudes Test) that could measure symptoms of eating disorders in the community. The written test asked 40 questions, such as: Does it take you a long time to finish a meal? Do you throw up after? Have you stopped menstruating for more than three months? Do you feel anxious after eating? It was a quick test, so we could give it to thousands of young women and then interview a few hundred high scorers to get a better idea of the prevalence of this disease. It turned out that just under 12% of the women who took the test were high scorers, but when we interviewed them, less than 1% had anorexia nervosa and just under 1.5% had bulimia in their full forms. These results were similar in many settings, including different social classes in Western societies.

To answer the question of whether the media was driving women to be anorexics, we wanted to find out whether women in the media were getting thinner. One obvious place to start was

Playboy magazine. In 1976 the American Psychiatric Association was meeting in Chicago, so it gave us a great chance to introduce ourselves to *Playboy*. The magazine gave us data on height, weight, and measurements of all the centrefolds since the magazine was first published. Sure enough, the *Playboy* models were getting thinner and thinner. Later we checked up on the Miss Sweden contestants, and they too were becoming thinner.

We were seeing, in other words, a thinning of the world's great beauty queens over the 1960s and 1970s. Then we looked at the image of Lady Liberty that Columbia Pictures used as its logo, shown at the start of its movies. Even Lady Liberty got thinner during the 1980s. It was so peculiar. Just as North American women were getting heavier (because of better health care, nutrition, and education), the female ideal was shrinking. Dieting and exercise were everywhere: Jane Fonda was showing women how to lose weight with exercise and the "right" foods—but she was also well-known to have controlled her weight through bulimic purging.

This told us that the idealized form for women in our culture was getting thinner. Then we looked at settings that required an extra-thin body size: ballet and other dance schools, as well as modelling schools. Most of the ballet school directors insisted on a thin body type. Many of the more rigorous ones followed George Balanchine's model of an ideal size for a dancer, and if your body didn't fit this mould as you went through adolescence, you either had to change your body or drop your dream. This was an extreme example of how a culture, the ballet world, pressures women to be thin. So, we wondered, how many ballet dancers suffered from anorexia or bulimia? Was the percentage higher in the ballet world than outside it? If so, it might give us more evidence that a culture can tip people toward anorexia.

Not surprisingly, the ballet schools had significantly elevated rates of eating disorders in their students. In some settings, 15 to

20% of the girls were afflicted. We also gained important insights. The girls who starved themselves were under the greatest pressure to perform, to succeed, and to achieve. They had to please others, not themselves, and to deal with the gap between these expectations and what they themselves might have wanted, they had to present a false front, and put their own aspirations in cold storage. They worked to please; and to make their parents happy.[14]

A classic example of this dynamic was found in a young ballerina I treated. She was burdened by tremendous expectations to succeed. So much hinged on her success—her scholarship, her social status, her entire dream of her future. She was being groomed to replace a particular performer in the national company. The same scenario was repeated at home. Her mother had been a ballet hopeful who had pressed the patient's older sister into a ballet career. When the sister rebelled, the mother turned up the pressure on the young ballerina. She dieted over 14 months and dropped from 106 pounds to 80 pounds.

When I first saw her, she insisted on pursuing the ballet career that had been carefully planned for her; but she also yearned for a broader world. At first she tried to accommodate the ballet world and her own desires, but after many months of therapy, she quit the ballet school to travel for a year. When we met again 10 years later, she was married, with a successful career in business and two daughters. She was a normal weight. As we talked, she emphasized how important it was to be able to follow her own pursuits. Once she could do that, her life became much more satisfying, even though she knew she was disappointing her mother.

The case for media causing women to starve was gaining ground. In Fiji, anorexia and bulimia nervosa were once hardly ever seen. In fact, obesity in women was admired as a sign of health, fertility, and social status. Then satellite television was beamed into Fijian homes in 1995, and suddenly women wanted to be thinner. A decade after our ballet work, Anne Becker, a Harvard psychiatrist and anthropologist, reported some startling evidence.[15] Three years after satellite TV was introduced, 75% of the Fiji women said they felt too fat, and 69% said they had been on a diet. And 11%, versus 0% in 1995, had induced vomiting to control weight. Furthermore, 29% in 1998 scored as at risk for an eating disorder, compared with 13% in 1995.

Studies from other countries, including Pakistan and Egypt, have evaluated students who go to Western countries such as the United Kingdom or the United States to attend university. These women display an increased drive for thinness and more frequent eating problems than their counterparts who attend university at home. One researcher has reported the same effect in Iran, from the opposite perspective.[16] Western television shows and DVDs have been banned in that country. Women on Iranian television are depicted with much of their bodies covered. Iranian women at the University of Tabriz were reported to have higher body satisfaction scores than their American counterparts. In China, the more urban and affluent the setting, the higher the frequency of these eating disorders. Similar studies of young women in westernized Hong Kong compared with a growing and affluent area, Shenzhen, and with a rural part of Hunan province have found that the prevalence of eating disorders exists on a gradient of westernization.[17]

Why, in the last 40 years, have women viewed their bodies so critically? To be sure, family and friends play an important role both in emphasizing what is desirable and in setting up a process of self-criticism. But family are really "culture bearers"—the culture of criticism and dissatisfaction is all around us. We found that fashion magazines, with their heavy emphasis on thinness, have an impact. Women with more maladaptive eating attitudes tended to overestimate their body sizes after being exposed to images of female fashion models. Women with disordered eating displayed an increase in anger and depressed mood immediately after viewing images of the models.[18] This heightened negative feeling and self-criticism can, and sometimes does, contribute to a cycle of deprivation followed by binge eating or even a syndrome of bingeing and purging.

The representation of the perfect female body is often used to elicit fears and insecurities in adolescent girls and women. Advertising relies heavily on images of unattainable female beauty in order to sell products, supposedly making such beauty within reach. Diet advertisements featuring celebrities and weight-loss articles have been found to be greatly overrepresented in women's magazines. In one study, more than one-fifth of advertisements in Spanish women's magazines directly or indirectly encouraged weight loss. Of course, this is predominantly for aesthetic rather than health reasons.

The media is only one risk factor. Another is the lack of connection to one's own feelings and the physical cues in the body. For people with anorexia and bulimia nervosa, the body does not feel natural or a source of comfort; instead, it feels artificial and distinct from the self, as though it has to be controlled by one's cognitive state. Part of the therapy must involve having the person develop an increased sense of ease with her body. The body needs to be a source of pleasure, not a thing to control.

Another key risk factor for eating disorders is low self-esteem. In the face of a job loss, or some other experience related to self-worth, most people can offset the blow with a store of good self-regard. But typically, people with an eating disorder are unable to call on this positive self-regard. They lack a sense of inner self-esteem, so to maintain their self-worth, they rely heavily on the external trappings of success. This makes them vulnerable in the world, particularly when the body has become the projection of a personal image. These days, people develop themselves and increase their self-worth by improving their bodies. Fatness is now equated with self-indulgence, lethargy, and slovenliness; thinness is associated with self-control, success, and attractiveness.

For people who go on to develop an eating disorder, cognitive styles from earlier in childhood, especially a black and white stance, or superstitious thinking, predominate, and these represent risk factors. A patient may say, for instance, "I walked into the work presentation and everyone could see that I am 5 pounds heavier, so I gave a poor presentation." Or "I lost 1 pound yesterday when I didn't have juice for breakfast so I'll never have juice again." Or "If I diet harder, these feelings will go away; when I reach 99 pounds, all will be wonderful." Two digits are better than three. These and other irrational beliefs feed into the disorder. Working on distorted cognitions is a slow but essential part of the therapy. Cognitive behaviour therapies have been shown to be effective for both anorexia and bulimia. At the same time, there is good evidence that, for younger patients, family therapy is effective. The treatment goal here is to establish clear boundaries between parent and child, but also to have the parent step in as a parent in specific areas. This aids in later permitting separation between parent and child, and the later independence of the child. The best work on this has been done at the Maudsley and has three phases to the treatment: weight restoration, returning eating control to the adolescent, and establishing a healthy adolescent identity.[19]

In 1979 Garner and I were working at top speed, developing new insights into this mysterious illness, when I was affected by an intense drama inside the Clarke.

It had begun in 1974, when Robin Hunter, after almost eight years, had left both his university and Clarke roles to become associate dean of postgraduate affairs in the Faculty of Medicine, a job he did not enjoy. After a couple of years, he left.

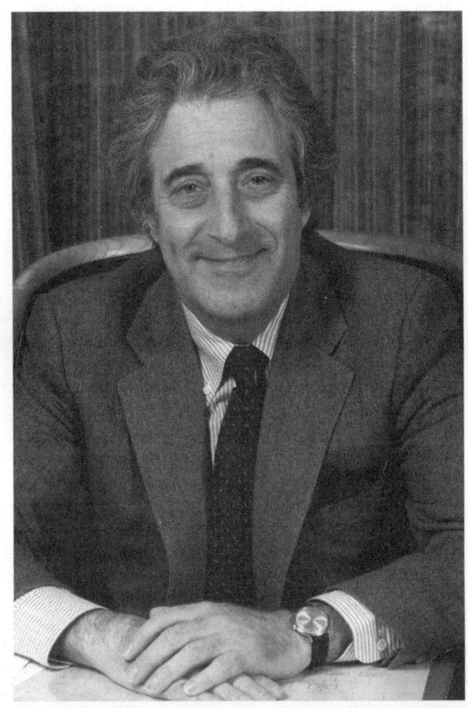

Fred Lowy, director of the Clarke and chair of psychiatry, 1974 to 1980, and dean of medicine, 1980 to 1987, at the University of Toronto. Lowy later founded the University of Toronto's Centre for Bioethics, and in 1995 became the president of Concordia University in Montreal. He was named an Officer of the Order of Canada in 2000. Courtesy CAMH Archives.

The search to replace him was a tumultuous one, and the successor was Fred Lowy, a Vienna-born, McGill- and US-trained psychoanalyst who had been at the University of Ottawa and head of the Ottawa Civic Hospital. Fred spent seven years at the Clarke and as University of Toronto chair of psychiatry before becoming dean of medicine in 1980. He later set up the Joint Centre for Bioethics at the University of Toronto. When Concordia University was having difficulty, he was recruited to be its president, a position he held from 1995 until 2005; he then took on this same role in an acting capacity in 2011. A remarkable man, Fred is cautious, smart, and a survivor in all circumstances. Peter Harris, one of the board chairs at the Clarke who worked with Fred, once remarked, "I have never seen a man lead so effectively from the rear." Lowy has had a distinguished career and was named an Officer of the Order of Canada in 2000.

Lowy, as head of the university's psychiatry department, appointed Moldofsky, who had been leading the Clarke's Psychosomatic Medicine Unit from 1975 to1979, to be chief of psychiatry at Toronto Western. It was a great challenge for Moldofsky: he was going to change a mid-level, undifferentiated general hospital group into one that specialized in mind-body problems and tied into the needs of the hospital itself.

Moldofsky asked me if I wanted to come with him to the Western; I declined. He then quietly approached Garner to join him. Garner by then had been working with me for six years, mostly with funds that we had to scramble for, but now, with his success on body image and psychometric scaling, he had landed longer-term funding through the Medical Research Council. Moldofsky offered Garner a secure salary at the Western, as a research psychologist. He asked Garner not to speak with me about it but, of course, Garner told me right away and refused the job offer. My friendship with Moldofsky ended, and although we were colleagues at the same university, our relations were never the same.

At the Clarke, I was appointed head of the Psychosomatic Medicine Unit, replacing Moldofsky. I quickly did two things. I appointed a new head nurse, Jean Simpson, a lovely Montreal-trained nurse who was heading a nursing unit at Women's College Hospital. Jean was like a breath of fresh air. Energetic, smart, personable, and direct, she helped craft a team on that floor that we could be proud of. She was never one to be intimidated by the physician, but she didn't flaunt her strength either. And she and I developed a relationship of mutual trust that would serve us both well in years to come. I also appointed Dublin-born Padraig Darby as junior psychiatrist. We formed a good little team—Jean,

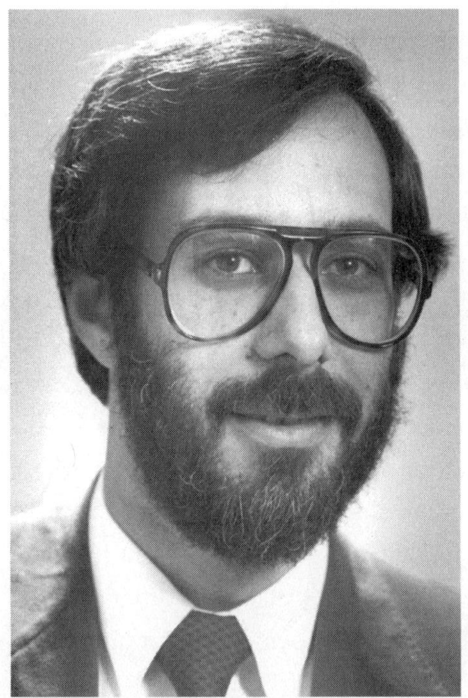

Paul Garfinkel when he worked on the psychosomatic medicine unit in the late 1970s. Courtesy CAMH Archives.

Padraig, David Garner, and me—and closed the week each Friday with a brandy in my office.

Meanwhile, Gerald Russell, a British-trained Belgian working at the Royal Free Hospital in London, came out with a paper that defined bulimia nervosa for the first time. This involved the powerful intractable urge to eat with loss of control, compensatory behaviour, and the morbid fear of fat. Often these are people at a normal weight. Just as Russell was finishing his manuscript on bulimia nervosa, he visited us in Toronto. We were on the same track, with research showing that anorexics with bulimia differed significantly from people who only restricted food.[20] Anorexics have a tendency to be perfectionists and withdraw socially, or to be inhibited. People with bulimia are more outgoing and impulse-ridden (and many become involved with drugs, theft, or promiscuity). Many of them have features of a borderline personality disorder. Bulimics much more commonly have a history of being obese, and of more obesity among family members. Anorexia has a much larger genetic component than does bulimia; people with bulimia are more influenced by culture. A large subgroup of bulimic patients purge (via vomiting and laxatives); we found that they have a young age of onset, and a very higher likelihood of sexual abuse and addiction, than do people with other eating disorders.[21]

Cases of bulimia nervosa skyrocketed. By the late 1980s, 70% of our patients had bulimia, and only 30% had anorexia nervosa. Bulimia is now twice as common as anorexia—1.1% of females suffer from it, according to an Ontario survey we did in the early 1990s. In addition, there are partial forms of this disorder that still result in impairment to the life of the person, occurring about three times as commonly.

Bulimia quickly gained a high profile. From the perspective of the physician, it was easier to treat. Big pharma supplied some promising medicines. The antidepressant SSRI medications proved to be useful in bulimia, but not in anorexia. Allan Kaplan and Tim Walsh found that these drugs don't prevent relapse in weight-recovered anorexic patients, for reasons we don't yet understand. When these drugs are combined with cognitive behaviour therapy, they lead to the best results in bulimia. We also have good evidence that three forms of focused psychotherapy—cognitive behaviour therapy, interpersonal psychotherapy, and dialectical behaviour therapy—are all effective.

Soon a whole industry evolved around bulimia nervosa. Bulimia even had a glamorous patron: Diana, Princess of Wales. In the late 1980s, the princess agreed to be honorary patron for an eating disorder conference to be held in London, England. Before the meeting, the four or five keynote speakers were invited to meet

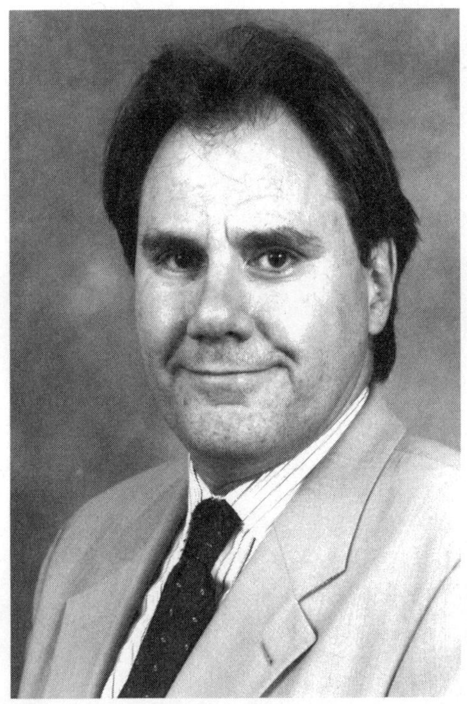

Allan Kaplan was a resident on the psychosomatic medicine unit in 1979. He went on to hold the first Loretta Rogers Chair in Eating Disorders, and was vice-chair, research, for the Department of Psychiatry. Courtesy CAMH Archives.

with her; each of us would have our picture taken with the princess. Most of the others eagerly accepted, but I hesitated. It wasn't just because of my anti-herd mentality; I really disapprove of the cult of celebrity. Rather, I was acutely uncomfortable with having Diana as our spokesperson when she was clearly still ill but so glamorous at the same time. I didn't want to do anything to enhance the glamour of the condition. She had a devastating illness, but what people saw was the thin and attractive. She spoke against bulimic behaviour, but looking at her made it hard to believe that her slender form was a healthy one.

After all, it's not the first time that society has glamorized the sick. In her book *Illness as Metaphor*, Susan Sontag describes how fashionable it was to look sickly when it was thought that tuberculosis indicated a gentle, delicate, and sensitive individual.[22] It became not just a sign of a so-called artistic personality but of a romantic individual, a sensitive, creative person. Pallor became a fashionable attribute. As a result, men would find pale women attractive, and women would try to whiten their skin with powders. So was I subtly condoning a fashionable condition by posing with the princess, I wondered. How would patients react? Might they want to adopt her bingeing and purging regimen? I politely declined.

I've been treating anorexics for 40 years, and it's been a fascinating and perplexing journey. Yet if you look at what has changed, the numbers are only mildly encouraging. In 1970 the mortality rate for anorexia nervosa was over 10%, with 20% of patients who survive having seriously impaired lives, including chronic underweight, social isolation, depression, and anxiety. Today the mortality rate is closer to 5%, but still 20% of patients are experiencing significant symptoms 8 to 12 years from diagnosis. On the other hand, three-quarters of treated patients do very well over time. Bulimia nervosa is a more positive story. The mortality rate is extremely low (0.3 to 0.5%), and a dozen years later, only 10 to 15% still have the disorder.

We also know more about the impact of starvation on the human body. That research began in the 1940s when Ancel Keys, a prominent nutritionist, enrolled 36 men for an experiment at the University of Minnesota campus.[23] They were put on a radical diet that caused 25% weight loss, comparable to that we see in our patients. These otherwise healthy men began to exhibit many of the symptoms of an eating disorder. Their sleep became fragmented. When they did sleep, they frequently dreamed of food, as our patients do. In the daytime they thought and talked about food often; some began to collect or exchange recipes. They became more socially withdrawn and most experienced a narrowing of interests. Their moods were characterized by irritability, anxiety, and extreme swings. They were unable to concentrate. Several developed binge eating when food was available. When we rediscovered this data in the 1980s, we realized why anorexia nervosa frequently develops into a self-perpetuating problem. When an anorexic patient experiences these starvation effects, she feels more helpless and out of control and increases her dieting and the consequent effects of starvation. Many symptoms of starvation also closely resemble those of depression—it is often hard to tell the two apart until the person's starvation has been reversed.

We have also learned more about the complications of starvation: electrolyte and water imbalance effects, cardiac abnormalities, and many gastrointestinal illnesses. Osteoporosis is common and a frequent contributor to impaired quality of life in the chronically ill. Among bulimic patients, erosion of dental enamel leading to loss of teeth is common. We also studied women who became pregnant while still ill and not surprisingly found that they had small sickly babies requiring special attention.

The study of eating disorders has contributed to the understanding of the regulation of hormones. Starting in the early 1970s, working with neuroendocrinologist Greg Brown, we found that when a patient increases her food intake, levels of growth hormone improve even before her weight is restored.[24] This is in contrast to her estrogen levels, which are very low and return to normal only with weight restoration. Patients who are starving generally have signs of hypothyroidism (low heart rate, low body temperature, low blood pressure, dry skin, and reduced metabolic rate) and some thyroid hormones in the blood may reflect this, but these changes respond to weight gain. High plasma levels of cortisol are typical of people starving from other causes and are also seen in anorexia nervosa. We have determined that muscle function comes back to normal after eight weeks of weight restoration. We've learned that medicines that promote stomach emptying can help patients deal with feelings of fullness and early satiety when they begin to eat again.

We now know more about the role of metabolic and hormonal changes in people with an eating disorder, and about the nature of recovery. This is helpful because we can tell patients what has occurred, why, and what to expect as they restore their weight. We have learned, for example, that the hormonal and structural changes can be reversed when patients maintain a good restored weight. Many women, once they recover their weight, can have normal fertility and become pregnant.

We have also found that 40% of the people with anorexia suffer from depression. This is a far higher rate than found in the general population. Anxiety disorders are equally prevalent. Why this is so

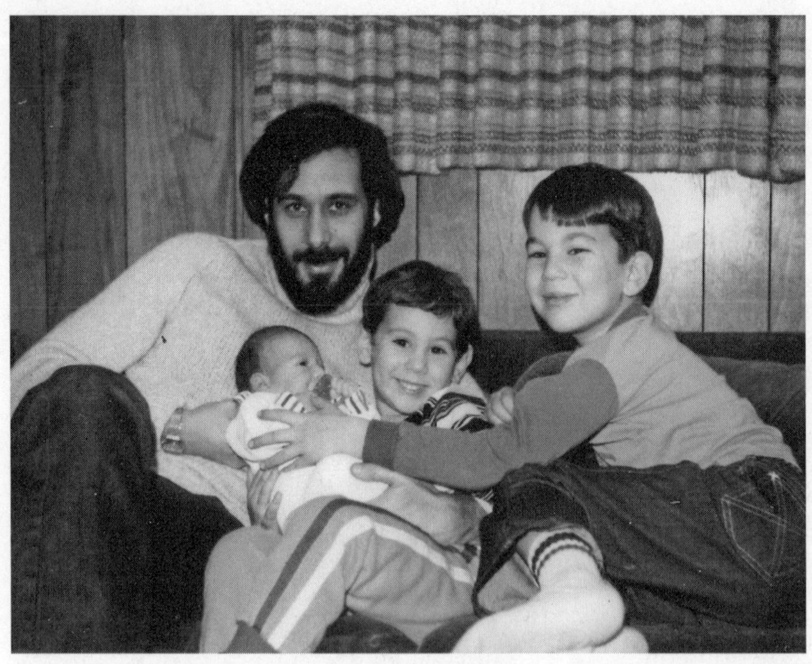

Paul Garfinkel with Joshua, Stephen, and Jonathan (1980).

is not clear. The lifetime risk of substance abuse among bulimics is close to 50%, again for reasons unknown. It may be related to family history or to a need for soothing and difficulties controlling one's impulses. In people with anorexia nervosa, the rate of substance abuse is about 20%, compared with less than 10% for the general population. The legendary British musician and composer Sir Elton John is a good example of someone with both substance abuse problems and bulimia.

By considering many factors that contribute to anorexia, I feel we've been more effective in dealing with patients. Consider Cathy, the patient who puzzled and infuriated us back in the 1970s. Many years later, she came back, and the differences in treatment were striking. Cathy had returned to university in another Ontario city, and I heard nothing from her for years. But I was asked to see her again when she was 28, married, and the mother of a nine-month-old daughter. Since the baby's birth Cathy had dieted and exercised, and she was down to 88 pounds. She told me her story. She had graduated from university and was working in accounting when she married a colleague. It had taken her several years to get to 115 pounds, and although she felt uneasy with this size, she could tolerate it. She believed this was because of her success in her career, in her enjoyment of playing piano, and in seeing men respond to her attractive appearance. But then her mother died a few months before the baby was born. Her father withdrew, angry with everyone, but especially with her.

Cathy's husband was eager to be involved in his wife's care. He appeared befuddled, eager to make a good impression but, as it turned out, jealous of Cathy's success at work and in her musical life. We admitted Cathy, along with her infant, to the hospital and started her on bedrest and with a graded diet beginning at 1,500 calories and increasing weekly. This was supplemented with a lot of nursing support, relaxation and breathing exercises, and, when her anxiety continued, a small amount of a minor tranquilizer at meals. This time emphasis was placed on her psychological state—on her grieving her loss, and dealing with her anger at her father and with her feelings about becoming a mother. We helped her recognize how she felt, and be comfortable with it. We talked about competitiveness and achievement, and issues of worth, dependency, and trust, as well as about her cognitive distortions. A big part of the treatment involved the couple, and although her husband balked, Cathy engaged in therapy. She was able to gain weight more comfortably, and she left the hospital at 110 pounds.

Over the next 18 months in treatment, Cathy realized her mother had been denigrated in the marriage and squelched in her artistic career. She confronted her father's infidelities. These insights became important themes in her ongoing healing. Over the years, Cathy has done well. She and her husband had two more children, both boys. Cathy gained reasonable amounts of weight and maintained it after these pregnancies. She is far more comfortable with her body size and shape. Cathy is successful in her work, with her children, and with friends.

Since the mid-1970s, the mortality rate of anorexia nervosa has been cut in half. But in other ways, not much has changed and we as doctors have to get used to modest success: your patient survives, even if she is still radically thin. I thought about this while I was rereading the early Toronto papers by Ray Farquharson and Francis Hyland written in the 1930s. Following up with their 15 patients after 20 to 30 years, they found that many had done well in spite of some ongoing symptoms.

One patient of mine who had suffered from anorexia nervosa for 20 years reached a plateau. Although significantly underweight, she was no longer in danger medically. She led a rather restricted life. But when she began to develop an interest in children, she seemed to find enthusiasm for and meaning in her life. She obtained formal training and successfully operated a kindergarten, which became a source of great pleasure to her.

For some of our patients, the sensitivity and growth associated with recovery led to a desire to help others clinically. One person who I helped treat in the 1970s came back from university one summer to describe all that we had done wrong in her therapy. As a result, I asked her to stay for the summer and work on designing an improved hospital program for patients; she did so, and found it satisfying and a way of repairing a rather unpleasant termination of her treatment a few years earlier. Another person who created considerable clinical difficulty during treatment is now on the medical faculty at a nearby university, and a highly esteemed teacher. Others have described their experiences movingly or humorously in theatre, literature, or poetry.

Farquharson and Hyland knew this back in the 1930s, and they had good advice for clinicians: "The most important factor in treatment is to gain the patient's confidence, which enables the doctor to help her change her attitude. By reassurance, patient explanation and firm but kindly encouragement, it is often possible to help patients change their attitudes, so that they gradually increase their intake of food and recover."[25]

In other words, warmth and genuineness, understanding and acceptance, openness and honesty are all essential components of effective and competent long-term care. What's more, clinicians must be prepared to accept the possibility that their most important function is to provide genuine human contact that focuses on quality of life and removes the sense of isolation and aloneness patients feel.[26]

If anything is to be learned from our history with these illnesses and indeed with all illnesses, it is that true compassion must be the foundation upon which any attempts to help and to heal must be made. Effective treatments are a relatively new domain for medicine, and in many arenas of human disease we have yet to find them; however, the role of the clinician is much more than purveyor of interventions; it includes the provision of comfort and hope. This can be hard for the therapist trying to treat someone with anorexia. One has to be willing to dedicate a large amount of time and effort, and be prepared to accept frustration and failure.[27]

Denial runs deep in some patients. One time I showed a patient in deep denial the results of a CT scan of her brain. Starvation produces an atrophy of the cortex, and a widening of the fissures, which is visible. I was sure this would frighten a young woman who so valued her cognitive abilities. But it had no effect: "I must be so intelligent to have my brain shrink and still be so smart," she said.

When a patient runs the risk of dying, the therapist feels helpless, angry, and resentful. For some very ill patients, all the therapist can do is provide a holding environment that keeps them alive so that their own healing and maturation may occur. You can never predict whether they will recover or not. In one of our studies on course and outcome, I realized that we really couldn't tell how people would do 5 to 10 years after treatment. Many people who I thought would do well were still struggling with an eating or mood disorder, while others—the ones I thought didn't benefit from treatment—described how a few weeks in hospital, or six months of therapy, had made a profound impact on their lives. They were doing well, despite all our predictions. These experiences have truly inspired me to work harder to help the chronically ill people who appear as if they will never improve.

I've also learned that people may need very different treatments during different periods of their lives. One young girl who I first treated when she was age 13 had to be admitted to hospital for profound weight loss that placed her life in danger. She had to be fed by a nasogastric tube to help restore her nutritional state. She had developed the eating disorder in part because of intense confusion around growing up. Her parents had come to Canada at considerable sacrifice for the future benefit of their children. This young girl felt that she had to "make it" in the new world in order to make her parents' struggle worthwhile, but she also feared that she would lose them if she became too removed from their traditions.

After her discharge from hospital, a course of six months of family counselling, together with support from the pediatrician, provided stability and good health for over five years. However, when at a university in a neighbouring city, she experienced the loss of a love relationship and developed a mixed picture of bulimia with major depression. My treatment now consisted of individual psychotherapy and a tricyclic antidepressant (it was before SSRIs were available). She did well and several years later married and went on to have two children and a satisfying career.

Then, during her early 30s, some of the features of the eating disorder recurred in response to feeling helpless in her marriage. On this occasion, marital counselling was the central component of the treatment. She had begun to feel trapped, in part because of her husband's professional success and the constricting burden she felt this forced on her. This recreated the old sense of helplessness she had felt in her adolescence. This woman, whom I have known now for over 20 years, has required different forms of care as her life circumstances have changed. There is no such thing as a one-size-fits-all treatment for individual patients or for all the various periods in a person's life.

I've also come to believe that we have to see beyond appearances. We have to appreciate people for who they are, not for who they should be. It's harmful to push people to fit a mould and to perform, to live up to the expectations of others, rather than to grow and develop according to their own potential. All of our work on the sociocultural aspects of the eating disorders has revealed this: It's not just the pressure to attain an idealized size that leads to anorexia. It's also the pressure to perform, to live up to the demands of others.

Too often in our current worlds, life feels like a race. We want our children to go to the right schools and the best universities, where they can meet the right people and get the best jobs. People with eating disorders often represent the extreme of what is wrong with this approach. They have been programmed to do all the "right" things, only to find that these things are not for them; they have felt empty living only for others. Often they will say, after recovery, that they were so preoccupied with the race to succeed that they forgot that life is a set of experiences to be realized, rather than an outcome. When we work with women who deny themselves nourishing aspects of food, we see that denying the body is really a denial of one's belonging in the world. "Winning" the race comes at the expense of what makes life worth living, and sometimes at the expense of one's own life.

This is a perplexing time for women, especially those with low self-esteem who need exterior trappings of success to feed their self-worth. They are expected to compete and be successful in the male world, and at the same time to measure their sense of themselves by their physical appearance and their ability to attract. It's a real dilemma. Often women are required to be active, decisive, and independent during the working day, only to be rewarded for the opposite behaviours in their personal relationships.

It is a strange conundrum: just when women in the developed world are finding jobs and liberating themselves from the restrictions imposed by earlier times, they've become fixated on the unattainable goal of extreme thinness. I see the idealization of thinness as a form of repression of women, like foot binding in ancient China, which severely limited mobility. Foot binding, although unbearably cruel, was a status symbol for women of the upper classes, until the practice died out in the early 20th century. Now society has a new form of repression: extreme dieting. I believe the promotion of dieting, self-control, and extreme thinness is fuelled by fears of female sexuality and power. Now that women are expanding their roles, it is as if they cannot be trusted. They have to be controlled through endless demands to perfect themselves.

This leads me to feel that any approach to understanding and treating someone with an eating disorder must have a base in principles of feminism. I'm convinced that the biggest challenge in conquering anorexia is to change social attitudes that equate thinness with goodness, desirability, and group acceptance. Truly exciting opportunities exist for studying how to prevent eating disorders through various approaches directed at schoolgirls when they are age 9 or 10. Such interventions would have to deal with issues of self-esteem regulation, attitudes to the body, and efficacy in relationships, as well as with attitudes to food and weight. In doing this we are facing the powerful and hugely influential media, fashion, and entertainment industries. These have not changed course in 40 years: the thin and the beautiful are revered and have many more opportunities in life than do those who are not thin and beautiful.

Dealing with people who have eating disorders on an ongoing basis involves a series of challenges. We are dealing with people who often have life-threatening illnesses, at a time when both they and members of their families are confused and feeling helpless. It is gratifying to see someone who had struggled so hard, for so long, reach an autonomous adulthood, come back years later well, and appreciatively describe a full life. But it is also extremely sad to consider the anguish, pain, and loss when the course of the illness leads to chronic illness or to death, as happens all too often.

CHAPTER 9
What Are You Doing in a Mental Hospital?

In the spring of 1982, I got a surprise call from another Winnipegger, Gary Rodin. Gary, the son of a prosperous grain merchant in Manitoba, had studied medicine in Winnipeg and then came to Toronto to do his residency in internal medicine. In an unusual step, Gary switched to psychiatry and then psychoanalysis. Now he was working at Toronto General, the largest and most powerful teaching hospital affiliated with the University of Toronto. The hospital was looking for a new chief of psychiatry to replace the departing Alistair Munro, and after many months, they still hadn't found anyone. I hadn't even thought of applying. Why would I? At 36, I was happy with my career at the Clarke. My book written with David Garner, *Anorexia Nervosa: A Multidimensional Perspective*, was getting favourable reviews, and I had been assigned new managerial responsibilities. But then Rodin invited me for lunch, at which he encouraged me to seriously consider it: "Why are you wasting your life working in a mental institution rather than in a general hospital?"

Rodin's attitude was similar to what most well-trained and enthusiastic psychiatrists of the early 1980s felt—the mental hospital was a place of custodial care; slow moving, not a place for discovery and "crackle." Psychiatry had been moving into the general hospitals for two decades, as part of the reunion with medicine. In the general hospital, psychiatrists were individual private practitioners. Their views carried more weight than their counterparts in a mental institution, and they were central to any planning and change. In the mental hospital, they were employees of

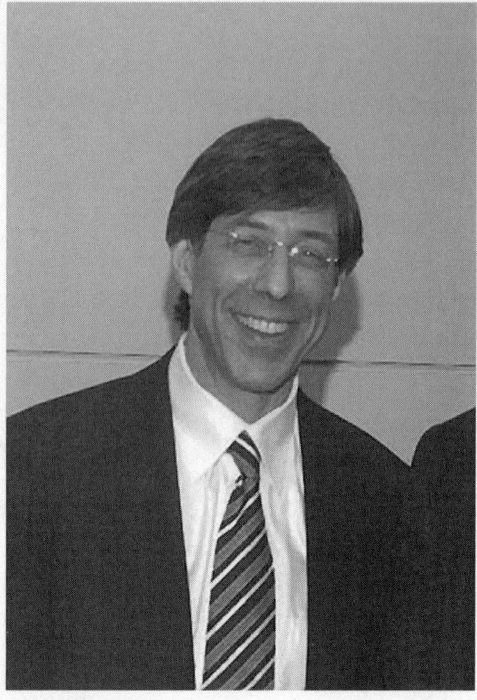

Gary Rodin being awarded a chair in psycho-oncology in 2005. Courtesy University of Toronto Department of Psychiatry.

the province, on a salary and unionized—more a part of a slow-moving bureaucracy.

When Rodin's call came, I had been heading up the Clarke's research department for the past year, and the job had given me my first taste of a management role. And I was thriving. I had developed an inclusive style, inviting Nicholas Mrosovsky (a zoologist interested in hibernation); Franco Vaccarino (a research psychologist studying pleasure centres in the brain); and Janet Polivy and Peter Herman (psychologists who had just worked with Stanley Schachter in New York on obesity) to rounds or to research seminars on the Psychosomatic Medicine Unit. I often asked opinions from a psychoanalyst like Doug Frayn or from a senior general psychiatrist like Abe Miller. If our attitude is we don't know but want to learn, it's easy to ask others.

I was flattered and surprised. If I did go for this job, I would probably be the youngest chief of psychiatry in Canada. I would be managing the same psychiatrists who supervised me only 10 years earlier. Yet I had no actual training in the art of management, let alone the management of psychiatrists. This would be a whole new ball game.

This prime spot had opened up because of a series of quick moves begun two years before on the chessboard of Toronto psychiatry. First, Fred Lowy, the gentle Viennese-born psychoanalyst who had been running the Clarke since 1974, was appointed dean of medicine in 1980. Lowy had been a steady leader who deftly handled the factions vying for minuscule or imagined advantages. As dean, he could now apply his subtle diplomatic and leadership skills to the entire Faculty of Medicine.

With his departure, a search committee was struck to fill Lowy's twin roles as university chair of psychiatry and director of the Clarke. Before long, the candidates were narrowed to two. One of them was my brilliant but polarizing mentor Vivian Rakoff. Since 1977 Rakoff had been working as chief of psychiatry at Sunnybrook Medical Centre, where he focused the group on geriatrics, adolescence, and mood disorders. Although he did an excellent job, his larger-than-life personality was controversial. Others didn't appreciate his art-and-science approach, although I think they failed to realize that real science and art are very much aligned through the creative process.

The other contender was Alistair Munro, chief of psychiatry at Toronto General Hospital. Unlike Rakoff, Munro used his considerable charm and humour to deal quietly but effectively with many people at all levels. He was an excellent general psychiatrist, well respected by doctors throughout the hospital. As a sign of that respect, Munro was named chair of the hospital's Medical Advisory Board, an unusual role for a psychiatrist. Munro was a popular figure, but after several rounds of voting, Rakoff narrowly won the competition.

Now, just one year later, and perhaps not surprisingly, Munro announced he was moving to Halifax to be Dalhousie University's chair of psychiatry. And then came Rodin's call.

A few days after my lunch with Rodin, I got a call from Vickery Stoughton, the hospital CEO who had come from Boston two years earlier. He asked to meet.

Bold and driven, Vickery was an attractive man my age, and he made a strong pitch for me to apply for the job. He made it clear that he had not one ounce of prejudice against mental illness. On the contrary: Toronto General, he told me, was raising the bar on both care and research of the mentally ill.

The psychiatrists at Toronto General were good, and they clearly felt that they were the best general hospital group in the city. They represented a European evidence-based approach, in contrast to the "impractical and foolish" group of psychodynamic psychotherapists practising across the street at the Mount Sinai Hospital. But they were going to have to change. The Toronto General was now emphasizing research in the clinical setting. A new research building, the Max Bell Research Centre, was being built, and research would be integrated into clinical care. My mission, then, would be to turn a department of experienced and effective psychiatrists into a hot spot for clinical research and teaching.

What's more, the hospital was going to develop nutrition and metabolism as a priority. It had brought experts from gastrointestinal medicine and endocrinology together with general surgeons. My passion for eating disorders would fit in perfectly. Besides, the women with eating disorders would be safer at the General if they had a heart attack or other life-threatening physical problem. I was sold, and I agreed to apply for the job.

A few weeks later, I found myself in the boardroom of the General's Bell wing, where I faced a dozen men and women on the search committee. The chair of the committee was George Ryerson Gardner, a Canadian philanthropist who made his money in the stock brokerage business, oil and gas, and Kentucky Fried Chicken outlets.

I talked about how important it was to integrate research into a clinical setting, and I used a tried-and-true approach from my teaching. I had found that medical undergrads were fussy, wanting to hear only the key points necessary for exams, and no more. If I added any unnecessary but interesting details, lots of them would open up their student newspaper, the *Varsity*. It wasn't so easy to talk over a wall of papers. So I lectured by enumeration: "These are the four things you need to know about anorexia nervosa," or schizophrenia, or whatever. It improved my ratings by students, but made the talks much less interesting to me.

I decided to use the same approach in my presentation. I suggested four priorities for the General's Psychiatry Department: nutrition and behaviour, women's mental health, depression, and consultation/liaison work, which involved caring for the psychiatric needs of the medical and surgical patients of the hospital. Soon after I left the room and was back in my office, the phone rang. I got the job.

I was looking forward to developing the eating disorders program in a general hospital. We would get support that wasn't available in a mental hospital. On a human level, though, it was challenging. I was able to take some members of my team with me: David Garner; an outstanding student, Marion Olmsted; and Allan Kaplan, a bright young American who had studied in Toronto and been a resident on my unit.[1] Barbara Dorian would join us in 1984. Barbara had worked on my unit at the Clarke in 1979, did a fellowship in immunology and its relationship to stress, and then worked with Barr Taylor and Stewart Agras, excellent psychiatrists at Stanford, before coming to Toronto General.[2]

But I had to leave others behind, and I found that difficult. My coping mechanism, I'm sad to say, was to get angry and criticize them. Now I realize this anger was just a cover for my genuine sadness about leaving a team I had created. As I have learned in my practice, it is often easier, especially for men in our society, to express anger or rage rather than sadness. I was experiencing a loss, but turned it into a fight.

At my farewell party, Rakoff spoke perceptively and with great generosity when he said that I was the adolescent who fights with his parents and leaves home, but then takes an apartment six blocks away and comes home twice a week to do the laundry. As usual, Rakoff hit just the right note.

Moving to Toronto General would take me into the heart of medicine, and I suspected it would be a different world. This was a tertiary care centre, after all. C.K. Clarke and Campbell Meyers had disagreed over the role of hospital-based psychiatry publicly and vocally, 70 years earlier. Was that split between the mental hospitals and the general ones still a problem? How would the doctors receive someone like me?

The rift between psychiatry and medicine had been around for a long time. Before World War II, the business was fractured: asylum-based alienists, private practice neurologists and general practitioners, and psychoanalysts were all vying for authority. Psychiatry was still physically and to some extent philosophically separated from other branches of medicine.

Then, in 1930, Dr. David Edsall, dean of Harvard Medical School and a director of the Rockefeller Foundation, wrote a report complaining that psychiatry was too removed from mainstream medicine. This report convinced the foundation to give out grants that would support a greater collaboration between psychiatry and other medical specialties. A few years later, with the large number of casualties from World War II, there was a new need to care for veterans with brain injuries, trauma, shell shock, addictions, and depression. Facilities for these veterans started to spring up, often in close proximity to general hospitals.

Despite this, traces of that old tension were in evidence back when I worked as chief resident at the Clarke in the 1970s. Robin Hunter, then chair of the University of Toronto's Department of Psychiatry, would visit Toronto General once a year. As chief resident, I'd go with him, and it felt like we were stepping into enemy territory. Hunter was a perceptive and accurate diagnostician, and one year he interviewed a young male patient whom he diagnosed with a personality disorder. In the ensuing discussion, it turned out that the man had had psychotic symptoms that a staff member at Toronto General had actually told the patient not to divulge in the interview. Hunter was incensed that his colleagues at Toronto General would try to deceive him, and despite my attempts to smooth things over, he got up and left the meeting.

By the time I arrived at Toronto General in 1982, psychiatry had been geographically well accommodated into the practice of medicine. The department shared the eighth floor of a large new building on Elizabeth Street, the John David Eaton Building, with some surgical departments. It was connected to the older Norman Urquhart Building, where the beds for psychiatry patients were located.[3] Although psychiatrists were complaining about the cost of the new wing (and its effects on their incomes), I was thrilled: psychiatry was right in the hospital, and treated like any other specialty group.

When you entered the General, it didn't take long before you were reminded that it was here in Toronto that Banting and Best discovered insulin. This great discovery was in the early 1920s, but for many years everyone at the General felt like they were the greatest, just by turning up. There was an arrogance among the doctors that was palpable. By the time I arrived, though, that arrogance had modulated to cockiness, but it drove a real desire to work hard, be measured against others, and excel on the world stage.

This was in large part because of the physician-in-chief, Charles Hollenberg. He came from Winnipeg, but he had the "disadvantage" of growing up in the more prosperous part of town, South Winnipeg. His family was renowned in medical circles in Manitoba; his uncle Jake, my former teacher, was a successful surgeon who smoked constantly. His father was also a doctor, and the family had formed the Hollenberg Clinic. Such was its fame that Charles used to say that non-Jewish patients thought Hollenberg was a Jewish word for doctor.

The family's success didn't dull his drive. Charles received his medical degree from the University of Manitoba in 1955. Five years later, he went to McGill to study endocrinology and metabolism, especially the fat cell and obesity. When he came to the General in 1970, the Toronto establishment was concerned. He was Jewish, after all. He had been selected to be the Sir John and Lady Eaton Professor of Medicine and chair of the Department of Medicine at the University of Toronto, and physician-in-chief of Toronto General Hospital; but only after university president Claude Bissell consulted the Eaton family did Hollenberg get the job.[4]

Hollenberg was the ideal Jew to break in. He was good-looking, tall and broad, light skinned and fair haired. He spoke with confidence. He loved to argue and to express his views vigorously about anything, even the university's ogling swimmer (a University of Toronto controversy in the 1980s when a male swimmer followed a young woman in the pool incessantly). His wife, Mimi, a character herself, playfully called him "Attila." As physician-in-chief and university chair, and later as vice-provost of the university's health sciences and then founding president of Cancer Care Ontario,

Charles was consistent. He clearly defined the goals to be pursued and the roles people had to perform to achieve them. This clarity was a huge advantage. He also had a great and uncompromising love of the academic enterprise: he believed in his bones that the academy in medicine was a noble enterprise.

Hollenberg built a superlative Department of Medicine. He recruited top people from Montreal and elsewhere, and soon Toronto was producing graduates of the highest quality. It encouraged the brightest students to combine medical residencies with graduate studies at the Institute of Medical Science, where physicians could learn science and research as they completed their residencies. He understood that an academic group required different types of skills: those of clinician-teachers and clinician-scientists, as well as of basic scientists.

On the down side, Charles always had to be in control. He understood power and used it. When as university chair he met with the chiefs of medicine from the eight other teaching hospitals, he lined their chairs in a row facing him—there was no question who was in charge. If you came into a crowded room, you could predict where Charles would be: talking to the most powerful person there.

A highly unusual man in academic medicine, dedicated to integrity, standards, and courage, Charles had a huge impact on me and on my career. I sought his advice often, particularly when I first arrived at the General. I sorely needed it.

Outside the department, I could still feel signs of the old medical prejudice against psychiatry. On the first day of my clinical work, I was at the nursing station of one medical unit reviewing a chart when a cardiologist introduced himself and his entire entourage of students and residents. He said to me, "You must be the new head of Psychiatry that I've been hearing about … I am so and so; I want you to know I believe in psychiatry." I said I was delighted to meet him and his team, and told him, "I believe in cardiology." He later asked me to see his wife in consultation.

Another time I was meeting one of the clinical chiefs to learn about areas of mutual work. "Oh, I get it," he said quickly, and then brushed me off to the program's head nurse. She would be "the one I would relate to." Two years later he asked me to see his partner for a serious psychiatric illness. It was a pattern I was to see regularly over that decade: whenever someone denigrated psychiatry or one of our patients, that person would usually call soon after to ask for help for a family member.

I was hired to put greater emphasis on clinical research and teaching, and I knew this would involve a big shift in culture, and I knew I would need every means at my disposal to accomplish it. The General had about 16 full-time psychiatrists and 20 part-timers, and their reception of me, especially in those early days, was chilly at best. They were hurt and angry that Richard Swinson, a British behavioural psychiatrist and their choice for chief, hadn't got the job. Swinson himself felt hurt, as if I had deprived him of his rightful post.

"Just which Garfinkel are you?" one colleague said. "I always get you and your brother mixed up." (My brother Barry had been a resident there in the mid-1970s—not remembering "which one" I was, was quite a putdown.) Another senior psychiatrist said what I feared: "Chiefs may come and go, but I'll still be here."

Frankly, the job was intimidating. I wanted the psychiatry group to fit the new academic core of the hospital. I wanted the hospital and the university to value psychiatry. To meet these goals was going to be a challenge, but I knew I had three key levers of power.

The first lever was the bully pulpit, and I used it repeatedly to drive home four key issues: (1) standards, measured not by ourselves, but by others; (2) people, which means recruiting and motivating the best clinicians and scholars, and being clear about what we ask them to do; (3) programs—what our priorities will be, and will not be; and (4) value to the hospital.

I must have recited these four points about a thousand times in that first year. People must have been thoroughly sick of hearing it. But I believed in them and I instinctively knew that, in order to compel others to listen, and to command leadership, I would need to repeat the same message over and over.

I told staff how important the academic enterprise is to the hospital, the university, and ultimately to the public. This was, I said, the best environment for training the next generation, not only of academic clinicians but of those who were to become the clinicians for our communities. Done well, our group would also become a magnet for the very best residents. Clinical care thrives in these academic settings.

The second mechanism I knew I had available was that of bringing in people with similar values to gradually change the culture. To my great relief, I didn't start this new job entirely alone. From the beginning I had an important ally in Gary Rodin. He had finished his psychoanalysis and had just received his first peer-reviewed research grant on the topic of depression in the medically ill. Gary was in charge of the program for the medically ill and did a great job—he's an excellent clinician, deeply interested in people and what makes them tick. He went on to study diabetes and eating disorders, and ended up with a chair in psychosocial oncology. He has loved his career, mixing clinical care and research, and has mentored many good people.

When it came to hiring, I started with the eating disorders program and stress and immune function, where Barbara worked. Within a few months, I was able to recruit Sid Kennedy, a bright and determined psychiatrist who came to Toronto from Belfast via studies in Newcastle. He developed an expertise in mood disorders and ended up as the chief psychiatrist of University Health

Network 20 years later. These new people mixed well with several staff who could appreciate the new model for an academic-clinical centre. Gail Robinson, a resident at Toronto General in the 1960s who stayed on staff and became the lone woman in the full-time group, had built a national profile in the field of women and abuse. Bob Buckingham, an excellent generalist and teacher, came onside, which was important because he wasn't a researcher. By the end of that year, the group was beginning to move in the right direction.

The third lever was money. In those days, the full-time psychiatrists got $40,000 or more from either the university or hospital, on top of the fees for service they received from government for treating patients. This was a significant piece of their revenues. This hard money, as they called it, was supposed to pay for teaching and research, yet many psychiatrists in my group did little of either. They got the money anyway, and they felt that they deserved it.

When I understood this, I was angry (and more than a bit self-righteous): How could they misuse public funds like this? I spoke with Rakoff, Lowy, and Hunter. Their advice amounted to the same thing: don't touch this issue, it's not worth it; just wait these people out. Then I spoke with Hollenberg. He provided a clear plan: make the medical staff as a group agree on a definition of what constitutes a full-time staff member. Then, once everyone signs off on this definition, get them to agree on job descriptions for each person, in consultation with me. This would include clear requirements for the "hard money." Then, once a year, review performance based on the job definition, rather than on what people felt like doing.

It was a good idea. When all agree to the process and the job definitions, people who don't like the new circumstance can go to another community hospital, go part time, set up a private office down the street, or continue to work at the hospital, without the hard money. This is exactly what happened. Most people accepted the change, apart from one or two psychiatrists who insisted on

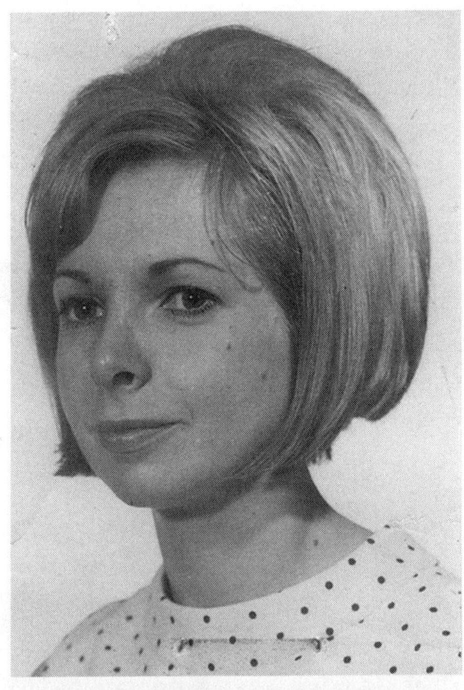

Gail Robinson in the 1970s. She went on to be a professor of psychiatry who has spent her entire career at Toronto General Hospital. She has worked with and written about women who have suffered abuse. In 2013, she received the Order of Ontario for this work. Courtesy CAMH Archives.

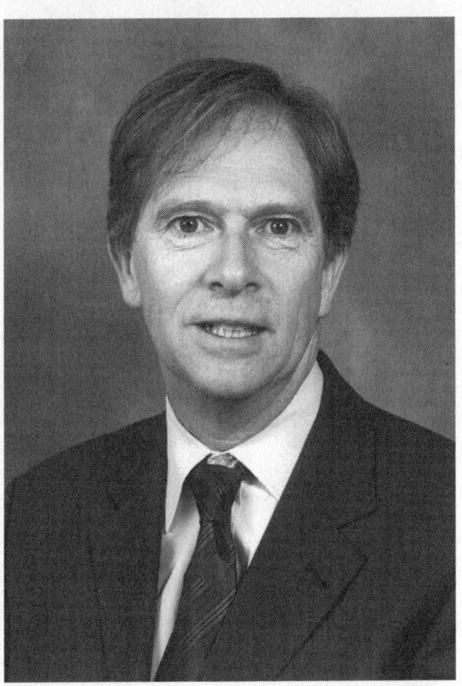

Sid Kennedy studied psychiatry in Newcastle before coming to Canada. He was psychiatrist in chief at Toronto General Hospital from 2000 to 2013, and has developed an international reputation for the pharmacotherapy of mood disorders. Courtesy University of Toronto Department of Psychiatry.

long, protracted discussions. These cases turned out to be useful. When I refused to back down, it was clear that the new financial arrangement was tangible evidence of a new culture.

Gail Robinson proved an important ally in this particular fight. Not only was she a good psychiatrist, mentoring and publishing on an important subject, but she had another critical role as president of Psychiatric Consultants, the partnership that handled all compensation for the Toronto General group. She was the only one sophisticated in financial affairs (often it felt to me that when it came to distributing the "draw" to each partner, she was more like a mother giving the boys their allowance).

In my first year, I was looking after Munro's eight beds, in addition to my administration duties, so I got a first-hand view of the wide range of patients you see in a general hospital. We saw people with deliria—acute confusional states due to drugs, surgery, or illnesses. Others had preexisting psychiatric disorders, or new ones related to the illness, its treatment, or being in hospital. In Toronto General's busy emergency room we saw people in crisis, often with an intent to commit suicide. People with personality disorders wreaked havoc on the wards by pitting staff members against each other, picking up on even the slightest inconsistencies between them.

Life at the General showed me, day after day, how important psychological and social factors are in human disease. A great deal of research, both then and now, confirms this link. After a stroke, depression is common, partly because strokes damage the brain controls for mood. It's common for people with medical illness to think about suicide. Dr. Amytis Towfighi of the University of Southern California found that about 8% of stroke survivors reported such thoughts; 6% of heart attack survivors, 5% of those with diabetes, and 4% of those with cancer contemplated suicide too.

And the reverse is true: mental illness can lead to physical illness. Depression is a significant risk factor for dementia, for example (by some estimates, it increases the risk fourfold).[5] Cynical hostility can be a risk factor for cardiac disease. Psychological stress or loss, and chronic hyperarousal of the autonomic nervous system, can be linked to the onset of disease. Depression significantly increases the risk of having a stroke and dying from it, according to a 2012 study published in *JAMA*. The study showed that depression was associated with a 45% increased risk for stroke and a 55% increased chance of dying.

Mental illness can alter the course of a physical illness. After a heart attack, for example, a major predictor of outcome is whether the patient becomes depressed. Some people do well after a diagnosis of cancer; they often emerge with a sense of mastery and an ability to live more in the moment. But for others, the illness is very difficult and leads to depression and bitterness. There is a 12-fold increase in suicide in the first week after a diagnosis of cancer is made.[6] This is before there is severe pain or side effects to treatments, so suicide at this time relates more to the person's internal state. People who are highly self-sufficient and never want to lean on others fear being vulnerable and dependent; this is the group that has most difficulty after a diagnosis like cancer.

Psychological treatments can be very helpful in dealing with chronic disease. For example, mindfulness (focused attention that can be practised anywhere), meditation (the application of mindfulness in a structured fashion), and yoga can all ease hypertension. Specific psychotherapies in people with advanced cancer improve quality of life, even if they don't extend it. They can help the patients talk about death and dying. It can give them a safe place to process the experience of cancer, reduce the strain of dealing with loved ones, and produce a sense of being seen as a whole person.

The scope of work was far broader than what I had seen at the Clarke. Yet some of the pressures on me, as a practising psychiatrist, were just the same. One memory exemplifies for me just how

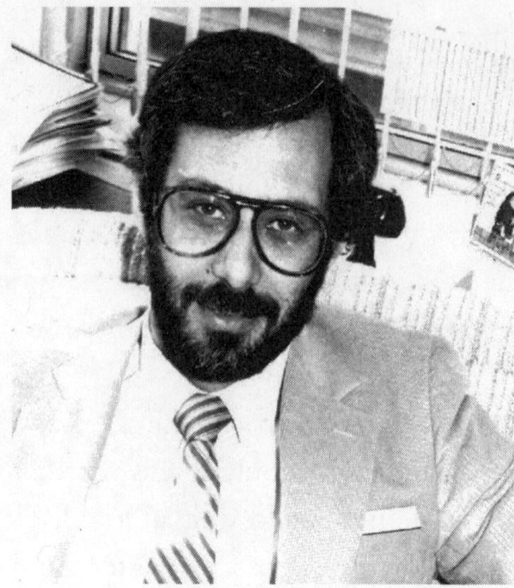

Paul Garfinkel while at Toronto General Hospital (1985).

stretched I was in terms of my responsibilities. On the week I was to give my first public lecture as a full professor, one of my patients reminded me how hard a psychiatrist's life can be. She was in her late 20s, a professional, and had come in with chronic diarrhea, weight loss, and low levels of potassium in her blood. This tall, very thin, attractive woman had been using diuretics and laxatives to keep her weight low, but she insisted she had a terminal malignancy. By this time she had many people running errands for her, keeping her company, and taking care of her every need. On the day I was to give my first professorial lecture, the truth came out. She didn't have cancer after all. She had invented the whole story. Now she wanted to kill herself, so I had to make her an involuntary patient. I finally made it to my lecture, late and harried. But that's real life for a psychiatrist.

Years later, I bumped into this patient at an information desk of a New York hospital. She was friendly and upbeat and told me about her new relationship with a famous actor. I have no idea whether it was true or not.

CHAPTER 10

A Department with Crackle

The General was becoming a terrific place to work or to be a resident. Kennedy took over the nutrition program. Swinson took charge of Mood and Anxiety Disorders, while Robinson handled women's mental health. Rodin headed the program for the medically ill. With all this talent on board, the department's reputation was growing by leaps and bounds, which made recruiting a pleasure. Russell Joffe, a mood disorders expert from St. Michael's Hospital, and Dennis Kussin, a superb generalist and a clinician-teacher, both joined the department.

One of my most important recruits happened by chance. In 1984, when I was in Montreal to give a talk, I met a young psychiatrist, David Goldbloom. He was planning to go to Bethesda, Maryland, to the National Institute of Mental Health and study biological processes in schizophrenia. We hit it off, and he changed his plans to come to Toronto General to work with me on anorexia nervosa and take on eight inpatient beds.

Goldbloom is remarkable by any standard. He is from a prominent medical family. His grandfather Alton was chairman of pediatrics at McGill, and his father, Richard, chair of pediatrics at Dalhousie, is a leading national figure. (David and his father share a childlike delight and sense of humour. When Richard came back from medical conferences, he'd bring gifts such as fake vomit, or a pair of plastic legs to dangle from the piano in the living room.) David's mother, Ruth, a powerful figure within Liberal political and fundraising circles, was responsible for the remarkable historical museum Pier 21, in Halifax. David's older brother, Alan, has been an excellent pediatrician and administrator in both Toronto and Minnesota.

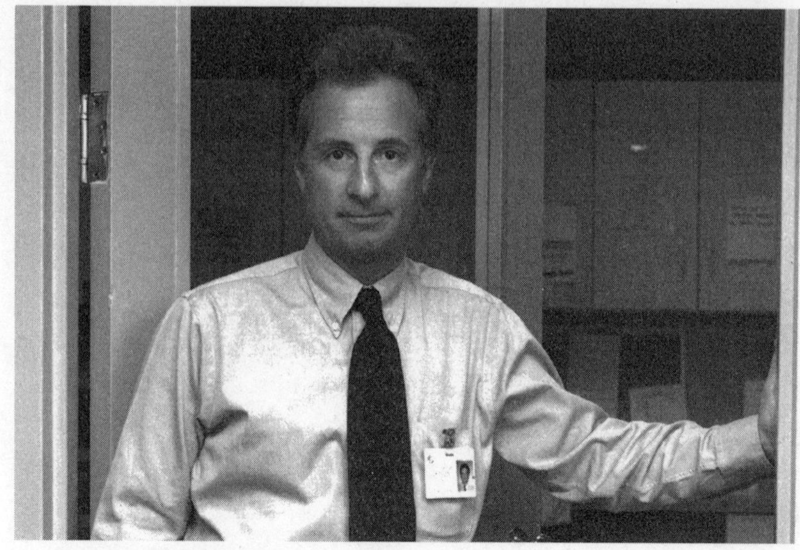

David Goldbloom was born in Montreal and raised in Halifax. He studied government at Harvard, became a Rhodes scholar, and studied physiology at Oxford. After medical and psychiatric training at McGill, he moved to Toronto General Hospital in 1985. He later was chief of staff at the Clarke. When CAMH was formed, he became its inaugural physician in chief. Courtesy CAMH Archives.

David clearly deviated by going into psychiatry, the field of his father-in-law Nate Epstein, the former chair at McMaster University and then at Brown University. (David's wife, Nancy, deviated from the family tradition even further by becoming an ophthalmologist.) Goldbloom was a pleasure to mentor. He is as smart and as quick as anyone. When I'd give him a grant or a journal article to review, his comments were always superb, and infused with humour and elegance.

We attracted research funds; we were actually bringing in as much research money as the Clarke was. I expanded the eating disorders program without taking beds from others (that would have been impossible). I did so by concluding that a day hospital program might be a better and less expensive way to treat these people, and with a lot of help from Stoughton, I made a successful pitch for money to the Ontario government. Allan Kaplan and Niva Piran, an Israeli-born psychologist, developed the program. It has been a gem, one that has won many awards and spawned similar programs around the world.

I was becoming more of a manager. After the first year at Toronto General, I was asked to chair a committee of the board of trustees on in vitro fertilization, a touchy ethical topic then. The committee held a wide spectrum of opinions, from anti-abortion on religious grounds to a free market attitude toward in vitro procedures on demand. I managed to bring them together with a reasoned moderated approach to permit in vitro into the hospital with careful regulation and accountability. Bringing this group together proved valuable in and of itself. It also helped me improve my team-building skills.

At the end of my first year, I became secretary to the Medical Advisory Board's executive. This was a step toward a position as chair, which meant I would be responsible for the group that oversees the self-regulating body of all the physicians, involving standards of care, recruitment, and planning. I would also get to serve on the board. I quickly found that the issues we were dealing with in Psychiatry were not dissimilar to the issues the hospital as a whole was confronting. What should a hospital like the General do in a city like Toronto? HIV was spreading fast. Did the hospital produce the right mix of clinicians to help people cope with a serious and at the time often fatal new illness? How do we account for the impact of every new clinician on other departments and labs? How could we improve the functioning of operating rooms? What about educating undergraduate medical students, who often get overlooked by professors, who would rather deal with super-specialized postgraduates?

Merging with Toronto Western

Late in 1985, Stoughton announced a real opportunity: merging with a neighbouring teaching hospital, Toronto Western, which was facing a significant financial crisis. Merging was an opportunity for us because we could save administrative costs and rationalize clinical services, and then use the extra money saved to provide increased care.

I agreed with him, but we faced a major hurdle: getting buy-in from the staff.[1]

I knew the Western slightly because I had been an intern there 15 years earlier. It was a century-old institution, and filled with doctors who despised the General. They thought we were elitist and arrogant, and that was why they had gone to a friendlier place. Merging with the General was their worst nightmare. The doctors at the General hated the idea too. They complained about how long it would take to go to the Western for rounds. They complained about everything. No one was happy, and one day the Western staff made that perfectly clear: its doctors and nurses wore black arm bands to signify the death of their institution.[2]

The merger was challenging—most mergers are. They suck up energy of creative people on a wide array of troublesome issues, from new telephone systems to committee memberships to the benefits of any savings. And they hurt some people; careers are changed and sometimes wrecked.

One of the trickiest issues was the composition of the powerful board of trustees.[3] We knew how sensitive this issue was, so we decided to start off by including everybody—all 54 original members of the two boards. The first few meetings took place in a lecture theatre, where we all sat in the audience. We eventually pared down the number of members to 28 (10 appointed, 11 elected, and 7 ex-officio). It worked out, as people meant well and Stoughton was a superb leader. The biggest problem was an interpersonal one—an ex-husband and wife, who were now seated around the same board table.

It was harder to handle the choice of who would lead the medical departments. We decided to keep leaders in place until their terms were ending. Then one department head would be chosen. My five-year term at the General ended in 1987, and since I wanted a second term, I had to stand for the position. I was up against my old teacher, Harvey Moldofsky, who led psychiatry at the Western. We had been on cool but civil terms ever since he tried to hire away my colleague David Garner from the Clarke to the Western. Now we were aiming for the same position. Fortunately for me, I got the job. This meant that my time was divided between the two sites for the next couple of years. I spent Tuesdays at the Western, and I really enjoyed the low key and relaxed environment. It was, in fact, a friendlier place than the General.

Eventually, the hospitals came together through the merger, and 25 years later it works beautifully, having added Princess Margaret Hospital (the specialized cancer facility) in the mid-1990s and the Toronto Rehabilitation Institute in 2011. Although the merger initially compromised the identity of the individual hospitals, which affected fundraising and public support, the combined board decided in 1997 to restore the hospitals' individual brands.

As a manager, my connection to scholarship was by 1985 through the fellows. Barbara Dorian was collaborating with Ed Keystone, a rheumatologist and immunologist, to assess the effects of stress on immune function and subsequent illness, and she was set to present her findings at the American Psychosomatic Society in Washington in April. This was one meeting I always attended, and this time I was planning to go with my son Stephen, then almost 10.

A week before the conference, Barbara suffered from a stone in the common bile duct. It turned into septic shock, and she was admitted to the Western in critical condition. There was no way she could present her data in Washington.

When we arrived in Washington, we withdrew Barbara's talk from the program. But over the course of the next two or three days, our colleagues insisted on an informal presentation. When I phoned Barbara, she thought that was a good idea and dictated some of the essential findings, which we put on an acetate roller, which Stephen managed as I spoke. The talk was a big hit—it had an urgency that a more formal talk with slides would have lacked.

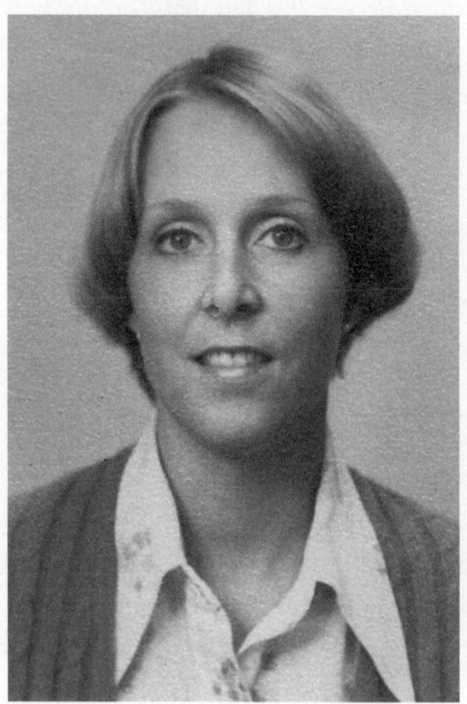

Barbara Dorian was a resident on the psychosomatic medicine unit in 1979. After completing her residency in 1982 (when this photo was taken), she was a fellow at Stanford and then on staff at Toronto General Hospital. Later she was psychiatrist in chief at Women's College Hospital. She developed programs for women who experienced sexual trauma and people who sustained work-related trauma. Courtesy CAMH Archives.

With the conference nearly over, Steve and I went out to do some last-minute shopping. We were in a hurry and jaywalking across one of Georgetown's wide streets when a small pickup truck, driven by an uninsured young driver, hit me. I have no recollection of the event, just of lying dazed in the gutter, my glasses broken, my face and good jacket covered in blood, and frantically looking for Steve. Fortunately, the truck had just skimmed Steve's toes, but he was weeping and being comforted by the police. An ambulance took us to Georgetown University Hospital (as it was then known), where I spent the next week under observation for extensive bleeding around my left kidney, and with a dislocated shoulder and broken fibula.

Stoughton knew the president of the Georgetown hospital and called him; he visited me regularly, and I received excellent care there. The staff were attentive to Steve too. While I was undergoing the diagnostic tests, a nurse sat with Steve in the ER and brought him a cheese sandwich, milk, and Kleenex.

My colleagues Gary Rodin and Jock Cleghorn took good care of Steve too. They even took him to the conference's closing party, and Gary then escorted him home to Toronto the next day. Dorothy waited until he was settled, and then she joined me. I received the best of American medicine; when the itemized $7,000 bill arrived, it included charges for a cheese sandwich, $2; milk, $1; and tissues, $1.

In June 1986, I was invited to be a visiting scholar at the Institute of Psychiatry in London. I took my whole family along. My friend Gerald Russell had become the professor and head of the institute. We stayed in a small but lovely apartment in Knightsbridge. We could walk to most of the sites. But I went in to the Maudsley about three times a week, taking the tube and then a bus, and got into the habit of doing the *Times* daily crossword. Halfway through the visit, we went to Paris for a few days, where we noticed that our son Jonathan was gulping huge amounts of water from every fountain he could find. The night we returned, I called Gerald, had Jonathan's blood sugar tested, and by mid-week had him admitted with insulin-dependent diabetes to the Royal Free Hospital, Gerald's old site. As I took Jonathan to the hospital, he wondered if he could have one last lunch at a Chinese restaurant before beginning what he was sure would be a lifetime of deprivation. I complied with his request, and so when we arrived at the hospital, his blood sugar was sky-high and I was scolded by the charge nurse. I left him there and went across the street to buy cigars, even though I had given up smoking about three years earlier.

Ten days later, for the boys' birthday (they share the same birthdate), we took Jonathan out of hospital for the evening, to a spot that had magician waiters. We tried to make it a decent evening, but none of us felt like a party. The next week we left London, three weeks early, and for our last night, we sat through *Les Miserables*.

Jonathan went to the Hospital for Sick Children in Toronto and began to see an outstanding clinician, Denis Daneman, and a wonderful nurse educator, Marcia Frank. He sounded so mature when at age 13 he returned from an educational session at SickKids and announced, "I'll have to make sure I have an extra starch whenever I have sexual intercourse."

Jonathan adapted well to his condition and its management. Today he is a disciplined man who has found an added sense of self-mastery through the good control of his body and blood sugars.

The next few years were not easy but had much joy. The boys were a handful, and we were busy with all the usual things young families do. Dorothy was devoted to all three boys, and she became extremely attentive to them, almost vigilant, following Jonathan's diagnosis.

When I think of my mourning for my parents in the early part of adulthood, I feel that it had created a curious split inside me. On the one hand, I was aware of loss, death, and finiteness, but on the other hand, I somehow felt that, now that I've experienced my grief, it's someone else's turn. This was, of course, superstitious thinking that was shattered by Jonathan's illness. But I felt that I had to be strong for Dorothy, which in some ways carved a distance between us. It was a prelude to the loneliness I experienced in the following decade.

I knew my time at the General was coming to an end. Rakoff's term as chair of psychiatry and director of the Clarke was ending, and I wanted that job. This would require me to move back to the Clarke. In 1989 I began to make my plans for the transition. It was time, and I was ready. I no longer questioned whether I belonged, or where I belonged. I believed I could do my work well, and that people responded positively to me and to my views. I was much more confident too. I could speak in public, which is critical for a leader. I still had an incredible capacity for hard work. Rakoff used to say I was diligent. I didn't mind spending long hours on planning strategy or helping a fellow on a study. In fact, I enjoyed it. I also enjoyed working with strong people, and I found I could motivate others. Helping someone who is ill is always satisfying, but at the General I learned that building a program or supporting others in the group was equally satisfying. I could convey this to others, and that helped motivate them.

I couldn't foresee that, on the heels of Jonathan's illness, which had been a severe personal trial, I was about to face the biggest crisis of my career.

CHAPTER 11
Crossing the Line

David Garner, the psychologist and head of research in psychiatry at Toronto General Hospital, was my professional partner in the study of anorexia nervosa, and one of my closest collaborators. Over 14 years, we had written books and articles together that would expand the world's understanding of anorexia nervosa. Two important tools, the Eating Attitudes Test and the Eating Disorder Inventory, which measure the psychopathology of anorexia and bulimia nervosa (fears of maturity, dissatisfaction with the body, awareness of inner feelings, and so on), came out of Garner's methodological expertise. Three of the papers we collaborated on, and a fourth, of his, are among the 20 most-cited papers ever written on eating disorders.

We did good work, and it was partly because Garner was a creative risk-taker. He even invented a successful board game, Therapy, which we played together. He didn't rely, as I did, on a steady university salary and billings from a clinical practice; he always managed to get money for his research from foundations and granting bodies. He knew he could get the money if his ideas were good, and they were. I trusted him, both as a researcher and as a human being. We became personal friends. David and his wife, Maureen, even spent a week with Dorothy and me in Dublin when I was there on sabbatical. My three young sons loved his playful manner, especially the way he loved to kid and tease.

In the fall of 1986, not long after we published our second book, this time devoted to the treatment of eating disorders, David came into my office at Toronto General. He said there was a problem: an ex-patient had complained that he had become sexually involved with her. It was all a fabrication, he assured me. This young woman had obviously distorted the nature of their relationship. In any case, he said, the Ontario Board of Examiners in Psychology was going to hold a hearing into the complaint, but there was nothing to worry about. Naturally, I supported him. Not long after, I sat with Garner and his wife at a social event, and Maureen said she thought the whole matter was ridiculous. She couldn't understand why David was so anxious about it. I comforted both of them, and I even agreed to be a character witness at the hearing.

A year later, on November 24, 1987, the day before the hearing, Garner came into my office, this time accompanied by a lawyer we both knew. He looked shaken, weepy, and agitated, in striking contrast to his normally confident, playful manner. "David has something he wants to tell you," the lawyer said.

It turned out that the young woman had produced hotel receipts from New York City that proved she and David had gone there together. It was true, Garner admitted. He had had sex with his patient.

I felt sick. This betrayal of trust—with me and especially with his patient—made me feel nauseated. I was angry with him, but he was so weepy that I felt I needed to protect him; I worried about his safety. I took him for dinner at a comfortable French restaurant just south of the university, but it was an awful night.

At the hearing the next day, the facts emerged. The *Bulletin* of the Ontario Board of Examiners in Psychology described what happened in some detail: Back in 1985, one of Garner's patients was an 18-year-old girl with anorexia and bulimia. On October 4, he "purported to terminate Ms. X's treatment," the *Bulletin* said, "without her knowledge or that of her parents, while she continued to suffer from and needed treatment for anorexia nervosa and bulimia." Eight days later, on October 12, "while she was subject to his continuing professional influence," Garner gave her a job as a mother's helper in his home. Then, between October and

December 1985, at his office and elsewhere in Toronto, Garner had had sexual relations with Ms. X, despite that she still viewed him as her therapist.

When Ms. X complained to the professional body, Garner initially denied "any sexual intimacy" between them. "It was only on the day before the hearing was to commence[,] when new evidence was presented[,] that Dr. Garner admitted to the particulars"—that he had had sex with Ms. X. At the hearing, though, Garner's lawyer said the sexual relations began only after Garner terminated her treatment.

The Ontario Board of Examiners in Psychology rejected that argument. Garner never held a formal session to terminate her care, and the board found that her records suggested she still needed treatment. What's more, Garner's secretary was still scheduling appointments for the young woman.

The board imposed a two-year suspension. "The issue of trust is paramount," it said. "Dr. Garner seriously breached this trust with his young client whom he knew to be dependent on him." This was, according to the tribunal, "unpardonable," especially since Garner for the previous 14 months had denied everything and "implied that the very fragile Ms. X was a liar."

From my point of view, this vulnerable young woman, battling bulimia nervosa, was in a compromised position, while Garner, using all the power and authority of the therapist, took advantage of her at the worst possible time.

That day, without waiting for the board to issue its penalty, I fired Garner from his job as head of research in psychiatry. I spoke with Rakoff, the head of the university's Department of Psychiatry, and he agreed that Garner should lose his position as professor of psychiatry.

Oddly, the university's Psychology Department did not agree. They let him keep his status as professor of psychology, and they even gave him an office for about six months. I don't know why they did not censure him.

I was furious. How could I have missed this? I blamed myself for not knowing, and when the Garner story became public, I felt betrayed and humiliated. When I told my family, I broke down. It was going to be in all the news, and I wanted them to hear first, especially since the kids were wild about David. I broke down again the next week when I spoke with the senior staff at Toronto General. The practical issues—the care of Garner's patients, his graduate students, as well as the granting agencies—were easy enough to handle. But I was filled with sorrow and rage.

The two-year suspension in 1988 was only the beginning of Garner's troubles. Just over a year later, he appeared again before the Ontario Board of Examiners in Psychology. Another patient reported that she had sex with him back in 1979 while under his care. The board revoked his licence to practise in Ontario.

By then, Garner had secured a job at Michigan State University. When the university found out that he had been censured in Ontario, it fired him. Over the next few years, he fought back and a judge reinstated him. That chapter ended in 1993 when the Michigan State tenure committee voted to fire him again. A year later, Garner gained the ability to practise as a psychologist in Ohio after colleagues confirmed that he had changed through therapy. In Ohio, Garner started his own eating disorders clinic, the River Centre Clinic, which seemed to be a real success. His wife, Maureen, by then a psychologist, quit her job at Toledo Hospital to join the clinic.

About 10 years after I learned of Garner's sexual misconduct, he contacted me. We had coedited a popular book on eating disorders in 1985, *Handbook of Psychotherapy for Anorexia Nervosa and Bulimia*, and it was time for a second edition. Did I want to coedit with him? If I didn't, he would go ahead with it, on his own. I felt uneasy about the situation. I didn't want to condone his behaviour, but the book needed updating and it could be enormously useful for practitioners and for the young women suffering from anorexia nervosa. I called Fred Lowy, then the director of the university's Bioethics Centre. He gave the bioethicist's advice: weigh the good of the new book for people in the field against the appearance of condoning Garner's behaviour. I felt that the book would be valuable. Besides, Garner had gone into therapy, and I thought he had matured. I went ahead and coedited the book, which was published in 1997. None of the original contributors withdrew because of Garner's problems, and the book did well. I even have a Japanese version on my shelf.

Over a decade later, in 2008, another patient in Ohio emerged to say she had sexual relations with Garner, from July 2005 to the spring of 2006, while he was her therapist. This was after he had received a five-month suspension for "a sexual boundary violation in his professional practice." This time, the board in Ohio cracked down with a permanent suspension, and the board in Pennsylvania soon followed suit.

The news shook me deeply. By coediting the book, had I offered passive approval of his actions? I questioned and have often regretted my decision.

As a result of these unsettling events, and perhaps as a way to better understand, I launched a study of the problem of sexual abuse in my profession. What I found was disturbing. This type of abuse is not uncommon, and therapists can slide down the slippery slope because of the nature of the therapeutic relationship and the lack of oversight, wilful or not, in the profession. Clearly, this is a serious problem, and one with a long history dating back to the beginning of medicine. One ancient paragraph of the Hippocratic oath makes this clear: "Whatever houses I may visit, I will come for the benefit of the sick, remaining free of all intentional injustice, of all mischief and in particular of sexual relations with both female and male persons, be they free or slaves."

Carl Jung, the Swiss psychiatrist who invented analytical psychology, had an affair with his patient Sabina Spielrein, vividly depicted in David Cronenberg's 2011 movie *A Dangerous Method*. Later he had a long-standing relationship with an ex-patient, Toni Wolff, who went on to become an analytic psychologist. Wolff effectively became Jung's second wife, visiting often for dinners and accompanying Jung and his wife, Emma, on many occasions.

Does the nature of the therapy tempt some people to cross the line? Jung's analytical psychology aims to develop a sense of wholeness by bringing the unconscious to awareness. To do so, the therapist uses symbols, dream analysis, metaphors, art, and religion. Therapist and patient often explore fantasies about sex and death, which may induce some therapists to cross the line and engage in a sexual affair with their patients. But to be fair, Josef Breuer, who worked with Freud on the famous Anna O. case, ran away when that patient aroused sexual feelings in him. Freud described this experience as "countertransference"—the process in which an analyst's emotions are aroused by the patient, based on his earlier experiences. Freud felt that this must be overcome in order for the analyst to do his job properly.

Some of Freud's collaborators were unsuccessful in this regard. One of Freud's disciples and closest collaborators, Sándor Ferenczi, had a sexual liaison with his patient, Elma Pálos. Ferenczi also had an affair with Pálos's mother, Gizella, who too was his patient. Freud intervened, worrying about the effect this could have on all of psychoanalysis. Eventually, Ferenczi married Gizella, and apparently they were happy together.

Freud had his own boundary violation, as described by Alan Stone, the eminent Boston psychoanalyst and authenticated by Professor Peter Gay of Yale, the author of the definitive biography of Freud. Hans Frink had trained in psychiatry at Johns Hopkins and moved to New York, where he began to practise psychoanalysis without any training. This was common at the time. Frink began to have an affair with a wealthy, married woman, but he took time off to go to Vienna for an analysis with Freud. Freud saw an opportunity. Since Frink was not Jewish, Freud thought he would be a suitable head of the New York branch of the American Psychoanalytic Association. After several months of Frink's analysis in Vienna, Freud instructed his patient to bring his lover to a meeting. Here Freud informed her that Frink would likely become homosexual unless she married him. The woman agreed and divorced her husband. Then she married Frink, her analyst. Unfortunately, when Frink subsequently began to display unmistakable symptoms of serious bipolar disorder, the marriage fell apart.[1]

Analytical psychologists and Freudian psychoanalysts are not the only therapists to fall into this problem. Surveys in the United States and Canada from the 1990s reveal that between 6 and 10% of psychiatrists engage in erotic activity with their patients. It is more common among psychiatrists than other medical practitioners—in Ontario, psychiatrists account for 21% of the complaints regarding sexual abuse, while making up only 8% of the province's physicians. Most cases involve a male therapist and a female patient, though approximately 20% involve a same-sex dyad, and in 20% of cases, the therapists are female.[2] About 8% of Ontario women acknowledge sexual harassment or abuse by doctors on surveys.

These figures are shocking because both psychologists and psychiatrists have a duty to care for their patients and to put their patients' needs ahead of their own desires. Physicians are taught early in clinical training to provide care according only to the patient's needs, not their own. They're taught to avoid harming the patient, to respect the individual, and to not exploit the dependency of the patient on the physician, while maintaining privacy and truthfulness. It is explicitly understood that an unequal power relationship exists between doctor and patient resulting from the physician/therapist's specialized knowledge and the patient's need. Trust, integrity, and a commitment to patients' well-being are essential to the provision of safety in the therapeutic environment.

This puts a clear responsibility on the clinician to make the patient feel secure so that healing can occur. The doctor also must clearly define the expectations of both parties, in a way that the treatment process is understood by the patient. These parameters of the doctor-patient relationship—the patient's feeling secure, and knowing that he or she won't be harmed by the clinician, who is there to serve the patient's needs—are at the core of the capacity to treat.

Clearly, having sexual relations with a patient violates this boundary and harms the patient, especially when the physician is in such a powerful position. This rule applies to any physician, from the heart surgeon to the internist, but it's especially important for the psychiatrist because he or she has the power to delve into the deepest, most vulnerable parts of a patient's psyche. People reveal to their therapists their most intimate thoughts, feelings, and fantasies. If the psychiatrist exploits a patient at that deep level, he or she can inflict awful, lifelong damage.

About 90% of patients have serious difficulties after a sexual relationship with their therapist. Even if sexual involvement begins only after termination of therapy, 80% of patients are harmed. This is one reason psychiatrists and psychologists should never have sex with their patients, even after therapy. The problems patients experience include anxiety, depression, flashbacks, a variety of physical symptoms (abdominal and pelvic pain, headaches), eating disorders, suicidal thoughts and attempts, and alcohol or drug abuse. Many patients are no longer able to trust medical practitioners again.

Psychiatrists still cross this line, not only by having sex with patients but in other ways too—by demanding monetary gifts from patients, engaging with patients in business relationships, entering psychotherapeutic relationships that have a dishonest financial premise, exploiting the confidences of patients for the personal and sometimes narcissistic gain of the therapist, soliciting funds for research from patients, and treating one's close colleagues and associates and other dual relationships.

The issue of therapists having sex with their patients wasn't on the radar screen when Garner was working in Toronto, but it flared up in the later 1980s, when a series of papers and books came out that revealed the extent of the hidden problem, the causes, and the reluctance of the profession to confront the issue. These studies and case reports caused the College of Physicians and Surgeons of Ontario to ask a lawyer, Marilou McPhedran, to chair a commission on this topic. Her 1991 report called for zero tolerance: there are no circumstances where such relationships may be permitted, the report said, and although due process must be pursued, erring physicians must be dealt with in the strongest possible manner. Shortly after the report was issued, the number of complaints to the college about abuse by physicians went up dramatically. In the nine months after the report, 149 complaints were sent to the commission, nearly as many as the total number of complaints in the four years from 1987 to 1991.

This suggests that before the report, a great many women were reluctant to complain about their therapists. Why? Some women may have had ambivalent and protective feelings toward their physician. This is an understandable response to the complexity of the therapeutic relationship, particularly the positive, engaging, and often flattering elements in which the therapist may appear to provide longed-for love and acceptance and in return be admired or even idealized. Patients who have been "seduced" by the power of the transference relationship with the therapist frequently become overwhelmed with guilt and shame.

Their self-blame is misplaced, as the therapist is the keeper of the therapeutic relationship and responsible for promoting and permitting any form of boundary crossing. Patients with a history of sexual abuse may be especially vulnerable because the physician may know that these patients have learned to keep secrets and tend to blame themselves when things go wrong. My colleagues at Toronto General, Melanie Carr and Gail Robinson, have described this well: "Women are often programmed to take responsibility for and feel guilty about relationships and their problems. The almost universal expression of guilt and shame expressed by women who have been sexually involved with their therapists is a testament to the power of this conditioning."[3]

Patients may also fear exposure and the possibility of further abuse and humiliation during the investigation and legal proceedings. Sadly, this was how the profession treated patients, especially before the widespread abuse was exposed. This reluctance on the part of patients to lodge formal complaints has been very convenient for deviant health professionals. They've been able to protest that, if there were truth to the rumours, the patient would have complained herself.

What kind of therapists cross the line? In their 1989 paper, S.W. Twemlow and Glen Gabbard identified three types of psychiatrists who become erotically involved with their patients.[4] A small group of them are psychotic. The rest have character disorders, or are what the authors called "lovesick." Typically, the latter group are middle-aged men, socially isolated and emotionally needy, who "fall in love" with women much younger than themselves. One-third of male psychotherapists who became erotically involved with their patients were in the midst of separation or divorce, according to one report. But most therapists even in the same situation restrain themselves. Nearly 9 out of 10 therapists acknowledged that they felt sexually attracted to some of their patients, but they still respected the boundaries. Yet some therapists, a surprising number, not only cross the line but do terrible damage to their patients.[5]

I met Samuel Malcolmson on my first day at the Clarke. He was the chief resident, an attractive, fit man of close to 30. He spoke forcefully about many issues, and I was always interested in his opinions. He had an odd habit of imitating Robin Hunter's gestures, such as the way he put his feet up on the desk, or running his fingers through his wavy hair. We travelled to Baffin Island together twice in the 1970s, as part of the Clarke's physician outreach program. He was a great companion when we were stuck there in a blizzard. We drank Scotch, played cards, and talked. Malcolmson eventually became psychiatrist-in-chief at the Queen Street mental hospital, on the site of the former lunatic asylum. He was an associate professor and always supportive of the university's role in the hospitals. We went so far as to name the lecture theatre at Queen Street in his honour to recognize his hard work there. By the end of the 1990s, he was chief of forensics at the Queen Street hospital. By that time, I was chair of psychiatry for the University of Toronto, and becoming the CEO of four hospitals that were to merge into one body, CAMH, the Centre for Addiction and Mental Health. Malcolmson wanted to be head of forensics for CAMH, and he was enraged with me when I offered the job to another candidate. In 1998, when CAMH was formed, he went into private practice, and two years later, in 2000, a 34-year-old woman struggling on welfare to make ends meet was referred to him. She became his regular patient in July 2001. Soon after, Malcolmson, who was married, induced his patient to have sex in his office and on various trips. She became pregnant and had his baby, a boy, in November 2003. The 71-year-old psychiatrist pleaded no contest to the sexual abuse and "disgraceful, dishonorable or unprofessional conduct." In 2009, the college revoked his licence.

Such outrageous transgressions can begin in a subtle way. Tom Gutheil and Glen Gabbard, prominent American psychiatrists who have written extensively on this issue, have stated that even well-meaning but inattentive physicians can take the first step down the slippery slope with a progressive series of nonsexual boundary violations. In the early stages, most boundary crossings are not sexual and may not constitute malpractice or misconduct; rather, they may reflect poor training, lapses in judgment, or variations in cultural conditioning, Gutheil and Gabbard suggest. They point out that gross examples of misconduct most frequently evolve from minor boundary violations. An early sign for physicians is when they catch themselves saying, "I don't normally do this but"(see people at this hour, or out of the office, or give a hug) with regard to one particular patient. Research in this area was so convincing that R.S. Epstein, R.I. Simon, and G.G. Kay of Georgetown University's Department of Psychiatry developed a test for physicians, the Exploitation Index, to evaluate their level of risk for boundary problems that could lead to serious violations.[6]

I was intrigued by this "slippery slope" phenomenon, but I had a question: Why do some physicians slide down the slope but not others? Perhaps the early boundary violations are a way for some kinds of personalities to test the waters, before progressing toward more significant transgressions. In a paper I cowrote in 1997, I suggested that the problem may not be simply one of inattentiveness or poor education, but rather the breakthrough of impulses rooted, in character traits that may be broadly termed as "narcissistic." This kind of character perceives him- or herself to be special, beyond the rules, and justified in whatever actions he or she takes. The narcissist claims "special things for special people."

Psychiatrists with this type of character function can take advantage of the intimacy of the psychotherapeutic encounter. It opens up dangerous opportunities for therapists who have poor impulse control, exaggerated views of their own specialness, strong needs for interpersonal affirmation, or unacknowledged longings for care, nurturance, and a sense of completion to mitigate an underlying sense of aloneness.

Working in relative isolation and with few external safeguards, some kinds of therapists can exploit the intensity and dependency of the relationship for their own emotional and sexual gratification. Patients in this position are extremely vulnerable. The disturbances that brought them to therapy and the inevitable emergence of historically based, infantile feelings can create a context in which boundary violations can easily occur. Not infrequently, highly sensitive patients involved in exploitative therapeutic situations are entrapped by an unconscious reenactment of a role reversal. They become the caretaker of the therapist and cater to his needs and wishes. In some situations, the therapist's wish to repair himself may include a merger with an idealized object, the patient.

Dr. Alan Parkin was probably the most powerful figure in Canadian psychoanalysis. He was an impressive sight. He had an air of sophistication, silver hair, and wore three-piece suits. He was dignified and formal in his appearance and speech, yet very stiff. But to me he always seemed driven, competitive.

Born in Toronto, Parkin completed his psychoanalytic training in London, England. When he came home in 1954, Toronto was a dead zone as far as psychoanalysis was concerned. Ernest Jones, one of Freud's close collaborators, had spent a few years in the city at the beginning of the century, but any seeds he planted in the city had withered long before. Although psychoanalysis was flourishing in Montreal under Dr. Ewen Cameron, the psychoanalysts hadn't yet migrated to Toronto. In 1956 Parkin moved to fill the void. He created the Toronto Psychoanalytic Study Circle with a core of 11 psychiatrists with an interest in psychoanalysis. He attempted to establish a psychoanalysis training program in the Department of Psychiatry of the University of Toronto. This activity soon was transformed into the Psychotherapy Section of the Ontario Psychiatric Society and, in 1961, the Psychotherapy Section held its first scientific congress.

Parkin later wrote *A History of Psychoanalysis in Canada* and clearly was the leader of the psychoanalytic movement that flourished in Toronto over the next three decades following his return to Canada. He personally analyzed many of the people who would go on to significant careers in this field. He had great sway in the decisions regarding who would be admitted to the role of training analyst. He was an associate professor at the university, but his main impact was as leader of the Toronto Psychoanalytic Society, which developed from the original psychoanalytic study circle. Psychoanalytic societies sprang up in all the larger centres as independent bodies, without the checks and balances of the university. Often they were home to great feuds and rivalries, in part related to people analyzing each other and their spouses.

In 1993 as complaints surfaced about doctors preying sexually on their patients, Parkin was summoned to appear before the College of Physicians and Surgeons of Ontario. The charge: professional misconduct for having engaged in sexual impropriety with four patients. He pleaded guilty. He admitted to having sexual relations with a patient while she was in therapy during 1986 and 1987. Further, he admitted to having sexual relations with a second patient in his office from 1968 to 1970 and for four more years subsequently. Both patients reported irreparable damage to their careers and to other relationships. The allegations with the other two patients were held in abeyance, since Parkin accepted revocation of his licence to practise psychiatry as the penalty.

Parkin's behaviour had been known to members of Toronto's analytic community since the 1950s, but nothing had ever been said or done publicly. Even when the college banned him from practising as a psychiatrist, he was still able to see patients as a clinical psychotherapist. Unfortunately, nothing prevented someone from practising outside the bounds of the profession as a psychotherapist, and psychotherapy hasn't been a self-regulated profession (this is now being corrected).

I had to confront this issue directly when I was chair of psychiatry at the University of Toronto in the early 1990s. We were looking to fill a senior post, and in the search process a female therapist wrote me to describe, in detail, her earlier relationship with a senior psychiatrist, who had been her therapist. That therapist was now being considered for this post. One of his nonphysician patients described a similar transgression. When I spoke with both of them, they refused to bring this forward to the College of Physicians and Surgeons, or to permit me to use their correspondence. I suspect they were afraid of being scapegoats and ostracized in the tight community of psychiatrists and their patients.

The hospital was swimming with innuendo and gossip, and some of the colleagues left the hospital department over the alleged transgressions, and the failure to address them. However, most of this man's colleagues over many years continued to work there and even honoured the man in public events, while complaining about his behaviour in private. It posed a real quandary for me: this psychiatrist, a well-known teacher of psychotherapy, was never able to confront the allegations in a proper hearing, and yet, after listening to the women's stories, I could not endorse him for the senior job. When I tried to talk to him about the situation, he became enraged; I felt more frightened and personally vulnerable then than at any time in my professional career.

Why does the profession not act quickly and forcefully to expose deviant practitioners? To answer the question, we need to appreciate what the charisma of a leader does to a group. Charismatic leadership, at best, can stimulate heroic, selfless, and altruistic acts beyond what rational expectations would support and, as such, is a force for enormous good in human endeavours. But it can also lead to the belief that the leader is not only superior but also above the normal rules that govern ethical or civilized behaviour. Innovative or unconventional actions may then evolve into patterns of conduct that are flagrantly opportunistic and unprincipled.

A charismatic leader can easily induce the people in his department to collude with his behaviour. He can seduce junior colleagues into friendships and collegial relationships by implicitly promising a special bond and a special place in the pantheon of professionals: *I'm special, and if you're with me, you're also special, and together we are a special family or fellowship.*[7]

In a situation like this, followers suspend their judgment of the leader's behaviour, and even when they're confronted by evidence, they're reluctant to face the truth. When they hear about sexual exploitation from a patient in therapy, they might dismiss the patient's account. That's often a mistake. Alan Stone of Boston reported that none of the women who consulted him about a case of erotic involvement with a therapist had fabricated their stories.[8] He describes the preoccupation with false allegations as "the profession's own wish-fulfilling fantasy."

So the followers close ranks around the leader. They may even get a sense of pleasure out of knowing about the forbidden acts. It's as if they're peeking through the keyhole. When other colleagues find out, and when people start to talk about it, in whispers and nervous laughter at meetings, they might feel uneasy or guilty. Yet they're paralyzed by the force of the leader's personality and by the fear of what would happen if they spoke out.

If these cases are ignored by the profession, it damages the students. As the news spreads, they become acutely aware of the double standard. The essence of modern psychotherapy is based on the integrity of the therapeutic relationship, but if the department (the hospital group, university, or analytic institute) does not deal with therapists who cross the line, students will see the hypocrisy—in other words, "Do as I say, not as I do." They will be disillusioned, or believe that they can violate boundaries with impunity also.

It's especially hard on analysts in training because of the deep relationship they have with the leader, who, as analyst, knows their minds as no one else can imagine. The young analyst can easily absorb the leader's attitudes toward breaking boundaries and repeat the same behaviour. But these young analysts run a real risk of permanent exclusion if they break away from the group. Relinquishing the relationship with the powerful leader can produce a devastating sense of loss, grief, and dissolution.

When transgressions can no longer be denied, the tables turn. The charismatic leader often becomes an object of derision, with the same intensity as he or she was previously exalted. This derision is often kept from the leader by his dwindling followers. They may continue to enable and encourage him in excesses and poor judgment with the fantasy that his fall from grace may be dramatic and definitive and will capture public attention in a way that sets him apart from the rest of the group. This stance also allows the disciples to maintain an ambiguous relationship with the leader out of pity and concern and a continued loyalty. As well, they may wish to avoid a true confrontation and the consequent retaliation. Or perhaps they experience a hidden pleasure in the reversal of power and transparency of the disgraced leader's need.

Susan Penfold is a psychiatrist who survived sexual and emotional abuse by her first psychotherapist. In her 1998 book, *Sexual Abuse by Health Professionals*, she argues that there's a "conspiracy of silence" stemming from a variety of issues, such as professional protectionism, a dis-identification with abusers, denial of sexual attraction to patients, rationalization of benefit, victim-blaming, and fears of retaliation by the profession and colleagues for exposing abusive practitioners.[9]

I'm not sure I would use the word "conspiracy." But I've seen professionals band together to protect each other, often because of past loyalties. This loyalty may undermine the sense of professional responsibility and fuel an ambiguous or avoidant stance about the aberrant behaviour. Sometimes the offending physician may behave coercively and force colleagues into an ambivalent collusion. In these instances, you may even hear colleagues say that the possibility of this behaviour must be weighed against the large amount of good the practitioner has done over the course of his or her career.

Health professionals have also tried to justify their transgressions by saying the patient was seductive or gave consent. They've even suggested that psychiatrists are drawn in by seductive borderline patients who provoke sexual acting out. These views have been refuted by data showing that no patient characteristic predicts sexual involvement with a therapist. In fact, as Australian psychiatrist Carolyn Quadrio noted in 1994, many professionals find relationships with patients more rewarding than they do their personal relationships. Quadrio speculated that it is the experience of power and idealization, not the patient, that is seductive to the abusive therapist.[10] The strangest rationalization of all is this: some practitioners think an erotic encounter with them is good for certain patients, by boosting their self-esteem or creating a "corrective emotional experience." To believe this, one would have to discount a large body of literature that documents the enormous harm to patients erotic involvement with a therapist causes. To discount this evidence, one would also have to wonder why the sexual liaison usually occurs between an older male therapist and a young, physically attractive female patient. The same erotic therapy is not offered to middle-aged or elderly women.

In the last two decades, we've seen real progress. Universities have developed educational programs to increase physicians' awareness of the damage done by transgressions. Students and residents learn about the dangers of the slippery slope. Encouraging people to get a second opinion early, when they feel they may be heading for difficulty, is helpful, though the people most likely to use this resource are the least likely to offend. The self-regulating colleges have been serious about examining, disciplining, and publicizing minor and major transgressions, which has both educational and deterrent effects. The zero-tolerance policy has been effective. Most important, the public is more aware of these issues. One side of this problem has not been addressed, however. We have no systematic means of determining which physicians are likely to have trouble with boundaries, or how this should be addressed. We do know that a significant contributor to this behaviour is the view that one is above the rules. A physician who thinks like this can easily slip into dangerous territory, where morality is relative and the rules that exist for everyone else don't apply to him or her.

Our profession must watch out for these types of physician behaviour, especially in academic surroundings where students can model their behaviour on them. Students above all need to respect the boundaries between them and their future patients. They will learn to do so if the teachers they admire practise what they preach.

CHAPTER 12

A Patient Commits Suicide

This is the story of a woman named Debbie, a patient of mine. A kind, sensitive soul, Debbie struggled to overcome anorexia nervosa and then depression. She worked hard to manage her illnesses, and for a few precious years she carved out a life for herself, with a job and nights out at the movies. She even found a sensitive boyfriend to escape the loneliness that had plagued her since childhood. But then the monster that is depression reclaimed her. Debbie ended her life by jumping off a balcony, at age 36.

Her parents and her sister were devastated, and so was I. I had treated Debbie for 17 years, from the time she walked into our anorexia nervosa clinic at the Clarke when she was 19 years old. When Debbie was referred to me by her local community hospital, she was completing her first year at an Ontario university. She was enrolled in a science program and had found it an extremely difficult year. She had to study exceptionally hard to obtain a B average. Toward the end of this first academic year, she began a progressive, restrictive diet, together with increased exercise. Her weight fell dramatically from 110 pounds (she was five foot five) at Christmas to about 72 pounds in the early summer.

Tall, thin, and unnaturally tanned, Debbie was also awkward, shy, and from her first comments, extremely self-critical. She hated feeling full—it was "being gross and bloated," she said. Being fat, she thought, was being lazy, and being lazy wasn't acceptable to someone who was a perfectionist with a strong drive to achieve. Like many young women with this illness, Debbie did not have an accurate picture of her body. At 72 pounds, she saw herself as being *somewhat* thin in her legs, but denied feeling *too* thin in her thighs, stomach, or waist. At 72 pounds, she thought most of her body was a normal size, and she felt comfortable wearing a bathing suit on a public beach. We did body-image testing to get a better idea of how Debbie perceived herself: Debbie saw herself as 18% larger than she was, and even at 70 pounds she wanted to be 7% thinner. "I'm bony but not thin," she said.

We put Debbie on a 1,500-calorie diet, with a gradual increase. We showed her how to do relaxation exercises, and we started a supportive type of psychotherapy, with elements of cognitive behaviour therapy. After four months in hospital, she was discharged at 99 pounds, still below the weight she had set for herself as the magic number: 105 (that is, she had to keep her weight below this number).

In January, Debbie went back to school, but within a few months, her weight dropped to 76 pounds. She came back to the unit about a year after her initial discharge. We put her on a high-calorie diet with modified bedrest to help her regain her weight, but we faced another profound obstacle: anhedonia, essentially a lack of pleasure in life. She enjoyed so little; her life had been only about trying to achieve, rather than about experience. It was sad.

Over three months, Debbie regained almost 30 pounds and her weight was about 110, her set maximum. She said she was comfortable with her new weight, and she got a job as a part-time clerk in a nearby general hospital. When she was discharged, Debbie continued in a daily program at the Clarke and seemed to be doing well. She maintained a steady weight over the next year but didn't yet trust herself. She was worried about losing control.

I learned a lot more about Debbie over the next few years, as we met twice a week, and latterly once a week. In grade six, Debbie said, she had to wear glasses and braces, and start a new school where she didn't have any friends. She felt shy and ugly, especially in comparison with her outgoing younger sister, Ann.

Ann made friends easily, whereas Debbie was a loner. She couldn't make friends, and she didn't participate in extracurricular activities. She never dated boys, nor did she experience any interest in sex. In therapy Debbie started to exhibit a pattern of black and white thinking—if she gained a few pounds, she felt that she'd lose control and be obese. Mostly she was critical of herself: *Did she say the right thing? Why was she angry at her sister, who was kind to her?*

Everything seemed to be so difficult for Debbie. Then things got worse. We learned she had Turner's syndrome, a rare genetic abnormality that would prevent her from having children. At first she believed that the Turner's confirmed everything she had always felt—that she was not really a woman. But with explanation of what Turner's meant for her and her life, and with replacement hormones, she seemed more accepting. She loved children, so after a difficult few months, Debbie agreed to train at a local community college, where she could learn to work with youngsters in daycare. She could earn an income and use this to rent a modest apartment. She tried to make friends, but it was still hard. She didn't drink, hated talking about clothes and boys, and was embarrassed to dance, even though she sometimes tried.

By the early 1990s, Debbie opened up a little. She started dating Bill, a shy, kind man who seemed to enjoy her as a companion and friend. Debbie began to experience real pleasure—she loved the movies and comedy, she enjoyed music, and she started having a life. She even took a course in cognitive behaviour therapy, which helped reduce the long-standing habit of criticizing herself.

Then Debbie's life changed again. First, Ann and her three children, whom Debbie adored, moved out of the city. Then her father, an accountant, was disabled by a stroke. Debbie had always loved him, and when he had trouble speaking, he fell into a depression that affected the entire family, which was extremely painful for Debbie. To make matters worse, Debbie was laid off from the daycare where she worked. This was a major loss, as her connection with young children sustained her emotionally as well as financially.

Debbie felt that her life was unravelling. She was forced to go on a government disability pension, leave her apartment, and move into assisted living in a high-rise. She had never been close to her mother, but now it felt like they were completely estranged because of her mother's attitude to public assistance (or so it seemed to Debbie) and because her father was not the active mediator he had been before. We tried to craft a schedule with structure for her—she volunteered at a pediatric hospital two days a week; did some crafts and yoga, and continued to see Bill. Then Bill said he was leaving the city, and Debbie. He could no longer handle her dependence and her depression. She had become a burden, and he needed to get away.

Devastated, Debbie felt suicidal, so we admitted her for a week. When the acute feelings had passed, we let her return to her apartment. Then the same hopelessness returned. Debbie came back to the hospital for a brief stay, before returning to her apartment. At some point in the next 48 hours, she jumped.

Debbie left a note explaining how painful the year had been. She was sad and guilty to let everyone down, especially her father and Bill. But at least now the pain and worry would end. She was jumping, she wrote, because she wanted to be certain the pain would end.

Debbie's death shocked and deeply saddened me. It was one of the most emotionally devastating moments of my professional life, and I was just not prepared for it. I had worked hard to free her, first from the vice-like grip of anorexia and then from the pit of depression, and we had made real progress together, or so I thought. I felt guilty. *Could I have done more? Had I been distracted?* Debbie's suicide had happened while I was focusing on the creation of CAMH, and I had cut back my practice during this time, but some patients I felt that I had to continue to see, and Debbie was one of them. *Could someone else have done a better job? Could someone else have saved her? Why jump rather than take the medicines she had in her apartment?* The hopelessness and determination to die must have been so awful for her.

As these questions circled in my mind, I noticed my grief was turning to anger, as if I had been betrayed. I had worked so hard for so long, and she had been succeeding. She had carved out a life for herself. I thought she would be okay. Why this?

The hospital did a psychological autopsy and found that the care Debbie received was appropriate. I had tried a variety of the newer antidepressants, saw her regularly, engaged the family, and attempted many rehabilitation techniques. At one point I asked for, and received, a second opinion regarding Debbie's depression. Debbie's parents were tremendously saddened but grateful for all we had done, and I attended the funeral, albeit awkwardly. I told myself not to feel defensive. I could learn from this, but that didn't make it right. I didn't recover for a very long while.

I tell this story because it is a not uncommon experience for psychiatrists. Although suicide is a relatively rare event, half of all psychiatrists will endure the suicide of a patient sometime during their career. It is not surprising: we're dealing with patients who have depression and schizophrenia and other serious mental illnesses that vastly heighten the risk of suicide. Even as psychiatrists we are not prepared for its impact. We are not prepared as human beings, in part because of our religious and cultural attitudes to suicide, and in part because medical schools and professional associations have not adequately tackled this sensitive topic. Hospitals are now conducting psychological audits, such as the one conducted after Debbie's death, to find out what happened and how such deaths might be prevented in the future. Supervisors are trying hard to connect with their residents about this topic, but we need to do far more, both for ourselves and for our patients and their families.

Many more people die of suicide than in wars. For example, in 2000 over 800,000 people committed suicide, versus just over 300,000 who died as a direct result of armed conflict.[1] In Canada, 4,000 people die of suicide each year, and 400 of these are youth. Suicide is the second leading cause of death for Canadians between the ages of 10 and 24, and the fourth leading cause of death for Canadians between the ages of 15 and 44.

In Canada the suicide rate has followed the pattern of most Western countries. It climbed in the 1960s and 1970s, peaked in 1978 at 14.8 suicides per 100,000, and then fell. The current suicide rate is between 11.0 and 12.5 per 100,000, with males closer to 20 and females at 5 to 6. Some populations are at much higher risk. Native Canadians living in northern Canada die of suicide five times more often than Canadians in the rest of the country. Inmates in correctional facilities and the elderly run a higher risk of killing themselves too, along with people who abuse drugs or live with a mental illness such as schizophrenia or depression. Mental illness is involved in 90% of suicides. For people with schizophrenia, for example, the risk for suicide is 20 times higher than it is for the general population. Not all people who kill themselves are mentally ill, though. Some people end their lives to withdraw from extreme pain or dependency. Social factors like unemployment, poverty, and social isolation also increase the rate of suicide. Recently, the Centers for Disease Control and Prevention has found that the suicide rates jumped in the United States from 1999 to 2010: the suicide rate among Americans ages 35 to 64 rose by nearly 30%, to 17.6 deaths per 100,000, up from 13.7. The most pronounced increases were seen among men in their 50s, a group in which suicide rates rose by nearly 50%, to about 30 per 100,000. For women, the largest increase was seen in those ages 60 to 64, among whom rates increased by nearly 60%, to 7 per 100,000.[2] These changes are thought to be related to the financial crisis of

2008. It has been suggested that falling community supports no longer protect people in a crisis and also play a role.

Before these events, the rate of suicide had fallen marginally. Whether the antidepressants have helped is a controversial issue: they may help some people climb out of depression, but they can also predispose children and young adults under 25 to suicide.[3] Recent data questions this latter conclusion: higher rates in youth may be more related to not receiving treatment than to taking antidepressants.

Nonetheless, suicide is still a very real problem for psychiatrists who have to deal with people who are at risk because of mental illness. We know this when we go into the field, and yet when we lose a patient, it is difficult to bear. Maybe this is because of the intimate relationship we have with our patients, or it could reflect the universal need to deny the possibility of death. Or perhaps the suicide of a patient stirs a deep sense of failure in the psychiatrist, as it did for me when Debbie died.

When I was a student, medical school did nothing to prepare future psychiatrists for the impact of patient suicide. We were taught how to assess suicide risk. We learned the individual risk factors (male, older, alone, white, a medical condition, no religion), and we were told to watch out for a plan and any previous attempts. We learned that a suicide in the family greatly increases risk, as does a physical illness or history of trauma. We learned that loss or a drop in self-esteem can precipitate a suicide, and we learned about the related factors, such as the presence of substance abuse. We were taught to ask whether the patient had the means to carry out the plan, such as having a gun in the house or a large supply of medicines. We took seminars on the Mental Health Act, so that we could understand what our responsibilities were to patients in danger and the limits of those responsibilities. We were also taught to be prudent: if in doubt, admit the person to a safe hospital bed.

In Toronto I would soon learn, though, that people with some forms of personality disorder, even though chronically suicidal, are often better treated out of hospital if at all possible.

We also learned about the impact of suicide on family members, and its historical significance, its epidemiology, and the psychodynamic theories. Suicide could represent rage turned against the self, or a hoped-for revenge, or a fantasy of reunification with a lost person. But we didn't learn much, if anything, about the impact of a suicide on the doctor.

In my third year of residency, when I was chief resident at the Clarke, Harvey Stancer, the head of the Clinical Investigation Unit, assigned a wonderful man, George Awad, to work on the fifth floor as his new resident. Awad had graduated in medicine from his native Cairo University and then moved to Russia, where he obtained a PhD in endocrinology. He and his Russian-born engineer wife, Lara, moved to work with a prominent pharmacologist, Ed Sellers Sr., at the Addiction Research Foundation. Two years later, as a man of 36—a bit older than most residents—Awad enrolled in psychiatry at the University of Toronto and was assigned to work with Stancer. The Clinical Investigation Unit was where patients with severe mood disorders who had generally been unresponsive to the usual treatments could be assessed, and hopefully helped with new treatments.

At the end of the first week, one of Awad's patients, a woman from a small town an hour from Toronto, hung herself. Awad, a sensitive and thoughtful man with good clinical judgment, felt guilty about the death, and he worried he would be blamed in formal processes. He was ashamed that, as an immigrant, he stood out in this unique way. He worried it was a reflection of his competence and esteem in the professional community. He felt that he should quit the program. Stancer explained that suicide could happen because they were dealing with the most severely depressed and most treatment-resistant patients in the province. I tried to offer support, both as a concerned colleague and as chief resident. The institute conducted an audit of the clinical care, which concluded that the woman had been at high risk and treatment-resistant, and that the care was at a standard to be expected. Both Stancer and Awad met with the families on several occasions. Awad settled down over the next few months and stayed in the residency program, which was fortunate for all of us because he embarked on a stellar career in both academic and later community psychiatry.

Awad's story shows just how deep the impact of suicide can be on the psychiatrist, and how poorly prepared for the significant impact of suicide, even though a significant percentage of psychiatrists will face their first suicide during their training period, when they're least able to handle it. This disturbing fact emerged from a study led by Ron Ruskin of 495 graduates and trainees of the residency program of the University of Toronto from 1980 to 1995.[4]

About one-third of respondents in Ruskin's survey experienced at least one patient suicide during their training program, a figure typical of studies reported on this subject. This number may even be an underestimate. A study of third- and fourth-year residents in the United States found that 60% had a patient commit suicide, though they had been unaware of it—the death notices had been published in the *Los Angeles County Medical Examiner*.

In the Toronto study, half of those residents who experienced patient suicide did so during their first postgraduate year. This is not surprising given the tradition of having psychiatric residents begin their training in inpatient units, where they are dealing with the sickest and most high-risk patients. Biologically oriented psychiatrists had a higher rate of suicide among their patients, which is also not so surprising given that their patients are suffering severe illnesses and psychoses. Even worse is that these young psychiatrists might have to deal with multiple suicides. Of those psychiatrists who lost patients to suicide, 20% had two to five patients who died by suicide.

The emotional impact is severe. Most of the young psychiatrists experienced a devastating emotional impact on first learning of the suicide. For 33%, the emotional turmoil lasted up to one month. For 7%, the disturbance lasted longer than three months. For many, it can be an isolated, lonely time. Some doctors feel they can no longer treat potentially suicidal patients. I have heard some psychiatrists describe an identification with the dead patient in their dreams; one spoke of how, for her, identification manifested in being accident-prone for some weeks after the death.

Many of the young psychiatrists said the suicide had a profound and enduring effect on them as individuals and as physicians. They experienced frequent and powerful feelings of fear related to their clinical practice, often feeling helpless, and with recurring images and feelings of horror. To get a better picture of the emotional impact, Ruskin asked respondents to fill out a questionnaire, the Impact of Events Scale. The results were striking: 20% of the psychiatrists who had a patient commit suicide met the clinical criteria for posttraumatic stress disorder.

For beginning therapists, the sense of shock is intense. Wayne Fenton, a psychiatrist at the National Institute of Mental Health, treated a young schizophrenic patient in his first year of residency. The patient had started taking the antipsychotic drug clozapine, an experimental treatment at that time, and he seemed to improve remarkably. When Fenton met with him late on a Friday afternoon, they spent the session discussing the future, including the possibility that the young man could return to college. At seven thirty that evening, the hospital called to say his patient had not arrived at the outpatient program, where he was supposed to spend the evening. A few hours later, there was another call:

the police had found a body and wanted to show Fenton photographs to identify it.

"This suicide was unexpected by everyone," Fenton said. "Particularly insofar as there was a feeling that here was a patient who was really improving tremendously." For years after the death, Fenton indicated that he became anxious every time the telephone rang at night, with "the feeling of your heart going into your throat, when you're afraid it's the worst."[5]

Experiencing a patient's suicide is worse for the doctor in training than it is for a psychiatrist later in his or her career, but the impact on a seasoned psychiatrist is nevertheless profound. In a large national survey of randomly selected psychiatrists over two decades ago, Claude Chemtob and his colleagues found that one-half of the psychiatrists who had experienced the suicide of a patient suffered from traumatic stress symptoms in the weeks following the event.[6] The psychiatrists, in other words, showed the same symptoms as anyone else seeking therapy after a major loss, such as a parent's premature death. Although the symptoms declined over time such that most psychiatrists were not affected at the clinical level six months after the suicide, all reported an ongoing negative impact on their professional and personal lives.

We always remember the patients we lose. "It was a nurse whom I had been seeing in intensive psychotherapy," one psychiatrist reported in a 1999 study I did with colleagues. "It was at the beginning of my career, and she was a very, very disturbed woman, and I admitted her to the hospital because I sensed that she was suicidal. In the middle of the night she got it into her head that she wanted to leave, and because she was not certified, she was able to go. She signed out. She left at four in the morning and went to a pharmacy and got insulin and injected herself. She changed her mind and came into emergency, but they couldn't reverse the effects of the overdose. She died in her late 20s. I learned a critical lesson from this: I had brought her over to the Inpatient Unit and had turned her over to its care; because I was only an outpatient psychiatrist, my formal contact ends once I hand the patient over. But I could have said, 'I'll pop in to see you tomorrow' or 'I'll keep in touch with you,' and I didn't. I often wondered if I had made that explicit, would it have made a difference? But I think she felt abandoned. It tortured me for months."

Even for the most seasoned psychiatrist, the suicide of a patient can have long-lasting emotional impact. Herbert Hendin, the former medical director of the American Foundation for Suicide Prevention, led a study based on in-depth interviews with psychiatrists, psychologists, and social workers. He found that over half of the therapists were shocked to learn of their patient's suicide; some didn't realize their patient was in a suicidal crisis. Others were aware but, like combat soldiers, didn't believe that it could happen to them. Some 70% of the respondents grieved, several for a very long time. In one case, the therapist and a cotherapist visited the patient's parents in a distant city three years after the suicide. Talking with the parents and visiting the patient's grave helped both therapists achieve some degree of closure with respect to the impact and meaning of the event, which until then had remained unresolved.[7]

After suicide, many of the therapists felt guilty. Hendin described one who wrote that her office was flooded by melting snow leaking through the roof the day after her patient's funeral, forcing cancellation of her treatment sessions. She imagined that the flood was punishment for her failure to prevent the suicide, the water representing the tears of the grieving relatives she had met at the funeral.

Many of the therapists said they were angry after their patient died. They felt that they had been rejected or even betrayed. "I felt angry at her rejection and destruction of the work we had done together," one therapist wrote. "I felt betrayed that she had done something so lethal without giving me forewarning." These therapists had made suicide contracts (agreements about the steps the patient should take to prevent acting on suicidal impulses) with their patients, as did one-third of all the therapists who lost their patients. Although none of the therapists gave up on these contracts, they felt less confident about their usefulness.

Suicide can shatter self-confidence in many therapists. Many of the therapists in Hendin's study were gripped by self-doubt, felt inadequate, or both. Seasoned therapists assumed that their years of professional experience would protect them from fear and self-doubt, and they were shaken to find that it did not. Therapists in training questioned their ability to help anyone or even whether they were suited to their profession. As one put it, "It scared me, terrified me, and left me doubting everything I did."

"I had a series of 'examination dreams,'" one therapist reported to Hendin. "In these, I was striving to overcome obstacles to my arrival at, or competence in, college or internship duties. I was recurrently getting lost in a series of Kafkaesque corridors, stairways, or meandering trains, hopelessly late, woefully unprepared, or—in one dream—only partly clothed."

Some therapists feel ashamed when a patient dies by suicide. One therapist in the study, whose patient was hospitalized shortly before her suicide, was ashamed of his response when the patient discontinued her therapy after discharge. He felt that he had not made sufficient efforts to persuade her to continue therapy, or to recontact her. After the patient's death, shame and fear for his professional reputation led him to neglect reporting her suicide to the hospital.[8]

Michael Gitlin offered a classic case in his 1999 study: "Along with numbed feelings, Dr. G began to feel an overwhelming sense of shame and embarrassment. While objectively knowing it was not true, Dr. G felt as if he stood out as the only psychiatrist among his colleagues and friends who had ever had a patient commit suicide."[9]

The suicide of a patient in active treatment is sometimes taken as prima facie evidence that the therapist mismanaged the case. Many therapists are afraid of being blamed, particularly for not hospitalizing the patient, and most are afraid of being sued by the patient's family. However, psychiatrists may be surprised by the family's reaction. In the Toronto study, over half of the respondents contacted bereaved families; in Hendin's study, just over three-quarters of the therapists saw their patients' relatives after the suicides, either at their own or the relatives' initiative. With discomfort, some attended patients' funerals. Most of these contacts with relatives were made with some trepidation and the expectation of anger and criticism. In almost all cases, however, the relatives did not criticize the therapist and instead expressed gratitude for the help their family member had received. In the Toronto study, therapists faced lawsuits in only 9% of suicides.

For most therapists, having a patient commit suicide is "the most traumatic event of their professional lives," Hendin said. "It is troublesome how long the difficulty stays with people." There doesn't seem to be the kind of working through you would imagine in a professional situation.

I think psychiatrists have a harder time dealing with the death of a patient than other specialists, like cardiologists or oncologists, when the death is by suicide. Skilled therapists tend to develop intense, close relationships with their patients. They care deeply about their progress and survival. A therapist may take it upon himself or herself to act as the saviour of a particular patient. This can set the therapist up for a devastating personal loss should the patient choose death over life.

The therapist's attitude toward death can also affect his or her response to a patient's suicide. Like many of us, some psychiatrists suffer from anxiety or even dread about death, leading to avoidance of the discussion. This can hinder therapy because if you are frightened about your own mortality and have never come to terms with it, you will be impaired in your ability to deal with a patient who is contemplating suicide—and to deal with the suicide if it happens. One might presume that psychiatrists are better able to deal with these issues than others, but it is clear that psychiatrists display a whole gamut of abilities in this area and, in fact, the opposite might be true.

One key issue that psychiatrists have to grapple with is the role and the responsibility of the clinician. To what extent do we need to protect our patients from their suicidal impulses? This issue has been debated throughout my career. In 1972 there was a famous debate in San Francisco on the ethics of suicide prevention between the pioneering suicidologist Edwin Shneidman and the iconoclastic psychiatrist Thomas Szasz. Shneidman argued that doctors should have a sense of responsibility for suicidal patients because those patients who talk about suicide are, by definition, ambivalent, and suicidal ideation is usually a symptom of a treatable frame of mind. Szasz countered by arguing that suicide is a civil right. He said that the therapist-patient relationship should be one of equals. If the therapist meddles in the patient's personal liberty, it represents an inappropriate interference. Patients, in other words, have a right to end their own lives, and doctors have to respect that right. Most therapists today would reject Szasz's extreme view. I don't agree with him either. We all have the right to make choices about our lives, but to make a true choice, you need to have intact judgment, and if illness impairs that judgment with a sense of despair and hopelessness, the patient is in no position to make a choice about ending his or her life.

This is fine in theory, but in everyday practice, handling a patient who might be suicidal involves agonizing decisions. Do we admit the patient to hospital for their protection or not? For a therapist, it's not a straightforward decision to make.

In Ontario, we have the right to detain a patient in hospital for 72 hours if we think the patient is in imminent danger of death. A doctor in the hospital can renew that 72-hour order for up to two weeks, and this can again be renewed for longer periods until the patient is out of danger. One might think that we should detain the patient if we feel any doubt about the potential for suicide, but it's not that simple. If we keep detaining the patient against his or her will, how will this impact the patient's trust of further treatment? If the patient spends a lot of time in hospital, what kinds of problems will that cause? If we're trying to get the patient to live a more independent life, how will a constricted life in hospital help? We see many people who contemplate suicide without ever forming a plan. We also see many people who do develop plans to die but either we intervene or they improve before they act. So do you admit? Or not?

The hospital route can be counterproductive. I recently consulted to a hospital in another country that had just experienced three patient suicides over two years. The hospital had responded by keeping patients there for longer than necessary, harming both patients who could have been treated at home and those waiting on admission.

But sometimes we have no choice—we just have to admit the patient to protect his or her life. These decisions are tough, however, and psychiatrists feel a heavy burden in making them.

Psychiatrists reflect our culture and its attitudes toward suicide, and in our culture, suicide ruptures a deep taboo. When someone dies of an accident or a natural cause, many people console themselves with the idea that it was meant to be. When someone commits suicide, the assumption may be different; in this case, a wicked act has destroyed our sense of order, and someone must be blamed. In 18th-century England, suicide victims were tried posthumously in a coroner's court to determine whether the victim had been insane and, therefore, innocent (*non compos mentis*)—or not. If they were deemed to be sane, the suicide victims were guilty of a crime and subject to forfeiture of property to the Crown and to desecration of the body. These attitudes lasted a long time. Suicide was not decriminalized in Canada until 1972, and I still remember a harrowing scene when I was an intern at Toronto Western. A young woman had survived a suicide attempt and instead of getting sympathy or concern from the resident, she got a lecture. "You're lucky I don't report you!" the resident said.

In the last 30 years, our profession has improved the teaching on the topic of suicide, as well as on what to do to help both the family and the psychiatrist in the aftermath. Now when suicide occurs in a hospital setting, the hospital will routinely conduct psychological audits—such as the one conducted after my patient Debbie's death—to find out what happened and how to prevent such tragedies in the future. Doctors can now talk about the case to patient care committees without fear of being subpoenaed in a lawsuit.

But this process is only for suicides in hospital; it doesn't cover suicides in private practice. These psychiatrists are all alone when one of their patients commits suicide, and that's unfortunate—for them and for our understanding of suicide. Audits need to spread to private practice so that we can learn more about why suicides happen and how they might be prevented. Reviews should not be designed as a trial to potentially blame the psychiatrist, but rather as a key learning opportunity. They ought to be driven by a critical, enquiring approach and need to start at the beginning: What was wrong? What was the personality structure that made the patient sensitive to what went wrong? What about the family history and friends—was suicide considered a reasonable option? What were the factors that sustained the illness? What treatment helped, or didn't? These questions and more should be posed in an autopsy to investigate why the patient died. This should be the focus of the enquiry, not the question of whether the psychiatrist was to blame. We need to do far more—for therapists, for their patients, and their patients' families.

We need to reach out more to psychiatrists, to help them deal with the emotional fallout of a suicide under their watch. In Ruskin's study in Toronto, 70% of young psychiatrists said that they "pretty much kept to themselves" after the suicide. One-quarter couldn't bring themselves to ask for help, even though they knew where to find it. The psychiatrists said it helped when colleagues and supervisors shared their own experiences of suicide, but they didn't appreciate the reassurances that the death was inevitable or even that the treatment had been a success. Nearly all therapists felt these assurances to be empty gestures.

It was the residents at the University of Toronto who asked the Psychiatry Department to add lectures on what to do after a suicide. Not surprisingly, the lecture focuses on how to deal with the intense feelings that suicide provokes in the young doctors. This kind of course is helpful, and I hope it will spread to other universities and to private practice. Psychiatrists everywhere need to find ways to work through their feelings after a suicide.

Suicides, sadly, are all too common in the patients we treat, and we need to act forcefully to prevent future suicides and to treat the people who are left behind. Psychological autopsies can help, so our professional bodies should make sure they happen in the private practice sector. If psychological autopsies are embedded in a process of learning, they can relieve guilt and self-doubt and help the therapist deal with the isolation that so many suffer after a suicide.

CHAPTER 13

Burdens and Satisfactions

The therapeutic relationship ventures often into intimate and hidden territory: the secret life of fantasy, dreams and their meaning, thoughts about sex and death, painful memories from childhood and life's most embarrassing moments. For the success of this therapy, the makeup of the psychiatrist is key. The doctor's personality is fundamental to success or failure. The treatment may include medication or changing the patient's environment but usually requires the patient to develop a new understanding of his condition and, often, of himself and his life circumstances. This can happen only through a trusting relationship between psychiatrist and patient.

There has been a lot of research on characteristics of the therapist that may bring about therapeutic change, independent of the therapist's specific techniques. The personality of the therapist, as well as his or her interest in helping the patient, have been found to be regularly and positively associated with therapy outcome.[1] These attributes permit the development of a working alliance with the patient. Therapists who are flexible, respectful, trustworthy, and interested are more effective than those who are not, regardless of the style of therapy. Most of all, therapists must be engaged with their patients and invested in the outcome of treatment. One person I know was lying on the analytic couch and saw a reflection of her therapist in a new brass plant stand. He was reading the *Globe and Mail.*

The personality of the psychiatrist may even be more relevant than the type of therapy offered. Hans Strupp, an influential figure in the psychotherapy field, conducted a famous study that compared experienced therapists with university lecturers who were not trained therapists but could form understanding relationships.[2] Each group treated about 15 patients with mild depressions or anxiety disorders. The professors were as effective overall as the therapists. An earlier study showed that experienced, highly regarded therapists from different schools of thought were actually quite similar and less doctrinaire than less experienced and more rigid therapists.[3]

However, the very characteristics that might define a positive therapeutic outcome—attentiveness, sensitivity, psychological insight—are not necessarily indicative of the psychiatrist's own mental health. In fact, the attributes that make for a good psychiatrist can also make for one who is vulnerable to emotional problems, including burnout and depression. The psychiatrist who is sensitive, who can empathize with the patient and feel the patient's pain can also be the type who invests so heavily in troubled patients that the burden may be difficult to bear and he or she may fall into depression, an anxiety disorder, substance abuse, divorce, or even suicide.

We need to do more to protect both our psychiatrists and our patients from this problem. We can improve our selection processes for psychiatrists, and we can educate them to look for signs of burnout or impairment. We can also ensure they receive appropriate help when they require it. And we can increase public awareness of the standards of good clinical care. But first, we need a better understanding of the mental health of psychiatrists.

Psychiatrists, the studies tell us, tend to be excessively negative or neurotic. We are sensitive by nature, eager to please, and not as likely as other doctors to be self-disciplined and oriented toward achievement. We also have more flexible, easily influenced intellectual interests than do our peers.

And most of us, at least in Ontario, find our jobs highly satisfying. In the late 1990s, we wanted to find out how psychiatrists in Ontario were doing, so Mike Bagby, Christine Dunbar, Barbara

Dorian, and I launched a survey. Our survey went out to all 1,574 Ontario psychiatrists, and over 800 responded. One of the aims of the survey was to assess how successful (defined along several dimensions) the province's psychiatrists felt. If they felt successful, we thought, they would probably be in a better position to help patients than were psychiatrists were who unhappy and regretful about their choice of career.

The results were reassuring.[4] It turned out that about 90% of the psychiatrists were satisfied overall with their careers. Psychiatrists experience tremendous satisfaction in caring for others. They value psychotherapy and the expanded range of treatments currently available—from evidence-based psychotherapies to newly developed medications that offer a greater probability of success. To possess the ability and perseverance that one needs to treat patients in serious emotional distress is for many psychiatrists a reward all by itself.

Ontario psychiatrists are far more satisfied than are psychiatrists in the United States, where over 20% are dissatisfied with their careers.[5] I think there are clear reasons why. In Ontario, psychotherapy is funded by the government, so Ontario psychiatrists are able to use it routinely to help their patients. In the United States, psychiatrists are increasingly trained as diagnosticians and psychopharmacologists. They can end up missing the personal human connection with their patients. Moreover, the ongoing reimbursement battles with insurance companies make US psychiatry more onerous.[6] Differences in rates of litigation also likely contribute.

It's revealing that psychiatrists in Canada were more satisfied with their jobs than surgeons were, according to a 2006 study from Western Canada.[7] Surgeons often complain about the difficulty getting time in the operating room. They have to deal with physical exhaustion, and they often face conflicts between their professional and personal lives. Psychiatrists, although generally satisfied with their jobs, nevertheless have to deal with the demands of distressed patients, and the emotional exhaustion that can cause for them. Surgeons can achieve almost instant results if the surgery is successful, with the appreciation that ensues from patients and others. Psychiatrists see progress slowly. The steps may be tiny from month to month. When progress occurs, it's confidential. You're not likely to hear a patient say, "Dr. X helped me get over my depression, or helped me to live with my schizophrenia. She's the best!"

Although our survey showed that most Ontario psychiatrists were satisfied, we found important clues about the conditions that might lead a professional into emotional trouble when we looked at 70 psychiatrists who were not satisfied. They represented 9% of the total. Four factors were reliable predictors: the perceived intrinsic value of psychiatric care, the degree of perceived emotional burden, the perception of financial success, and one's satisfaction derived from psychotherapeutic work.

Nearly all psychiatrists believed in the intrinsic value of psychiatry. Presumably, people who enter medicine and any of the helping professions have a strong desire to care for and offer treatment to others; 2% in our survey did not value psychiatric care—a terrible sign for these people and especially for their patients in a clinical practice. One-quarter of our sample, mostly men and young women, were struggling with the emotional burden from patients. They did say, though, that family and friends and the psychiatrist's financial compensation helped them deal with the emotional burden.

Of Ontario psychiatrists, 9% actually regretted becoming a psychiatrist. Most of them were men who were isolated in private offices, far from the creative juice of the research- and teaching-oriented hospitals, where they might have had an intellectual outlet and contact with colleagues. Working alone, it was harder for them to reach out to colleagues when they were confronted with difficult emotions that arise in the clinical psychotherapeutic endeavour. This group also complained of a lack of respect from other medical specialists.[8]

Still, psychiatrists are overwhelmingly content with their career choice. There may be several reasons for this. It is widely believed some people enter the mental health field because they have a history of psychological difficulties and are trying to understand or overcome their own problems. Another large group display compassion for people who are suffering; for some, their having grown up with a person with mental illness may push them toward a desire to help or even to rescue. Some people enter medical school with an interest in the whole person, or in the person in the context of his or her world. These students have long been a source of psychiatric residents (but many now go into family medicine). These days there is another group selecting the field: many are motivated by a desire to understand the workings of the brain. A recent Australian survey noted the most common reasons for choosing a career in psychiatry were an interest in psychological issues and the promise of intellectual stimulation.

There is, however, a dark side. A number of psychiatrists suffer terrible emotional consequences. Physicians commit suicide more often than people in general do—it's one of the leading causes of potential life lost, according to Daniel E. Ford, a professor at Johns Hopkins University School of Medicine.[9] The suicide rate among psychiatrists is even higher.[10] The American Psychiatric Association's Task Force on Suicide Prevention study concluded in 1980 that "psychiatrists commit suicide at rates about twice those expected [of physicians]." It also found that "the occurrence of suicides by psychiatrists is quite constant year-to-year, indicating a relatively stable over-supply of depressed psychiatrists."[11] No other medical specialty yielded such a high suicide rate. Ford's team also found that psychiatrists had the highest risk of all physicians of dying from suicide. But a recent review of all suicide deaths by doctors in the United Kingdom showed four groups with high rates: community health, anesthesia, psychiatry, and general practice.[12]

Too many doctors do not seek treatment. This might surprise you; after all, doctors live in a world surrounded by health care professionals. Surely they would have no problem finding the medical help they need. And yet they often don't seek it out. Doctors with suicidal thoughts are less likely to consult someone than is a member of the general public. Why don't these doctors ask for help in a world full of doctors? They may find it hard to reach out when they're feeling less than adequate. Sometimes they treat themselves instead, especially if they believe the consequences of seeking treatment might subject them to shame, or worse. They may have a reason to be wary. This is a difficult area: physicians who are depressed and report this to their licensing boards or hospitals have experienced consequences. These have included increased supervision, licensure and practice restrictions, discriminatory employment decisions, and hospital privilege limitations. These consequences are often appropriate but perhaps less so, for example, if the doctor is responding well to treatment.

As perfectionists, doctors can magnify an error and move on to extreme self-criticism. If they don't know how to turn off the stress through social support, a hobby, or a sport, it may overtake them, and when they do try to kill themselves, they usually succeed: doctors learn a lot about the body, and if they are going to attempt suicide, they are more likely to make it lethal. Also, doctors have available to them large quantities of highly lethal substances and may be more likely to use these in an impulsive moment.

So why do some doctors—400 per year in the United States—kill themselves? What particular kind of problems do they suffer? An important insight comes from the Grant Study of Adult Development, begun at Harvard University in 1938. The study began by asking 268 male sophomores, average age 18, to meet with a psychiatrist for eight interviews (among many other tests performed). They then followed these men, who had started out life on such a promising note, to see what happened.

In 1972, the average man in the study was age 47. Some 25 years after college, when compared with their classmates, they were healthy and successful. A quarter of the class became lawyers or doctors; 15% became teachers, mostly at a college level; and 20% went into business. The remaining 40% were distributed throughout other professions such as architecture and accounting, or engaged in advertising, banking, insurance, government, and engineering.

After 30 years, the Grant Study director, George Vaillant of Harvard, followed up again. At that point, 17% of the physicians had been hospitalized with a psychiatric illness, 34% had undergone psychotherapy, and 36% used recreational drugs, all much higher rates than for the nonphysician colleagues in the study.[13]

Probing further into the research, Vaillant found that the doctors in trouble shared some characteristics. They showed a higher level of dependency, pessimism, passivity, and self-doubt than other men in the study. They were the type who asked themselves to give more than they had been given.

Childhood counts. When the physician from a barren childhood becomes overly burdened by the demands of dependent patients, trouble arises, according to Vaillant. This type of physician resorts to drugs to alleviate fatigue. Working late is not the primary issue. In the Grant Study it was not the physician who worked late who got divorced. Instead, physicians in unhappy marriages worked late to avoid their spouse.

The personality of the doctor, then, is a big factor in determining whether he or she gets depressed on the job. What about the job itself? Does listening and working to reduce others troubles lead to emotional trouble? Being a psychiatrist can be a hard job. Psychiatrists have to deal with the everyday fear that patients might harm or even kill themselves. As we've seen in the previous chapter, psychiatrists mourn that loss as a family member does and frequently feel guilty and self-critical. Could we have prevented it? Did we do the right thing? Did we miss something?

Many mental health professionals believe that they will experience violence in their work. Even if we brush it off as a normal occurrence, dealing with violent patients is stressful for all psychiatrists, no matter what their level of experience. One story we heard from a psychiatrist participating in our survey is typical: "Just after my residency, when I had started on part-time staff at the hospital, I was seeing a patient in my office in the early evening—I had seen him three or four times previously and knew he could get angry but was surprised when he jumped up and started to hit me with his fist. It felt awful, I was powerless, but a colleague heard the noise and came in the room—we called a code … For a while I blamed myself for provoking him; but whether I could have been more careful in my language, I still had to deal with him and his divorce. For a very long time I felt very tired by my work—I must have been very on guard. I was careful about who I accepted into my practice. I still am."

The disdainful attitude of other doctors toward psychiatry compounds self-critical attitudes. Although the profession is gaining respect from other specialists, largely because we've developed a more scientific approach to dealing with mental illness, some psychiatrists still complain that they aren't treated with the respect they deserve. Old attitudes still linger, as we heard from another psychiatrist in 1999: "Other specialty areas frown on psychiatry. I hear it all the time, either directly or hearsay, through other parties. It's still disappointing to hear it. Either it's not proper medicine or it's not effective or they're all crazy or they really don't help anyone or they screw people up more than they were before they came in or they're not real doctors. They say things like that—everything that is degrading, which is one of the reasons I never really wanted to go into this field." This lack of respect from others was found in our study to be a contributor to career regret.

The job is stressful in ways that the general public may not understand. An insight into this came from a study of 75 psychodynamic psychotherapists in San Francisco.[14] They provided a useful list of the problems that a practising psychiatrist faces: isolation was the most frequent problem, followed by the need to control emotions, ambiguity in the field, struggles with their professional identity, and the need for personal connection, which cannot be satisfied in the office. Some complained that they were unable to share their patients' problems with other people, which only increased their sense of isolation. Ten of them pointed to difficulties dealing with countertransference, involving the feelings they developed toward their patients, and five said that the practice of psychiatry opened up deep emotional issues in themselves. One-quarter of respondents admitted that their frustration in fulfilling omnipotent wishes was a significant problem. Therapists are often people who have a great need to help and rescue others, which may be a response to a deeper need to receive love. When the all-powerful rescuer is thwarted, he or she can feel helpless. A further problem identified was the exaggerated internal demands for performance, and the guilt the psychiatrists felt when they were unable to meet such standards. There were other frustrations as well—the long delay in achieving results, the need to maintain a particular image in the eyes of the community, and the tension in dealing with hostile patients.

Coping with all of these stressors can lead to burnout, a syndrome introduced in 1974 to describe features of emotional exhaustion. People who are burned out feel overextended and tired, with nothing left to give. They can become negative and cynical, and lose feeling for other people, including patients. They often feel incompetent and inadequate and may become depressed. Studies of psychiatrists in the United Kingdom have demonstrated that they display greater emotional exhaustion as a result of work than a comparable group of physicians from other specialties.[15]

But the odd thing about psychiatrists is that they can show signs of burnout at the same time as they score high on personal achievement and satisfaction.[16] One study sent a questionnaire to 55 psychiatrists and found that 52% scored highly on emotional exhaustion and 48% on depersonalization. Nevertheless, 80% of them rated themselves favourably on professional accomplishment. In other words, psychiatrists are satisfied with our professional achievement, even though we often feel depleted.

Some psychiatrists get burned out and suffer emotional troubles, while others do not. How do we make sure that psychiatrists of the future are in a favourable position to cope? I think we have to look at the kind of people we admit to the profession, and evaluate how they are trained.

To choose residents, we have traditionally relied on grades, test scores, and lengthy interviews. But therein lies the problem: not all of psychiatric practice is about how smart you are and how much you know; it's also about how you communicate, work with others, and respond to unforeseen problems or criticisms. Do we recruit for the characteristics that will lead to good-quality psychiatrists who are satisfied with their work?

When I first applied for a psychiatric residency, I didn't have to take a test, write an essay, or even do an interview. Although our profession now does a better job of evaluating applicants, we still shy away from entry tests of personality or emotional makeup. Currently, the only way we have to detect people who will be indifferent to the pain of their patients, or who will take advantage of their power to satisfy their sexual desires, is through interviews and references, and then performance in the residency. The personality tests inspired by our line of work have been used to vet corporate leaders and airline pilots, but not the people whom society trusts to help people deal with their deepest fears and problems.

The traditional lengthy interview may be a poor way to choose. Interviewers typically select their scores in the first five minutes, and there is little consistency in the scoring. These days, some Canadian universities at the level of medical school entry now give prospects 8 or 10 mini-interviews in which they have to evaluate a situation or an ethical problem, and say how they would approach it. Scores on these types of interviews are predictive of results on licensing exams that test doctors' decision making and patient interactions, five years later. This is an effective means of selecting medical students, and I believe a similar approach could improve our ability to choose psychiatric residents.

Once a person has entered the field, we can do a much better job of educating him or her about the importance of connecting empathically with patients, even if one is not primarily a therapist. We can inform the new psychiatrist about the value of collegial support and about the significance of maintaining a balance and of personal relationships outside a practice. We can discuss how to prevent the temptation of making patients the major source of life gratification. We can help psychiatrists practise self-care.

All this may help, but what do we do about the psychiatrist who slips on the job? How do we know who is on the other side of the proverbial couch? Is the psychiatrist in good shape, or depressed, addicted to drugs, or even at risk of committing suicide? Might the psychiatrist be inclined to cross the line and have sex with a patient, or use the patient for other purposes? Any of these scenarios would have a huge negative impact on a patient in an intimate therapeutic relationship.

Ultimately, it may be up to the patient to detect the problem. If you are that patient, this must sound odd. After all, you are going to see the doctor because you are suffering in some way; you don't think it's your role to see whether the doctor is unwell. But from the start you should be assessing the clinician to see whether he or she is right for you. Hopefully, you've based the initial meetings on a referral from a GP, internist, or some other person you trust, someone who's benefited from treatment, and because word-of-mouth reputation has been positive. You shouldn't be hesitant to ask questions early on regarding area of expertise, theoretical frame, and methods used. But you might also look for signs of emotional trouble: Do they seem interested? Are they always late? Forgetting important details week to week? Do they appear red-eyed, smelling of alcohol? Do they seem to touch you inappropriately? Do they want to see you at odd hours or socially? Do they talk too much about themselves or their past? If you feel concerned about an issue, raise it with your psychiatrist or the referring physician, or consider finding a new doctor. If it is a very serious concern, raise it with the professional licensing body for the province.

Can You Tell in Advance Whether a Psychiatrist Will Have Trouble?

Is there any way to tell in advance whether a psychiatrist will suffer mental problems, which then might affect his or her therapy with patients? When I was a resident, Ted Waring and I decided to find out. We enrolled 70 residents (out of 120 eligible) at the University of Toronto and the University of Western Ontario and asked them to do a series of psychological tests before finishing the first six months of their residency program. We gave them the General Health Questionnaire, a good screen for emotional problems. We also gave them the Minnesota Multiphasic Personality Inventory

(MMPI), one of the most frequently used personality tests in mental health. This tool identifies personality structure, which is stable over time, and psychopathology, related to various emotional problems or disorders. Since the MMPI was launched in 1939 it has been used to measure everything from the preoccupation with health issues; to how strongly one holds certain sex stereotypes, like the Marlboro Man; to the level of one's anxiety and the ability to trust, or the need for control or rebellion against control. We also used the Eysenck Personality Inventory (EPI), which measures two dimensions of personality. One is the outgoing extrovert versus the inward-looking introvert. The other is the stable person versus the neurotic, the kind of person who experiences negative emotional responses when confronted with very minor stressors. The third test we administered was the Strong Interest Inventory (SII), which is often used by career counsellors to assess a person's level of interest compared with those of others in a specific career.

As might be expected, psychiatric residents reflect a range of personality types. But about 15% scored as having emotional problems at this time, their first residency year, according to the General Health Questionnaire. We found that the emotionally disturbed residents differed in some significant ways from the others. The Eysenck test showed they scored high on the neuroticism subscale. The MMPI showed they scored high on the depressed, isolated, and confused scales. The vocational test showed that their interests aligned not with the field of medicine, but rather banking or accounting.[17]

Our study did not involve a treatment or even informing the individuals of their results; the university's ethic committee would not allow us to disclose this information. Years later, in the mid-1990s, we were interested in what had happened to these trainees. Most were doing very well in their careers. It turned out that 2 of the 40 residents we studied had had their licences revoked, both because of sexual involvements with their patients.[18]

Was there any advance warning from all the personality tests we had given them when they started their residency? As it turns out, yes. In the MMPI, both psychiatrists scored high on the psychopathic deviancy and mania scales, a profile code type known as 4-9/9-4, which measures antisocial tendencies or psychopathic behaviour. Individuals who score high on this scale often have difficulty incorporating the values and standards of society and are likely to engage in lying, cheating, stealing, and sexual acting out. They also show poor judgment, take risks, and typically do not learn from past experiences. Such individuals typically have great difficulty with authority and are also described as having poorly developed consciences and fluctuating ethical values. They are seen as selfish and self-indulgent, and are not very successful in delaying the gratification of their impulses. The Ma scale of the MMPI was developed to identify psychiatric patients manifesting hypomanic symptoms. Individuals with high scores on this scale are likely to be energetic and talkative, and prefer action to thought. They have great difficulty in inhibiting expression of impulses. It is not uncommon for these individuals to have an exaggerated appraisal of their own self-worth and self-importance. We found other disturbing facts about these two residents from their scores on the MMPI test's K scale, which measures the extent to which a person attempts to deny psychopathology or to present things in a favourable light. They both scored high on this scale, which suggests they had little or no awareness of their character problems.

In sum, MMPI profiles of the two psychiatrists who would eventually lose their licences showed evidence, at the outset of their psychiatric careers, of antisocial attitudes and behaviours, as well as of a defensive cognitive-perceptual style. The tests in the first six months of residency showed this, and yet these two residents were given high marks by supervisors. They clearly presented themselves in a favourable way in order to gain approval, and the senior psychiatrists supervising them didn't recognize their character problems.

When we saw these results, we were stunned. It looked like we had a battery of psychological tests that could show, in advance, whether someone was likely to break the rules, cross the ethical line, and abuse the trust of vulnerable patients. This could be a good reason to administer psychological tests to all medical residents contemplating a career in psychiatry. As it turned out, two other residents had a similar profile but didn't break the rules. In fact, they were doing well and making significant contributions to the field.

This raises an issue on screening prospective residents for psychiatric programs. The interview and questionnaire process, supplemented by references, is much more rigorous now than it was in the 1970s, and the candidates have improved. Nevertheless, we should consider whether personality and emotional vulnerability tests could be useful for screening, both for admission purposes and to help those who are struggling.

Obviously, a high test score does not mean that the person will get into trouble; in our circumstance, there was a 50% false positive rate. Would we deny good people a career helping others because of the personality test? Or would we say that the harm done by the 50% who crossed the line is worth denying people with these profiles entry to psychiatry? There is no clear answer. But one way to deal with this issue is to have residents take these tests and then give them the results, with a good explanation, so they can get help early to avoid problems. Coming to know yourself is a lifelong process, and in a profession like psychiatry, where the personality of the therapist is so crucial for the success of the treatment, it's important to get to be self-reflective. Are you impulsive and have problems with alcohol, or are you introverted and anxious? Are you afraid of intimacy, or do you long for relationships? Testing residents raises another question: Should other people (e.g., supervisors) know the results? My view is that this cannot be justified at this time. But it is important to ask whether the protection of the public and the preservation of the integrity of the practice of psychiatry are reasonable grounds to "wrongly" deny some physicians access to their field of choice? If so, then what would be an acceptable rate of false positives—that is, physicians who were denied who would not have had any difficulty? Clearly more study is warranted before this question can be addressed.

The Feminization of Mental Health

The gender makeup of the profession has changed dramatically in the last 40 years. In 1968, only 11% of medical degrees conferred by Canadian universities were to women. By 1999, more women than men received medical degrees. The huge numbers of women moving into medicine have changed the character of psychiatry. In 1982, only 14% of practising psychiatrists in the United States were women. By 1996, that number jumped to 25%. In Canada, about one-third of practising psychiatrists were women as of 2002. The field of psychiatry is becoming more and more feminized. At the University of Toronto, 80% of residents are now women.

Men currently earn only 20% of all master's degrees awarded in psychology, down from 50% in the 1970s. They account for less than 10% of social workers under the age of 34, according to a recent survey. And their numbers have dwindled among professional counsellors—to 10% of the American Counseling Association's membership today from 30% in 1982.

What impact has this had on the practice of psychiatry? Not much, according to the studies. A good therapist is a good therapist, whether male or female. Our surveys of Ontario psychiatrists show that men and women are very similar in most respects. We found some intriguing differences, however.[19]

Women worked slightly fewer hours per week, but they saw patients for longer periods. They were more likely than men to see patients with anxiety disorders, and less likely than men to do forensic work. Women were just as likely as men to teach or do research but—and this is of concern—women were less likely than men to publish in a scholarly journal or get funding from pharmaceutical companies.

As we studied the differences between men and women with respect to the burdens and satisfactions, we found a pattern. Women view themselves as less successful than men do. They are less likely than men to have research training, to become principal investigators on peer-reviewed grants, or be currently involved in research. They have fewer peer-reviewed publications. Women in psychiatry and in all of medicine still earn less than men. They are more critical of themselves as professionals, which may limit their striving for certain kinds of success.

At the same time, women have fewer regrets and would choose psychiatry again more often than men.[20] How can this be understood? Women more so than men are comfortable seeking support from other women, friends, and colleagues regarding the demands of their professional lives, and much informal support occurs through participation in related activities. These connections may provide an important buffer from the demands of clinical practice. It is difficult to be the recipient of the emotional needs of many ill and needy patients, and psychiatrists are often forced to face fears of their own vulnerabilities. It is easy to become overly involved with patients, leading to emotional exhaustion and burnout. Can women handle these demands better than men? We are unable to say for certain, but it's possible that women, by emphasizing relationships in their work and in their lives, may feel more satisfied than men, despite their rating themselves as less successful. It may also be a question of expectations. The older women in our study began medicine at a time when women didn't expect as much recognition and financial reward as the men, especially if they were married.

Younger women, on the other hand, have higher expectations in this regard, but they still don't see themselves attaining the same levels of success as men. These younger women are more like men in their attitudes: they had more regret in career choice, and they reported a less satisfying balance between professional and personal lives than the older women. They felt a greater emotional burden from their patients, perhaps because these young women were still doing the majority of the work in the home and with children.

Has the socialization of women equipped them more than the men to handle the pressures of psychiatry? Perhaps. Women may also have an important advantage given that the largest proportion of patients in psychotherapeutic practice is women. These factors may make the nature of the work intrinsically easier for women because of a more intuitive understanding of the other, as well as a decreased sense of isolation and a familiarity with accepting the emotional needs of others. Here's what one female psychiatrist told us: "I think I understood a lot about human problems well before I went into psychiatry, and so that helps a great deal. My personality style is that I tend to be patient. I tend to be understanding and receptive for sure. These are qualities that are important for a psychiatrist to have. I'm flexible, I'm open-minded, and those qualities are important in a psychiatrist. They're also important in any physician."

Yet some of the studies raise serious concerns about the mental health of women doctors. One study that sampled virtually all the female physicians in St. Louis in 2001 reported that between 39 and 51% had a history of depression. This is more than double the depression rate for women in the general population. According to data from the Johns Hopkins Precursors Study, the rate of suicide in women doctors is 130% higher than it is in the general female population, and 40% higher for men. Female psychiatrists are even more vulnerable than female doctors, according to the 2001 Women Physicians' Health Study, a US national survey of over 4,500 women doctors.[21] It compared female psychiatrists with other female physicians. Female psychiatrists were less likely to be married and were more liberal politically. They worked fewer hours than their other medical colleagues and were more likely to work in solo practices. They were similar to other female physicians in many significant ways, and most of them, over 80%, were satisfied with their jobs. But the psychiatrists had experienced many more difficulties in areas especially relevant to this discussion. Compared with the general population, more of them had a past history of depression (34% versus 17%) or abused alcohol (4.0 versus 1.5%), or were victims of sexual abuse (8 versus 4%). Their family histories showed much higher rates of depression, alcohol abuse, and earlier sexual abuse as well. In other words, they had significant emotional vulnerabilities, suggesting a need to attend to self-care and, when indicated, to seek treatment.

Does the high rate of depression among the women studied have an important bearing on the future? It is possible that there will be an impact on practice patterns, for example, time off work; but it's also possible that levels of depression may moderate in female psychiatrists trained recently if they have more opportunity and fewer pressures than their older colleagues from the 1980s. The profession also has an obligation to increase education for recognition of vulnerabilities and self-care, and to enhance efforts to provide support and early intervention.

How will the profession change as it becomes more and more a female domain? It is really difficult to predict, in part because psychiatry itself changes over time and the behaviour of female practitioners will also likely change—just as the younger women in our study differ from the older group. There will be human resource issues, however. Women do work a few hours less per week than men, and even the younger male psychiatrists work fewer hours than the older group; if women continue to see patients for longer periods, we can expect fewer patients treated by each psychiatrist.

Other areas where the profession may benefit from a preponderance of female clinicians include reduced rates of sexual boundary violations and a more collaborative approach to multidisciplinary care, which is essential for the future. The feminization of the profession may have an effect on research and scholarship, unless the female psychiatrists of tomorrow become more invested in the academic enterprise and more competitive in pursuing grants and publishing. Support and mentoring may be vital to encourage women to assume these roles, and this should be systematically addressed in academic settings to ensure promising young women fulfill their potential and that of the profession. One of the fundamental issues for the future of psychiatry will be the fusion of science with compassion, and female academics who remain committed to the relational side of psychiatry may be ideally suited to be leaders in this area.

CHAPTER 14
Science and Care

Vivian Rakoff, the chair of the University of Toronto's Department of Psychiatry during the 1980s and one of the legends of Canadian psychiatry, used to say that psychiatry was both a science and an art, and the essence was to balance the two. More than four decades later, his words ring as true as ever. In that time, I have witnessed a dramatic swing in our profession away from the art and toward the science.

When I started in 1970, psychodynamic thinking and practice dominated psychiatry in the United States and to a lesser extent in Canada. Patients spent a great deal of time lying on the couch, or sitting face to face with their therapist as they explored their internal world, their dreams and fantasies, their past, and their relationships. Psychiatrists tried to help them see meaningful connections and relate these to their distress or disability. Psychoanalysts dominated academic centres and it was difficult to challenge their views, particularly if your critique was seen as a form of psychological resistance. They believed their ideas and treatment evaluations were beyond reproach.

The intellectual heirs of Freud and Jung largely influenced diagnosis until 1980, and the DSM, or *Diagnostic and Statistical Manual of Mental Disorders*, was written in the language of dynamic psychiatry. The DSM guided treatment in some places and split the profession over whether it had any basis in science in others.

By the time I ended my term as chief of psychiatry at Toronto General in 1990, the pendulum was swinging the other way. New drugs could allow people with severe mental disease to live outside an institution. They could relieve the burden of depression and stop the delusions and hallucinations of psychosis. Science was clearly winning the war. The biologists, who believed drugs could cure or alleviate many mental illnesses were pushing aside the psychoanalysts, who still felt that therapy had all the answers. Scientists were legitimately demanding proof that treatments were effective. Overall, this was an incredible advance for mental health, but we would come to see that there was still value in talk therapy and that this was lost in the wholesale embrace of science.

Psychoanalytic thought was in freefall. Psychoanalysis might be a fascinating tool for illuminating the human condition and furthering the education of future psychotherapists, but it couldn't prove its value as a tool for healing. There was a concern that daily contact with a therapist may even lead some patients backwards—replacing the challenges of the outside world with an intense preoccupation with themselves and the therapeutic relationship.

In 1980, two momentous events hastened psychiatry's medicalization. The first was the 1980 landmark case of Dr. Raphael Osheroff, a successful nephrologist from West Virginia who fell into a depression after a difficult divorce. He had been admitted for seven months to a psychiatric inpatient centre, Chestnut Lodge, where he was treated with psychotherapy for what staff diagnosed as a personality disorder. This treatment did not help: he lost weight, was unable to sleep, and became agitated. Finally, his family transferred him to a centre that viewed his situation differently and treated him with medications. He recovered quickly. He sued Chestnut Lodge for negligence and won a large settlement.[1]

The second significant event was the 1980 publication of DSM-III. Introduced by the American Psychiatric Association in 1952, the *Diagnostic and Statistical Manual* had been dominated by psychoanalysts, who used concepts like reaction formation and neurosis to describe mental illness. Psychoanalytic theory, rather than observable symptoms, guided the diagnosis of mental illness.

Then, in the 1960s, Sam Guze, an internist who moved to psychiatry, thought psychiatric patients deserved the same scientific approach as other patients, and his colleague George Winokur, at Washington University in St. Louis, Missouri, felt the same way. The opponents of psychoanalysis began to gather together. There was Eli Robins, former chair of the Department of Psychiatry at Washington University School of Medicine and a leader of the movement to apply traditional medical and scientific standards to psychiatric research and treatment, and his wife, Lee Robins, a pioneer of psychiatric epidemiology. They and a few of their colleagues stood alone for years as they called for a scientific approach to psychiatric diagnosis, instead of those based on psychoanalytic theories. The American Psychiatric Association finally listened, and in 1974 it hired Robert Spitzer of Columbia University, a psychiatrist who had trained earlier in psychoanalysis, to work on a new approach to the DSM.

Under Spitzer's leadership, the association switched to an entirely new approach to diagnosis in 1980. It wouldn't rely on theories to explain why people got sick. Instead, the DSM would list symptoms and organize them into neat disease categories and checklists of precisely described criteria for more than 200 objectively described diagnoses. This would be published in the third edition of the DSM. When DSM-III came out in 1980, it was more than three times as long as the previous version. Spitzer and colleagues listed 265 diagnostic categories in 494 pages. They added bulimia nervosa and autism, which was previously called childhood schizophrenia. Instead of "hyperkinetic reaction of childhood," DSM-III renamed the condition "hyperactivity disorder" and introduced attention deficit disorder (ADD). Neurosis was dropped; personality disorders were added. They discarded the theories about repression and the unconscious. Mental conditions were described, but there was no explanation of why people suffered from them. Most of the committee members for DSM-III were descriptive psychiatrists. The analysts were no longer invited to join the committees developing criteria for disorders.

The new DSM had a big impact on the profession. Checking symptoms often dislodged the art of understanding and empathizing with the whole person who is suffering a mental illness or distress. Yet psychiatrists didn't complain; many of them thought this new approach would be beneficial to them. Long relegated to the back seat of medicine, they wanted the acceptance and respect of their profession, and the way to get it was to start talking about medical illnesses and chemical interactions in the brain, and to stop talking about abstract theories of the mind—chief among them psychoanalysis—that many could not understand. They stopped resisting giving antidepressants on the theory the drugs might reduce the patient's motivation to get into therapy. They took it for granted that medicine was part of the therapy. Some clinicians went all the way and dispensed with therapy altogether. Too many just reached for their pens and wrote prescriptions.

Psychoanalysis took another hit from research that aimed to answer the question, did psychoanalysis work? By 2002, the verdict was apparently in.

The Research Committee of the International Psychoanalytic Association reported this: "Existing studies have failed to unequivocally demonstrate that psychoanalysis is efficacious relative to either an alternative treatment or an active placebo."[2] In other words, psychoanalysis was deemed not to be an effective treatment.

The swing seemed to be complete.

The economics of health care funding, especially in the United States, also played a significant role in pushing talk therapy out of the practice. It didn't pay psychiatrists to do therapy; psychiatrists could make more money just prescribing medicines every 15 minutes. Funders could save more money by dispensing with psychiatrists for talk therapy; nonmedically trained therapists were a lot cheaper.

Big pharmaceutical companies played their part too in psychiatry's conversion to medications. They make far more money when depression is considered an illness requiring medication, as opposed to a problem of living or a response to adversity. The result is that, by the new millennium, psychiatrists had been pushed out of therapy: only 10% of US psychiatrists actually do psychotherapy for depression. It's a sad statement about the profession today.

Psychiatry had swung from the proverbial couch to the lab. In many ways, this was a good thing, but it raised a serious question for me in 1990 as I thought about my next move in the advancement of Canadian psychiatry: How do you balance science and caring?

Science, to be sure, was important for our field. For far too long, a significant part of psychiatry had considered itself to be beyond the rules of evidence, partly because it was impossible to look inside the human brain with any precision or confidence. As we've seen, asylum doctors and psychoanalysts usually operated outside the university. Untrained to the scientific method, the vast majority were not able to critically evaluate scientific evidence. Even when powerful new drugs to combat psychosis and then depression and anxiety were proven to be safe and effective by randomly controlled trials, these psychiatrists often ignored or rejected existing evidence, or relied on therapies that were not proven effective.

Opinion or intuition often guided clinical decision making, rather than proven evidence. Electroconvulsive therapy (ECT) provides another example. ECT had been proven to greatly improve the condition of people suffering severe depression in 80 to 90% of cases, and yet many psychiatrists refused to recommend it mainly because of prejudice (some theirs, some the public's). Starting in the mid-1970s following a public outcry and community lobbying action against ECT in the mass media, 35 US states passed laws restricting the use of shock treatments, and by 1980 ECT use had fallen by half. Some US states even banned ECT in publicly funded hospitals, which meant that only people with money could afford this powerful treatment. Canadian physicians followed this trend.

In this respect, psychiatrists are not so different from other doctors. When doctors diagnosed and treated patients for a physical illness, they have traditionally based their decisions on clinical experiences, or on the oral or written tradition of medical learning. Science is a relatively recent addition to medicine.[3]

I agreed that psychiatrists should use scientific evidence more to inform clinical decisions for diagnoses and treatment, and not just rely on subjective practical reasoning. I felt that this required three things: more science in our field, more people capable of interpreting the findings of science, and a willingness of clinicians to adapt new evidence into practice. However, I never thought that psychiatrists should turn into pure technicians who examine patients, check off a list of symptoms, and dispense pills. It is impossible to reduce an ill person to a checklist of symptoms. Diagnosis can never replace understanding. Who has ever sat with a seriously depressed patient and felt that this was merely a collection of symptoms rather than a unique individual immersed in a sense of hopelessness and lost meaning?

We can never forget that psychiatry, like all of medicine, is a helping profession that aims to improve the physical, mental, spiritual, and social well-being of human beings. Psychiatry is concerned with illness but also with the texture and drama of the human condition. Yet the art of medicine, the caring side, is easily dismissed in a scientific world. This was true then, and it still is true today. Caring in medicine can be neglected at a time when the pursuit of science has brought us powerful and effective new treatments. I believe this is a mistake for our profession. Practitioners need to be healers who connect to patients on a human level.

Rather than just focusing on the illness, they need to see people as they are—multidimensional and complicated individuals with strengths that can be fostered. They must tailor their treatments to individual patients, and never forget that the practice of medicine, while based on scientific evidence, is first and foremost a social interaction between someone who is suffering and a healer.

When we lose this caring side of medicine, we lose the ability to sit and be with people who are ill. A physician in one of our studies put it this way: "I think we have failed, somewhere along the line, to teach our residents how to cope with someone who is suffering. To sit in a room with someone who is crying, someone who is in pain, someone who is psychotic and confused and frightened of you, and I think we hide behind our pills. Because the pills become an interaction that says, I'll solve this problem for you quickly so that I don't have to sit with your tears."[4]

The challenge to balance caring and evidence-based science is not new. I've always been an admirer of Sir William Osler, the Ontario-born and McGill-educated physician who was the first professor of medicine at Johns Hopkins and later the Regius Professor of Medicine at Oxford. A great man and an outstanding doctor, he fundamentally changed medical teaching in North America by introducing the clinical clerkship and medical residency. The idea of the residency, with its emphasis on bedside teaching, was borne of his insistence that students learn from seeing and talking to patients.

I have collected the first editions of many of his books, and loved to quote him in my addresses to psychiatrists, especially when I was at Toronto General. The group there even came to expect it, and when I left they gave me a first edition of his *Principles and Practice of Medicine*. In his day, Osler used to complain that doctors relied excessively on treatments that had never been proven to be effective. Since they were not interested in proof, doctors often believed in a particular school of thought, which led to the growth of denominations. Members of denominations resisted the advances of knowledge because they were ideologically committed to particular therapies. Practitioners maintained their beliefs rather than applying new evidence when it was powerful, or testing or refuting it.

This description could fit psychiatry as it was in 1990. We had dichotomous value systems—clinical practice and scientific research. The clinicians were the humanists who tried to understand complicated human beings in all their dimensions. The scientists thought the cure would come from the lab and the thrilling new insights about the workings of the brain. As the pendulum was swinging from the caring side of the profession to the power of science, the two camps were deeply split.

This wasn't good for patients or for doctors, so I wanted to introduce a value system and an educational program that integrated both streams of thought. We need science and humanism together—together at the bench and together at the bedside.

CHAPTER 15
Return to the Clarke

In the fall of 1989, I was invited to a dinner hosted by H.T. "Mac" McCurdy. Once the deep morning voice of Montreal, McCurdy was now president of Standard Broadcasting, and he and his wife, Joey, had invited Andy Barrie, the much-loved morning man on CBC's morning show in Toronto, along with his wife, Mary. Just hearing McCurdy's and Barrie's voices would be a delight for Dorothy and me, and I knew we were in for an entertaining night.

I also knew that this dinner had something to do with my mentor, Vivian Rakoff, stepping down as head of the Clarke. McCurdy was the chair of the Clarke, and everyone at the dinner, Barrie included, were members of the Clarke's board. I suspected that I was a leading contender to replace Rakoff, for what I considered to be the finest psychiatric position in the country: the combined leadership of the University of Toronto's psychiatry group and CEO of the Clarke Institute. The University of Toronto trains one-quarter of all the English-speaking psychiatrists in Canada. Whoever got the job would be able to influence the practice of psychiatry for the next generation.

I was ready. I had been chief of psychiatry at Toronto General for eight years (and, more recently, at the Western as well), and I had just left my position as chair of the hospital's Medical Advisory Board. I had also turned over the leadership of the eating disorders program to Sid Kennedy the previous summer. I was turning 44 and eager for a new challenge. To compete effectively for this position, I needed to take a clear-eyed look at the state of the Clarke. What legacy would I inherit from Rakoff, and how would I enhance, improve upon, or even redirect it? What was my vision?

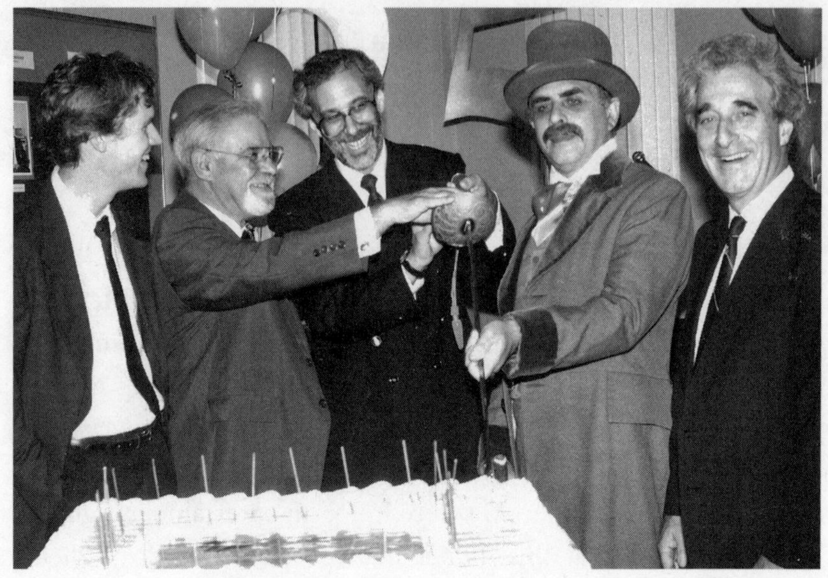

Celebrating the 25th anniversary of the Clarke in 1991 (from left to right): Jon Hunter (Robin's son), Vivian Rakoff, Paul Garfinkel, Joel Jeffries (playing C.K. Clarke), and Fred Lowy. Courtesy CAMH Archives.

Rakoff, a doctor who always stood on the humanistic side of psychiatry, who believed it to be a social interaction rooted in science, had nonetheless greatly enhanced the scientific side of the Clarke, scoring a huge victory when he convinced the provincial government to spend $7.5 million, an enormous sum then, on a PET (positron emission tomography) scanner. It was the first PET scanner in the world to be dedicated to a psychiatric institution. Rakoff was convinced that it would change psychiatry by offering us the first insights into the black box that is the brain.

Before this time, the tools we had that would allow us to see what was happening inside the brain were very limited. Animal studies and the behaviour of people who had survived head injuries or brain illnesses gave us a rough idea of the brain's internal geography relative to functions. We knew about the emotional circuitry that runs through the cingulate cortex on the medial side of the brain, the hippocampus and the thalamus.[1] We understood, from the study of people who get sick, the areas of the brain that governed some sensory or motor functions or some types of cognitive functions. But we knew little of the detailed circuitry that underlies so much of the brain activities, and we had no way of seeing the brain actually functioning in a living person. I encountered this roadblock every day during my early research on brain chemistry. We were unable to use a test of blood or urine or even of cerebral spinal fluid to determine the levels of a brain chemical like serotonin because so much of this transmitter was also found throughout the body—the quantities from the rest of the body would obscure whatever was happening in the brain.

The PET scan promised to reveal the brain's amazing secrets for the first time. PET allows you to watch the brain in action as it utilizes glucose that has been tagged by a radioisotope. The rate of glucose turnover is an index of the level of brain activity at a given moment. This technique also allows you to see which parts of the brain burn glucose in response to a stimulus over a period of time. Over the next couple of decades, the PET scan, along with other powerful scans such as the MRI (which measures the structures in fine detail but not function), functional MRI (which measures brain activity by detecting associated changes in blood flow), and SPECT (which measures how the brain functions using radioisotopes, like PET does), as well as molecular genetics, would expand our knowledge of the brain 10-fold.

In 1990 we were only at the beginning of a new voyage into the previously hidden parts of the brain, so it was a thrilling moment to be at the head of a research-oriented psychiatric institute. The operating costs of the PET scanner, though, were estimated at about $1 million per year, and there seemed no clear plan in place on how to pay for them.

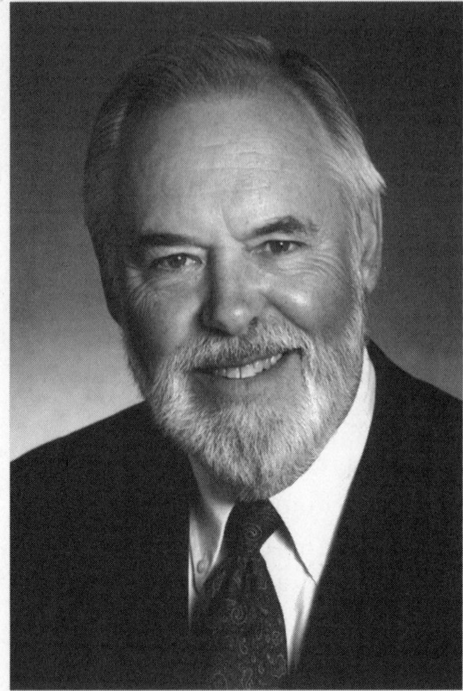

Ted Tremain was an outstanding mentor through his roles as board chair of the Clarke, chair of the nominating committee that formed CAMH, and chair of the CAMH Foundation. He was a selfless man who pushed strongly for improvements to the quality of patient care. Courtesy CAMH Archives.

In developing the scientific power of the Clarke, Rakoff had also hired some real stars, like Phil Seeman, who broke new ground on dopamine systems and the mechanisms of action of the antipsychotic drugs. There are a total of five different dopamine receptors (four of which were cloned by Seeman's lab group), but the dopamine D2 receptor is the primary target for all the antipsychotic drugs. He showed in his laboratory that the degree of blocking of the dopamine D2 receptor by a chemical predicted its strength as an antipsychotic drug. Seeman transformed antipsychotic drug design because his findings helped drug companies sift through thousands of chemical candidates to find potential antipsychotic medication. Today this is a billion-dollar business. In another important move for the university department, Rakoff promoted or hired a new team of psychiatric leaders. Mary Seeman, Phil Seeman's wife and an excellent, caring psychiatrist interested in the chronically ill, was installed at Mount Sinai Hospital as its new chief.

To head psychiatry at St. Michael's, Rakoff brought in Isaac Sakinofsky, an old friend from South Africa. He is a careful clinical psychiatrist and an expert on suicide. Joe Beitchman, an expert in speech and learning problems, was recruited from Ottawa as head of the Child Program at the Clarke. Don Wasylenki, chief at the provincial hospital in Whitby but previously at the Clarke, was brought back to be head of the Continuing Care Division, which looked after patients chronically ill with schizophrenia. Ex-Montrealer Saul Levine, an adolescent psychiatrist, became chief at Sunnybrook, and Ken Shulman, a Toronto-born geriatric psychiatrist who studied in the United Kingdom and then later at the Harvard School of Public Health, began to build a strong geriatrics program at Sunnybrook. Henry Durost, an outstanding clinician-administrator, originally from New Brunswick and then Montreal, was appointed clinical director at the Clarke.

Rakoff, never one for administrative detail, shied away from a key but sometimes unpleasant part of managing: holding people to account. As a result, the Clarke was a luxurious place for a researcher. Thanks to its generous and historic research funding, some researchers with a laboratory could be receiving up to $500,000 in research support per year, without having to compete for grants from government agencies. So, although there were a handful of great and productive researchers at the Clarke, such as Seeman, Kurt Freund, and Oleh Hornykiewicz, there were also a number of not quite outstanding people who needed the right kinds of incentives to be more productive. There were also some mediocre researchers who were still receiving public funds without producing much in the way of research results, year after year. In sum, the Clarke's research performance was surprisingly weak, particularly in light of the resources available. The Clarke's scientists did not have to compete for funds, so, human nature being what it is, they were not producing the research one would expect from such a significant institution.

These two concerns—holding people to account, and the reinvigoration of research—seemed to me the most critical for a new leader to take on at the Clarke.

• • •

I met with the search committee in February, about three months after that initial dinner hosted by McCurdy. In my presentation, I emphasized academic standards, quality research, and research productivity in an environment of superb clinical care and teaching. This vision was clear, as the Clarke had been established for this purpose less than 30 years earlier. The need for the institute had been based on C.K. Clarke's desire to have a Kraepelin-style university setting in Toronto. I proposed that programs would be determined by the populations we saw—schizophrenia, severe mood and anxiety disorders, severe childhood mental illness, sexual paraphilias, and mental disorders in forensic populations. The Clarke was to have research in all its important areas, and the university should train clinical and academic psychiatrists capable of critical evaluation and rigour in their thinking, and with skills beyond dynamic therapies.

I told the search committee that I wanted to boost the academic performance of this potentially great institution to where it ought to be, and that to do this I would have to make psychiatrists and basic scientists at the Clarke accountable for the research money they were receiving. I would encourage researchers to compete for funds from granting agencies, pushing them to be more competitive in the international research world. My new recruits would be people who were properly trained in research and could mentor others in their areas of expertise. Finally, at a time when our

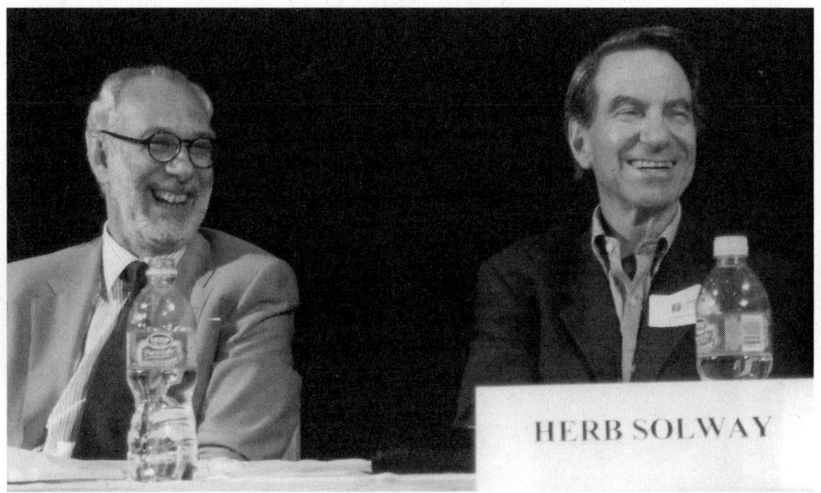

Paul Garfinkel and Herb Solway. Solway has had a long history of board and community service, initially through the Clarke Institute and later CAMH. A former managing partner of Goodmans law firm, he is an excellent judge of people and of backroom strategy—he was often at the centre of any important discussion. Courtesy CAMH Archives.

profession was swinging toward the scientific approach to mental illness, I spoke about how important it was to balance science and care. This to me was the fundamental challenge for our profession.

Shortly after meeting with the search committee, I was offered the job. I could not have been more thrilled. Within two months, however, the Ontario elections would turn my world upside down.

Bob Rae and his NDP government were unexpectedly elected to power: they weren't prepared to govern, and no one I knew in health care was ready for them. I was worried from the very start. This left-leaning government saw doctors as a financial burden, billing the government for their time and for laboratory and radiological tests. The Rae government wanted to reduce the number of doctors by cutting medical school enrolments, and soon it began taking aim at psychiatrists.

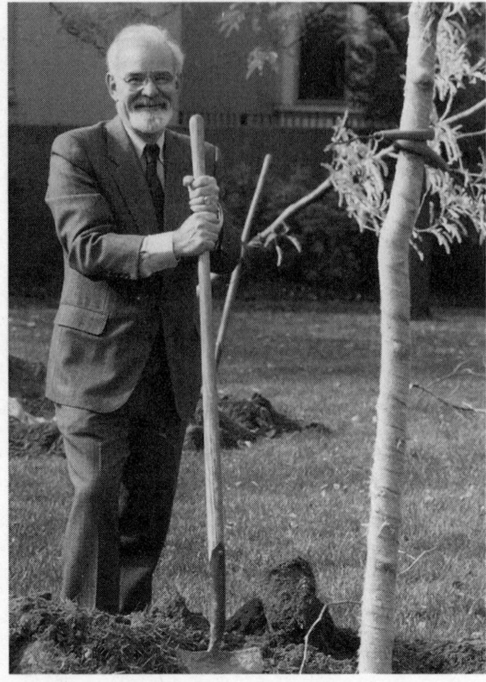

Vivian Rakoff in 1989, breaking ground to establish a PET Centre at the Clarke Institute. In 2008, he was awarded an honourary doctorate of science from the University of Toronto. Courtesy CAMH Archives.

Managing the Clarke

My new job was far more complex than anything I had tried before. I had to work with a board of trustees, and for the first time in my career, I was an employee of a board that had the power to fire me.[2] I was a bit wary of it at first. The board of 11 was dominated by successful business men. Three were government appointees, such as Libby East, a Liberal appointee who thought that the Clarke should focus on biological research and leave clinical care to other hospitals. The NDP appointee was from the other side of the spectrum: Pat Capponi, a former psychiatric patient and mental health activist who would soon publish her first book, *Upstairs in the Crazy House.*

I soon started to rely on two quietly powerful figures. Herb Solway, 15 years my senior, was managing partner at the Toronto law firm Goodmans. He was such an excellent judge of people that even at 80 years old he would still be called in to interview potential recruits for the firm. Solway had been on the Clarke's board on and off since 1969, when a relative of his had committed suicide on a weekend pass from one of the inpatient units.

Ted Tremain, an accountant by training, was vice-chair and head of the finance committee. As soon as he saw how little I knew about earnings statements and balance sheets, he gave me his own version of *Accounting for Dummies*. Tremain, a truly remarkable individual, soon became chair of the board. He had retired early and devoted himself to family investments and to giving back to the community, and he did so in a unique way, without any ego at all. He really wanted what was best for the institution, and he wanted to enhance his CEO, which made working with him a real pleasure.

For Tremain, patient care always came first, and he began the tradition of Christmas Day visits, so that every patient and staff member would get a warm greeting, a meal, and a gift on the holiday. He brought his quiet dignity to those who were so ill they had to be in a mental hospital at Christmas. This holiday tradition continues at CAMH to this day, and now with many people, their families, and pets all bringing comfort to others. A quiet, modest man, Ted never sought public recognition, but he always gave me great advice. Ted's modesty, ability to work with others, and strategic view would be crucial in the challenging years that lay ahead.[3]

As I started at the Clarke, one of the immediate priorities was to put together my senior management team. Herb Pardes, then president and CEO of Columbia-Presbyterian, and Tom Detre, dean at the University of Pittsburgh's medical school, both emphasized how important recruitment was, so I started on what can only be called a recruitment binge.

I asked Richard Swinson to join me as the Clarke's clinical director, effectively the institute's psychiatrist-in-chief. Some were surprised; Richard and I had clashed at Toronto General after I got the job he had wanted. But I knew Swinson was unhappy in his position at the General. He had been passed over again when Gary Rodin was appointed chief of psychiatry. As chair of the university's Department of Psychiatry, I saw this as a problem. We might lose Swinson if he didn't see a satisfying role for himself in Toronto. Swinson was a well-regarded clinician and an expert in anxiety disorders. I admired that he took care of very ill people on an inpatient unit. His treating the seriously mentally ill reflected a values system I wanted to promote at the Clarke and the university.

To head up the research program, I hired Greg Brown, head of neuroscience at McMaster University. He was a psychiatrist and neuroendocrinologist with an interest in the sleep hormone melatonin. We had worked together on some projects in the 1970s, and I had always respected his straightforward approach. For the crucial mood program, I recruited Russell Joffe from the Toronto General group. A South African–born psychiatrist, Joffe was investigating the role of the thyroid hormone in mood regulation. He was also a highly regarded teacher and mentor.

Jock Cleghorn joined us to run our schizophrenia program. His father, Robert, had been chair of McGill's Psychiatry Department right after Ewen Cameron. Jock had been trained as a psychoanalyst in Cincinnati and later was chair of psychiatry at McMaster. As his term ended, he undertook research training for a year in neuroscience and neuroimaging in Boston. Jock introduced me to Shitij Kapur, a resident in psychiatry studying in Pittsburgh, who then came to Toronto as a fellow and spent 16 wonderful years developing a stellar research career.

Phil Seeman, head of psychopharmacology, was moving back to his University of Toronto laboratory, so this gave me a chance to hire two of his former graduate students, Chaim Niznik and Hubert van Tol, as codirectors of a program in molecular biology.

They were superb, both for their science and for their ability to train younger people, and both died tragically young. (Niznik died suddenly of heart disease in his lab late one Friday in 2001; van Tol was hit by a car while riding his bike several years later.)[4]

Stan Freeman, who had been in charge of a large social and community psychiatry program, was retiring, so I promoted one of his former students, Dr. Paula Goering, to launch a program in health systems research. Dr. Morley Beiser came from the University of British Columbia to form a program in transcultural psychiatry, which led to important work on Native mental health, immigration, and refugees. Cleghorn introduced me to Bob Zipursky, a rising young Canadian psychiatrist in San Francisco who was studying PET images of people with schizophrenia. After we brought him back to Canada, Zipursky ended up taking over the schizophrenia program, and 15 years later he moved to Hamilton as head of psychiatry at McMaster.

Like many in academic psychiatry, I was convinced that the genetics of psychiatry was going to be the next big field. We had long known that some psychiatric illnesses, like many physical illnesses, have a genetic component. Children of schizophrenics, for instance, have a higher rate of the illness than other people. A Scandinavian study showed that an identical twin of a person with schizophrenia has a 50% chance of becoming ill, whereas a fraternal twin has a 20% chance and a sibling has a 12% chance of getting the illness. These rates are all substantially higher than the 1% rate you would find in the general population.[5]

When I began the job at the Clarke, the race to find single genes for mental illness was in full swing. A single gene for Huntington's disease had been discovered by the Hereditary Disease Foundation, working with the National Institute of Neurological Disorders and Stroke, and later in the decade Lap Chee Tsui and Francis Collins discovered the gene for cystic fibrosis. Around that time, Peter St. George-Hyslop began to work in the Azores with families who had a rare, very early onset form of Alzheimer's dementia, and through this he discovered a gene, presenilin 1, important for these families' illness.

These great discoveries were raising hopes that single genes might cause some of the mental disorders. Although we wouldn't find the holy grail, a single gene for mental illness (there isn't one), the scientists I recruited would discover many intriguing clues and insights.

I hired two young Canadian clinical psychiatrists who had been studying genetics at Yale, Jim Kennedy and Anne Bassett. Bassett went on to define a genetic abnormality in a subgroup of people with schizophrenia that is associated with cardiac defects and at times speech, cognitive, and language problems. This abnormality is due to a spontaneous genetic change rather than inheritance. Bassett also showed how genetic counselling for family members of patients with schizophrenia led to increased knowledge about schizophrenia and less fear of familial recurrence.

Kennedy became a leader in the field of psychiatric genetics, studying OCD, ADHD, and mood and eating disorders. His team would find a way to predict, based on the genetic profile, whether someone with schizophrenia or depression would suffer side effects from drugs.[6] Kennedy was also a terrific mentor to younger colleagues. He led us to a real superstar, Art Petronis, who has become a world leader in the new field of epigenetics, which looks at how the environment turns on and off our genes. Petronis came to Toronto from Lithuania as a young physician to visit his aunt. He dropped by the Clarke to see Kennedy too, and Kennedy immediately recognized his talent and found a place for him, even though there were no funds available. Since then Petronis has done groundbreaking research, for example, on the expression of genes influencing brain plasticity in learning and memory.[7,8,9]

To run our new PET scan, we wanted somebody with experience in imaging and nuclear medicine, and preferably a medical doctor with some appreciation of clinical matters. There were only a few dozen people like this in the world. I turned to Sylvain Houle, an expert in nuclear medicine at Toronto General. He has built one of the best PET groups in the world. He quickly recruited Alan Wilson, one of only a handful of radiochemists able to produce the radioisotopes for the PET lab. Gradually, this group has expanded and evolved in a spectacular way.

The PET scans have yielded important new clues about the function of dopamine in schizophrenia. Brain dopamine levels appear to be higher in people with schizophrenia. We still don't know how much these changes are state (after the illness has started) or trait (part of the person's makeup and maybe part of the predisposition), but unmedicated young people with schizophrenia and those with the very early features show elevated dopaminergic function. A practical side to this initial research emerged over the following decade: Kapur's team demonstrated that blocking 70% of the dopamine receptors relieved the positive (delusions and hallucinations) symptoms of psychosis. This finding has influenced clinical practice, as medications are now being given in much smaller doses, substantially reducing side effects.[10]

PET has also supplied tangible proof that addictions are a brain disease, not a symptom of moral decay. Dr. Nora Volkow, director of the National Institute on Drug Abuse, scanned the brains of people addicted to drugs such as cocaine and heroin. The scans show they have fewer dopamine receptors in their reward pathways than do nonaddicts.[11] There is a similar finding of altered brain function in alcoholism.

Beyond neuroscience, though, I wanted rigorous enquiry by thinkers who could critically evaluate current approaches, whatever the specific field. I was eager to see research in psychotherapy, so I hired Norman Doidge, a talented psychoanalyst from Toronto who had been training at Columbia in New York to work in the Clarke's outpatient program. Norman has since gone on to an outstanding writing career and a private psychotherapy practice. Zindel Segal, a psychologist who had worked with Brian Shaw on cognitive behaviour therapy, was promoted to lead our psychotherapy research group and has since published widely on this therapy, and more recently on mindfulness-based meditation.

In clinical research, there was a significant gap. The problem was not a lack of money but of training. I gave staff psychiatrists seminars on research design and methodology, but this only highlighted the lack of knowledge in clinical research. My goal became to develop a new generation of young clinical researchers. After my initial hiring binge, I felt more confident. But it didn't take long before I ran into trouble. At issue was the very identity of the Clarke, its meaning and purpose.

I thought my vision was clear: The Clarke should strike a balance between research and caring for people who were mentally ill. But the three key figures I hired—Swinson, the clinical chief; Brown, the head of research; and Joffe, the head of the mood program—pushed at every opportunity to make the Clarke more of a pure research institution where highly specialized scientists could study the mystery of the human brain and concepts in psychology. They wanted to change psychiatry for the next generation, through programs of advanced research, but went too far in wanting to restrict clinical care. This is not to suggest these three colleagues were not personally compassionate in dealing with patients—they were—but they had a different vision for the institute.

One day, I received a startling phone call at home from Swinson, informing me that the Medical Advisory Committee, which governs the doctors at the Clarke, was pushing to house the General Psychiatry program elsewhere and to ask the board to close the

Clarke's emergency ward. Mentally ill patients in crisis could go to the General Hospital for emergency care.

I thought that would be a big mistake, for a host of reasons. Psychiatric patients were not receiving good care in the emergency rooms of the general hospitals because of discrimination and lack of resources. If we closed our emergency ward, we would be closing the door to our community. And, under an NDP government that already thought doctors in general and psychiatrists in particular were not serving the public, we would be perceived as elitist and less relevant. Also at stake were areas of research. I believed that an emergency room and acute-care unit were important for treatment research.

What's more, I wasn't convinced that highly specialized neuroscience units were the best introductory settings to teach young residents general psychiatry. The psychiatrists on these units often saw their patients in a focused manner in order to probe a specific problem with the latest tools and medicines that science could and did provide. This one-sided approach didn't serve trainees well. A psychiatrist might be an expert on the impact of serotonin, or on the adrenal gland, but should still be able to sit with a person and give them hope, support, and caring. The caring side of our profession was being undervalued on the new frontier of neuroscience.

This was an important issue from the university perspective. We were training many specialist psychiatrists, but many of us began to think we had to produce very capable generalists as well. I strongly supported the view that we should form a General Psychiatry program and give it the same status as programs, such as mood disorders and schizophrenia. The only question was where the hub of the generalists should be: the Clarke or one of the general hospitals. I wanted the hub to be at the Clarke.

It was, in many ways, a clash of two visions. I wanted the Clarke to be a place where science was infused with caring and an appreciation of the complex humanity of individual patients, including those who walked into the emergency room. The psychiatrists who wanted to close the ER saw the Clarke as a tower of advanced research—clinical cases would serve research studies. Most ill people in our community would have to be treated in a general hospital, rather than at the Clarke.

When the issue finally came to the board, I made my case: if we closed the ER, we'd be taking the huge risk of isolating ourselves from the community. As well, our resident numbers would be reduced, and our research was not yet good enough to stand on its own.

The board agreed with me. Not long after, David Goldbloom, who was still on staff at Toronto General, came to the Clarke to take over as head of General Psychiatry, which included supervising the emergency ward. Goldbloom loved working in emergency, and he did a brilliant job as a teacher, a physician, and a leader in this important role. (A couple of years earlier, I had tried to recruit Goldbloom to run a program on impulse problems such as binge drinking and bulimia, but as he was mulling it over he suddenly developed a bad case of migraines. The headaches disappeared as soon as he declined. When he accepted the job as head of General Psychiatry, though, the migraines didn't return.)

The senior team never fully resolved our differences. Swinson and Joffe were polite on the surface, but they clearly didn't agree with my direction. Joffe left in 1995 when he was offered the position of chair of psychiatry at McMaster. I felt like part of me had been ripped out, not because he got the promotion but because of the way he handled his exit. He took the heart of the depression program with him—Trevor Young, Stephen Sokolov, and Anthony Levitt—all good young people. I accepted that as what academics do when they are building programs in a new setting. However, I was really hurt and angered by the manner of their leaving—remarks made that continuously put down their experiences at the Clarke. I recall that a physician wife of one of our board members commented that the Clarke's depression program had a new recording on the telephone answering service: "The depression program has moved to McMaster University."

A couple of years after Joffe left, he was appointed dean at McMaster. He then recruited Swinson to be chair of psychiatry.

As the dispute about our vision was simmering, the group suffered another terrible personal and professional blow. One day in the spring of 1992, I saw Cleghorn, our chief of schizophrenia, outside the Spadina entrance near the big garbage bins. He was pacing, which was unusual for him. When I went up to him, he told me that he had just seen his doctor and had learned he had pancreatic cancer. Sadly, he died shortly after that, at age 57. And professionally, it was a terrible loss: Jock had served as a bridge between my views and those of the three other senior colleagues.

It was a hard time. I thought I knew how to put together a team, and I thought that if I brought strong players to the Clarke, as I had, I would be successful, as I had been at Toronto General. Yet now, just a few years into my tenure, I was facing serious internal dissent. The most senior members of my team obviously didn't share my vision, and I was being undermined in a public way.

Getting my team aligned with my vision for the Clarke was only the beginning of my troubles. From the start, I tried to reward academic excellence and teaching, and I thought I knew how to do it. One key ingredient was to change the physician compensation system. I tore a page from what I had learned at Toronto General and focused on the financial partnership as a way of influencing physician behaviour. I proposed a new system that would reward the psychiatrists for their teaching and especially peer-funded research, all the while knowing that it would reduce the income of psychiatrists who did little academic work and earned most of their money seeing patients. I expected to run into resistance, as I did at the General, but I hoped that, eventually, after a few compromises, we would find a way to move forward as a group.

It was a much more painful process than I had imagined. The Clarke psychiatrists were difficult to budge. They moved slowly. They postponed meetings, or didn't turn up in sufficient numbers for a quorum. They liked the arrangements they already had, and they had the manpower to slow me down. They were four times larger in number than the psychiatrists at the General, and I had few allies. But I couldn't back down. If I wanted to promote academic rigour at the Clarke, I had to make sure the financial compensation rewarded the values of the institute and the university. The Clarke psychiatrists were so stubborn that I exploded more than once. I even told them at one point that I felt like firing the entire group of doctors and running the Clarke myself. Later that night, once I calmed down, I was surprised at just how angry I still was: *This is unbelievable! This isn't me talking*. (Besides, I couldn't fire them even if I wanted to.)[12]

In the end, the Associates Executive Committee, which governed the Clarke psychiatrists' financial partnership, came to the conclusion that the new compensation formula could actually enhance the culture and values of the Clarke. The deal was done. Once everyone cooled down, most of the psychiatrists decided they loved the new deal after all. It was a small satisfaction that buoyed me over the next few challenging years.

I found it hard to manage academic physicians who often felt hugely self-important. They thought that what they were doing was critical and didn't always want to participate in what were considered mundane events, such as teaching the students or talking to the public at a forum. Some of them would forget to show up at a scheduled lecture. I called this "academic narcissism," and many times I steamed about it instead of considering new ways to bring people onside.

As the clouds darkened, I felt like I was living my life in a fishbowl, and that I was doing it alone. Dorothy was busy establishing her career teaching English as a second language, Jonathan and Stephen had gone off to McGill and the University of Victoria respectively, and Josh had his own circle of friends. A synagogue that had once held meaningful relationships for me no longer did so, and my relationships at work were vastly different: as the boss, I was no longer one of the gang.

This role also brought me face to face with my own character, for better and for worse. I had to learn to deal with old friends and colleagues in a new way. Trying to be impartial was not always easy. I could be tough and stubborn about some things—the academic enterprise and funding priorities, for instance. I could stand up to a powerful donor who wanted to choose his favourite psychiatrist for an endowed chair. But at the same time, I could easily be swayed by old connections with deep roots. I had to put up with stories that travelled along the grapevine, stories that I felt distorted what I was doing. And now, unlike earlier challenging times, I was facing this alone.

CHAPTER 16
The Academy

When I was appointed CEO of the Clarke, I automatically became the chair of the University of Toronto's Department of Psychiatry. This was a big job that spanned both academia and the everyday workings of hospital psychiatry departments.

I would oversee the 500 psychiatrists, including the 150 full-time people in the then eight primary hospitals in terms of their academic work. I would participate in selecting the chiefs of the hospital psychiatry departments, and evaluate not only their personal performance but also the performance of their hospital departments. I would lead planning to set priorities and standards for the university department. In keeping with the standards of the university and Faculty of Medicine, the department would set up criteria and then follow these to determine who received an academic appointment or promotion. I would ensure fair processes that determined that the university's money was well spent. On the teaching side, I would ensure processes to determine where residents and medical students worked, and I had to make sure that our curriculum and supervision were of the highest quality. Over time I realized that getting more resources—money and space—was an important part of my role.

A high-quality research setting with excellent caring faculty is the best place to teach and treat patients. My goals were clear. I wanted to prod the University of Toronto's psychiatrists out of their comfortable jobs into the competitive world of international research. I wanted to broaden the definition of scholarship to encompass not only the thrilling new frontier of neuroscience but also the translation of science into a comprehensible language for practitioners, patients, and their families. Scholarship had to include the rigorous study of education for psychiatrists so that the standard of research and care for the public could be raised. Psychotherapy had to be studied in a scientific way. If this field was to be considered and funded as a branch of medicine, I saw no reason why we wouldn't test its effectiveness in the same way we would any other treatment. I wanted, in other words, to promote scientific thinking in the department but at the same time make sure that it was balanced with clinical care. A strong bridge needed to be built between the two.

I soon found out, though, that my powers were considerably less than one might think. As chair of psychiatry at the university, I didn't have nearly as much direct authority as I did at the Clarke

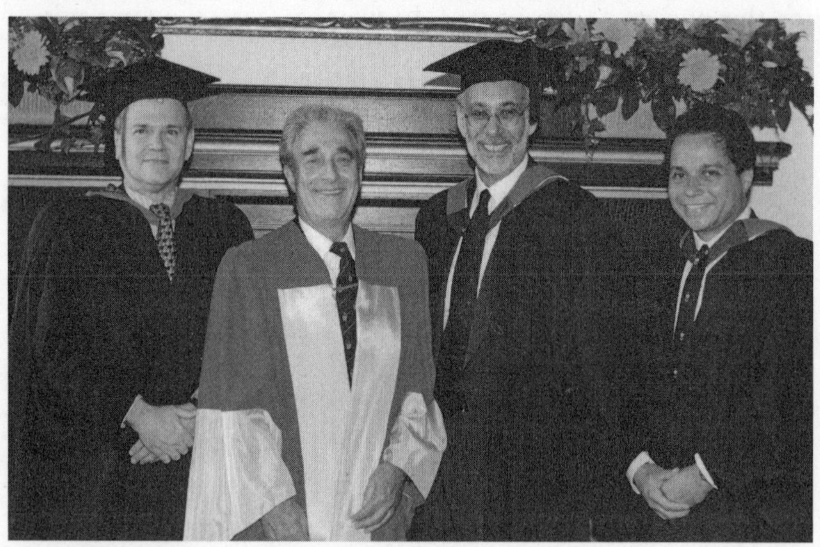

Fred Lowy receiving an honorary degree from the University of Toronto in 1998 (from left to right): Professor Arnold Aberman, dean of the Faculty of Medicine, Lowy, Paul Garfinkel, and Professor Peter Singer, director of the Centre for Bioethics. Courtesy University of Toronto Department of Psychiatry.

and the Toronto General. Everything was done through others. I couldn't fire the professors; they effectively had jobs for life, as teachers and clinicians, unless they crossed the line and had sex with their patients or ran into difficulty with the standard of their care. Taking away teaching roles didn't make much of a difference; it wasn't highly valued at the level of undergraduate medical students at the time. I had far less control over the finances than I did at the Clarke and Toronto General; the money was distributed to each hospital group by my executive committee, and at the Clarke, another committee handled the funds from the university to the institute. In the academy, I knew my powers of influence were limited. Physicians could just say "Go to hell," and sometimes they did.

I had one significant lever—the bully pulpit. I was an ambassador of our profession to the public, and to politicians at all levels who were making key decisions about mental health care that would affect both patients and practitioners. I could use this power to speak out on topics I really cared about. Nothing would change overnight. Progress would be slow, especially among some psychiatric clans in the hospitals that saw no reason to change. But I was determined to persevere.

At the outset, I felt that many of the academic staff were not performing at the international level expected of a major university. It wasn't enough to be a decent person and a reasonable clinician. The university is in the business of knowledge, and of people. We generate knowledge, transmit it to the next generation—our students, clinicians, the public—and we store it, through publications. We prepared a new generation of people for practice and for academia. So we wanted excellence in all these areas—in the group, if not in each person. So, for example, if one of the hospital units had twelve psychiatrists, I thought we needed to have two or three researchers, five or six good teachers, and three people who could translate the discoveries in the lab into a form that made sense for students and the public. And all twelve had to be good clinicians in order to be role models, demonstrating scientific knowledge and the art of the profession.

But this had not been happening. Too often I'd see psychiatrists with academic appointments produce a modest research paper every two to five years, or even less. Many staff never gave an academic talk or published at all. It was a nice, comfortable life, but nothing like the publish-or-perish world I saw at distinguished universities in the United States. I didn't want to recreate their system; it felt heartless. But in the United States, money was a huge incentive: professors earned a low base salary and had to scramble for research funds from granting agencies, including for their personal support. This naturally made them very competitive on the research front. Our researchers, on the other hand, enjoyed a relatively high base salary; if they didn't win research funds from outside granting agencies, it didn't affect their personal or professional lives in a significant way. The only way to change the culture was by using funding as an incentive. In doing this I did try to be more even-keeled than I'd been at the General. Still, my impatience with the resistance to change eventually crept back into the discussions, and this caused frustration for me and the groups from each of the hospitals I was involved with. So I tried my best to praise the benefits to individuals and to the group of maintaining high academic standards.

I emphasized the "noble" academic enterprise every time I could. Every year since Robin Hunter's time, the department had had a cocktail party after Labour Day, in September, on the 12th floor of the Clarke. Its purpose was to welcome the new residents and reconnect faculty and residents after the summer. I continued this tradition, and added a component of my own, an annual lecture to precede the party. Each year I spent weeks preparing it, so that the standard was high, and I covered varied topics—for

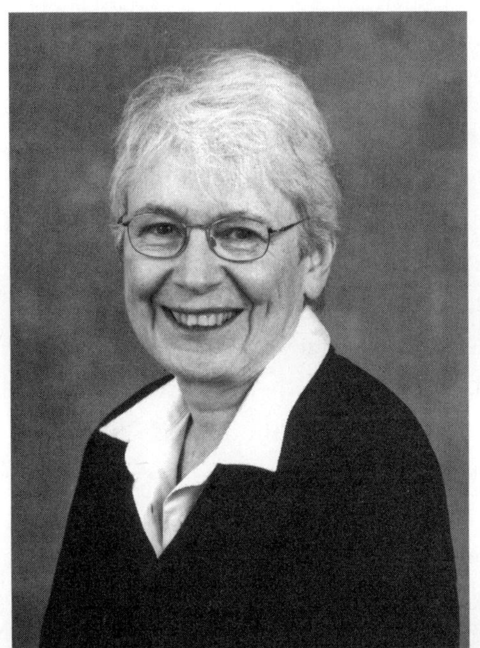

Mary Seeman, a professor of psychiatry, had an outstanding career working with women with schizophrenia. She was vice chair of the department of psychiatry from 1990 to 1995. She later became an Officer of the Order of Canada in recognition of her outstanding contributions. Courtesy University of Toronto Department of Psychiatry.

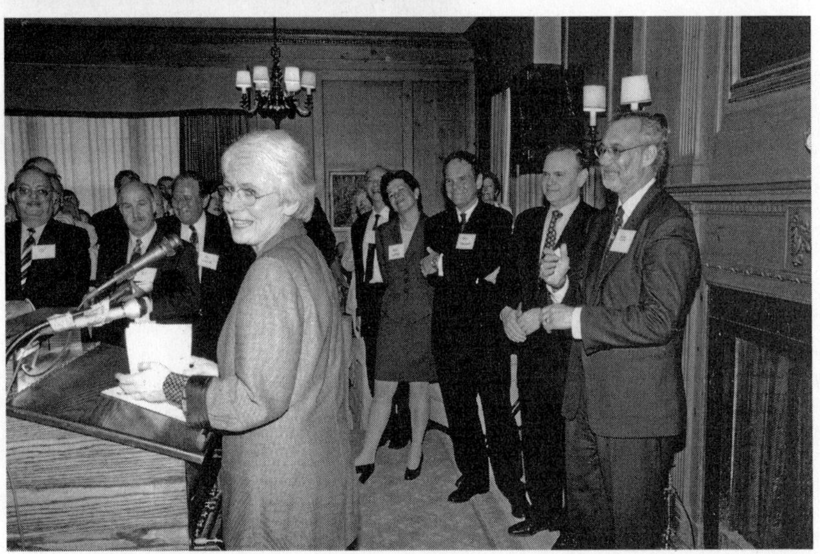

Mary Seeman being honoured with the Tapscott Chair in Schizophrenia studies. The five people behind Seeman are her husband Phil, philanthropists Ana Lopes and Don Tapscott, Dean Arnold Aberman, and Paul Garfinkel. Courtesy CAMH Archives.

example, the scholarship of teaching—to impress the fact that all aspects of the academy mattered.

At the lectern and at every other opportunity, I promoted the significance of the academic enterprise. Advances in patient care over the next generation depended on our ability to impart values, attitudes, and skills. Quoting Osler, I'd talk about how our world needs both science and art. I pressed my fellow psychiatrists to build bridges between science and the practice of psychiatry. Osler felt as relevant as ever, especially in a time when our profession had swung from an unscientific exploration in the realms of psychotherapy into an obsession with the laboratory and the chemistry and biology of the brain.

I tried to make academic promotions more meaningful. As had been done in our department for some time, we held public lectures for newly promoted professors. I made them special occasions. We held a book launch every year or two to celebrate books our faculty had written or edited, and we brought in prominent writers like Oliver Sacks or Hermione Lee as guest speakers.

To build bridges between science and caring, I expected all of the key people, apart from the research director, to be good clinicians; we were a clinical department, training future clinicians for Canada, after all. Mary Seeman, a compassionate psychiatrist who had built an international reputation studying women with schizophrenia, agreed to be my vice-chair.[1] All the key hospital chiefs—Gary Rodin at University Health Network, Ken Shulman at Sunnybrook, Susan Bradley at Hospital for Sick Children, Joel Sadavoy at Mount Sinai—were strong clinically. Shulman built a significant group of solid clinicians with exceptional expertise in teaching at Sunnybrook. At SickKids, Bradley developed the child program, with research on attachment, gender development, speech and language problems, and infancy. The Mount Sinai group under Seeman and later Sadavoy, continued its work on psychotherapies.

Rodin developed psychosomatics at University Health Network, where staff developed expertise on subjects like HIV, transplantation, oncology, and cardiac disease, which occupied the border between psychiatry and medicine.[2] While Goldbloom led the General Psychiatry program at the Clarke, Gail Robinson and Donna Stewart expanded the women's program and through their work with the medical school improved the training of future doctors.

I encouraged the study and evaluation of psychotherapy from many angles. At the Clarke, researchers like Zindel Segal and the team that developed around him tested and improved cognitive behaviour therapy. They showed how useful it was for depression and how refinements such as mindfulness-based cognitive therapy could play a role in preventing relapse. Shelley McMain started the newer dialectical behaviour therapy clinic for patients with borderline personality disorder so that they could learn distress tolerance and improve interpersonal functioning. She developed a superb clinical teaching program and became a leading teacher for younger colleagues. Interpersonal psychotherapies, based on dynamic theories and focused on relationship issues, were developed by Paula Ravitz, first at the Clarke and later at Mount Sinai. Excellence in group therapies was developed at Mount Sinai under Molyn Leszcz, a psychiatrist who had studied group psychotherapy in California. University Health Network did excellent work on psychotherapy for people with medical illnesses, helping them adjust to conditions like heart disease, cancer, and autoimmune illnesses.

If I wanted to make meaningful changes in the profession, I needed to promote the value of scholarship, including an attitude of critical enquiry, a capacity for self-scrutiny, and a desire to have one's work critiqued at a broad level. In a 1986 article, J.D. Burke, Harold Pincus, and Herb Pardes called this the intellectual orientation of science.[3] Learning what questions to ask and how to pursue them with rigour is much more important than any technical skills that are mastered. Scholarship implies intellectual tolerance, but with clear standards, and the relentless pursuit of scientific truth. It also implies a reflection on one's own activities and striving to make future endeavours meaningful both for oneself and for others.

Scholarship requires an acknowledgement that standards apply and that everyone plays by the same rules, the ones that force open debate, replication of findings, and distinction between a guess and a fact. The rules also involve review by our peers. It's true that the peer-review process has problems. For example, peer review can reflect an old boys' network, or a tendency to a conservative stance. Nevertheless, like democracy, peer review may not be perfect, but it's the best system we've got.

The standards of scholarship is not a theoretical topic. What we study and how we study determines new knowledge, which in turn creates new treatments. How we translate those treatments into practice influences the mental health of a large percentage of our population. I thought that we needed to broaden the definition of scholarship because it had become, by the early 1990s, a code word for neurobiology, that is, the work with animals in the lab or imaging studies of the brain or testing the response to new drugs. New technologies had made this a thrilling area of research, but I believed that it was essential to apply the highest level of inquiry to everything we did as an academic enterprise. We needed to ask: What is the best way to teach? What is the best way to translate psychiatric knowledge and make it more accessible for the students and the public? How do we make information broadly available?

To do this I encouraged the development of priority programs and appointed as their leaders people who were poised at the cusp of science and clinical care. David Goldbloom, for example, played a strong role in bringing new knowledge about our field into the public arena. Trevor Young and Arun Ravindran have educated the medical profession by translating developments in the pharmacology of mood disorders through their excellent consultations and presentations.

A prominent educator, Ernest Boyer, was the chancellor of the State University of New York and later president of the Carnegie Foundation for the Advancement of Teaching. He proposed four types of scholarship: (1) the scholarship of application, which includes building bridges between theory and practice, and showing theory and practice in vital interaction; (2) the scholarship of teaching, to transmit knowledge in a way that is applicable and inspiring; (3) the scholarship of integration, linking areas of study across disciplines and broadening the applications of research; and (4) the scholarship of discovery, for the generation of new knowledge.[4]

Just before he died in 1995, Boyer refined his ideal concerning the communal nature of the scholarship of teaching as the scholarship of sharing knowledge—"academics must continue to communicate ... in order to keep the flame of scholarship alive."[5] I took this new outlook to heart. I wanted to make sure all four forms of scholarship were practised at the highest level.

Overall, it is the quality of scholarship that counts, rather than the particular area of study. If the quality isn't maintained, standards gradually fall and, years later, the organization slips into mediocrity. Excellence, on the other hand, depends on the professional culture. People want to be excellent in a culture that values excellence, in a culture that celebrates it, rewards it, and hires for it. This includes the performance of superior clinicians; they are highly admired for excellence in clinical practices.

The Value of Mentorship

As chair of psychiatry, I was in charge of the teaching of psychiatry to residents, albeit from some distance day to day. I had been concerned about the training of physicians from the early days of my residency at the Clarke, when I learned that an unacceptably high percentage of young doctors fail their psychiatric exams, preventing them from entering the profession. Later on, as I became aware of the disturbingly high rate of depression and suicide among psychiatrists, I grew concerned that we as a profession were not doing enough to help our own—for their sake and for their patients'.

Now in my position as chair I had an opportunity to help by promoting mentorship. I was fortunate in my first years in Toronto and in psychiatry to have had exceptional mentors—Harvey Stancer, Vivian Rakoff, and Robin Hunter. My involvement with them occurred at a particular time in my life when I was not only developing as a professional but also losing both my parents and reflecting on relationships, generational issues, and the meaning of loss. I was incredibly grateful to have mentors at a time like that, and it made me think about the next generation and how I could do the same for them.

Mentors play a critical role not only in medicine but in business, sports, the arts, and other professions.[6] In a 1979 study of executives, Gerard Roche of Heidrick & Struggles found that people who have been mentored are generally happier with their careers than colleagues who have not.[7] The mentor is more than just an experienced colleague helping in career development; he or she is a trusted advisor with whom a close personal relationship develops. One identifies with a mentor, who in many ways is a model but also provides counsel and advice based on the best interests of the less experienced colleague.

People need different types of mentors for different phases of their careers. Early in your career, you may ask mentors to help you with specific skills such as interviewing, diagnosis, and treatment. Values and attitudes may also be imparted—getting involved in your community as an activist to improve the lives of the mentally ill, for example, or not trying to impose middle-class values on the underprivileged. But as you face mid-career challenges, mentoring is ideally tailored to your individual strengths and career goals. Mentors can increase access to career-advancement opportunities, or help you extend the skills honed in a current role and apply them to broader challenges. The way to attract mentors is by demonstrating experience and articulating eagerness for the next opportunity.

Young scientists need mentors of a special kind. They must learn to handle the frustrations and rejections of granting agencies, journal editors, and administrators; the feelings of rivalry and competitiveness of peers; and the multiple demands that eat into family life. It is so helpful to have regular contact with an experienced colleague who has been there. The problem, though, is the shortage of appropriate mentors. It can be a self-perpetuating problem. When R.A. Kirsling and M.S. Kochar surveyed senior medical faculty in the 1990s, they found that 90% had a mentor; among these, 81% who had a mentor indicated that they had served as a mentor to a younger medical colleague. By contrast, those not exposed to mentorship were themselves less likely to serve in this capacity later in their academic careers.[8]

I myself enjoyed being a mentor. Back in the 1970s, I started leading study groups to help residents prepare for their psychiatry exams. I held these study groups at my home Tuesday evenings, where we could relax and take whatever time was needed. Because I loved the historical literature on psychiatry, I insisted we review all the important literature and also cover specific topics for the exams. This mentoring quickly became one of the favourite parts of my job. Perhaps I was looking for a way to make up for the losses in my family life, but I also loved the collegiality and the discussions about controversial issues. Members of those groups have gone on to significant careers of their own. Gary Rodin, Charles

Marmor, Sid Kennedy, Allan Kaplan, Barbara Dorian, Christine Dunbar, Ken Shulman, Don Wasylenki, Art Sohn, Michael Rosenbluth, Dennis Weir, and Frances Frankenberg are just a few of the 40 or so people who made those Tuesdays so special.

Managing a Department

My responsibilities through the eight psychiatry departments in Toronto turned out to be so wide-ranging and complex that I needed to bolster my senior team. On the advice of a committee I formed in 1995 to advise me on governance, I expanded my leadership and management advisor from one person, Mary Seeman, to four portfolios. Shulman took charge of clinical affairs. Brian Hodges, a young and extremely energetic psychiatrist, would supervise education issues. Don Wasylenki, by then chief at St. Mike's, and Paula Goering, a health systems researcher at the Clarke, would oversee the development and coordination of programs. Greg Brown would run research.

Jean Simpson, my old friend and colleague, took over as chief operating officer of the Clarke. Simpson had successfully handled management jobs in industry and in the Ontario government, so I knew I count on her process-driven management style. I trusted her completely, and with this new team in place, I was ready to tackle several large issues.

One of the big challenges in our hospital network was the persistent overlapping of departments. Did it make any sense to have mood disorders specialty programs at Sunnybrook, Toronto General, and the Clarke? Tony Fell, the prominent Toronto business man who was at the helm of RBC Dominion Securities for many years, was also then chair of the board at University Health Network; he frequently said that if you could get competitive banks to agree on a common Visa card and bank machines, surely not-for-profit hospitals could collaborate on IT systems, clinical programs, and a great deal more.

I tried to get the psychiatrists to collaborate, but I often found that they clung to their fiefdoms. The Hospital for Sick Children, the Clarke, and the university, for instance, all had child and adolescent programs, so I persuaded them to search for a single leader after Susan Bradley retired. They complied and a leader was chosen, but only a few years later the hospitals went their separate ways (they have since reunited the program, in 2013). I had more success linking women's mental health programs at the Clarke and Women's College, through the appointment of a shared chief, Barbara Dorian. At the Clarke she consolidated an inpatient program for women who had been abused; at the Women's College site, she developed several outpatient and day programs for women who had been traumatized and for workers with physical and psychological injuries following industrial accidents. Yet I didn't have any success in getting the Clarke and Queen Street to collaborate on chronic schizophrenia. Why the differences? Usually they related to the people in charge of these programs and their willingness to collaborate and learn from each other.

The Axe Falls

I found myself in the uncomfortable position of handling the budget cuts foisted on me by the NDP government. At the start of the NDP mandate, I admired the party leader's determination to focus on the poor and the disenfranchised in our society, including the mentally ill patients who were left out in the cold, on the street. My admiration soon faded, though, when I saw how the government mismanaged its finances. The debt was becoming unmanageable. In the first five years of NDP rule, the ratio of debt to GDP had doubled; Ontario was spending nearly one-fifth of its revenues on interest payments alone. Ontario lost 40,000 jobs, and its finances were in such a mess that the NDP had to betray its own supporters in the public sector by freezing wages and giving civil servants extra days off without pay in order to cut costs.

Doctors were on the firing line. The government had from the very beginning insisted there were too many doctors costing too much money, and psychiatrists were deemed to be particularly expendable. To reduce the population of psychiatrists, the government cut the number of placements for residents. Over five years, the number of psychiatric residents declined from 120, to 105. This was painful for all of us and hurt everyone. Senior doctors lost their junior assistants, who had enabled them to accomplish much more, and also lost the pleasure of individualized teaching.

The budget cuts presented other challenges for the Psychiatry Department. We had to make some hard decisions. By the mid-1990s, we realized we were unable to support academic programs in all of our teaching hospitals, so we decided to merge two departments of psychiatry, at the Wellesley and St. Michael's. Staff at both hospitals were furious and vented their anger on me. By then I was used to it, but it wasn't exactly what I had signed up for. Nonetheless, I could see why they were so unhappy. The two departments did have distinct characteristics. The Wellesley was more interested in psychopharmacology, whereas St. Mike's prided itself on serving the needs of the downtown community, including the many homeless. Still, I convinced myself that this was for the good of the larger group. We had to make cuts or the whole psychiatric enterprise at the University of Toronto would be weakened. Of course, the merger meant there would be only one chief. The head of psychiatry at the Wellesley, George Awad, an excellent psychopharmacologist, was selected. This caused a great deal of uproar—people at both hospitals were angry. The head of St. Mike's, Isaac Sakinofsky, eventually came to the Clarke, but he was bitter. He had worked hard to build a good department, and I had killed it. It gave me another lesson in how painful these changes are for people who care for their local hospitals and their working arrangements. I had seen it at both Toronto General and the Western, and soon would see it again across the system.

As a psychiatrist, I know that endings are hard, and these types of decisions are exceptionally difficult. We are often afraid of making a mistake—maybe the problem is still fixable and we'll look foolish. We hate hurting someone or having a confrontation. People confuse hurting someone for a good purpose (having surgery, for example) with pain that is harmful and serves no higher purpose. When an organization is cut back, people might think *I'm a loser*—especially if compensation is tied to size and the strategy is geared for growth. For others, letting go might bring up hidden issues, like the fear of abandonment. Someone who has had many earlier painful losses may try to avoid endings. Many of us are afraid of the unknown.

For me, the key question was whether merging the departments of the two hospitals was necessary for the greater good. Coming to the answer required input from different people, but in the end I had to feel that this was what had to be done. One has to believe the change is necessary for the greater good or it will be too tempting to pull back rather than see colleagues be hurt.

Cutting departments or programs is one thing, but ending professional relationships is quite another. When Shitij Kapur told me he was leaving CAMH after 16 years to become the dean of the Institute of Psychiatry in London, England, I was upset, even though it was an amazing opportunity for him. He was in his early 40s and certainly one of the best people I had ever worked with. A week later, I realized it was a wonderful move for him and believed that the department should enthusiastically support him. I suppose I had evolved since Joffe told me 12 years earlier that he was moving to become chair of psychiatry at McMaster. That was also a promotion, and yet it felt like a personal hurt because of all the negative talk I was hearing from others about how he had felt poorly treated at the Clarke. Promotions can cause many types of feelings. We are proud of our colleagues' achievements and successes, but sometimes we feel left behind.[9]

There was one very awkward part of my job: the conflict of interest in being the CEO of the Clarke and being the university's chair of psychiatry. As chair, it was my job to decide how much money (out of a relatively small pot of $4 million) and how many students would be allocated to each hospital. But since I was CEO of the Clarke, I was determining some of the allocation of the budget of my own institution. I tried to get around this by assigning Swinson to represent the Clarke at university meetings, but there was no question that this was a conflict. Everyone scrutinized every penny that went to the Clarke during my time, and if anything, we took larger budget cuts from the Clarke (because it had other resources to draw on).

I was under pressure to split the two jobs, but I refused. The Clarke made a real contribution to the university. Its fundraising arm, set up under Rakoff, raised money not only for the Clarke but for the whole university. The Clarke needed the chair, I thought. It was vulnerable at this time, and I was worried that if I abandoned the top job there, it would be a further blow. So I kept the dual role. (The job was divided in two when my 10-year term at the university ended, but by then the Clarke had become part of CAMH.)

With the province in a serious recession, I knew I had to find other money for psychiatry. We ramped up our fundraising from philanthropists. Rakoff was a real pioneer here because he launched the Clarke Institute of Psychiatry Foundation, together with an energetic businessman, Arnie Cader, in late 1986. By 1988 the foundation had hired a director to raise funds to support the operation of the PET program. Then, in the early 1990s, the president of the university, Rob Prichard, began a large fundraising campaign. The other teaching hospitals were excelling in the fundraising business too. We began to use the Clarke Foundation to raise funds for academic chairs and professorships, first with the Tapscott family for a chair in schizophrenia studies in 1994, and then with former federal finance minister The Honourable Michael Wilson and his wife, Margie, for the Cameron Wilson Chair in Depression Studies in 1996. A determined woman, Doris Sommer-Rotenberg, raised funds for the first-ever chair in suicide studies, which we located at St. Michael's Hospital. Together with Women's College Hospital we developed the Shirley Brown Chair in women's mental health. We also obtained federal funding for a professorship in transcultural psychiatry. Later in the 1990s, Prime Minister Jean Chrétien's Liberal federal government began a process of funding chairs throughout the country, and we capitalized on this as well. Now more than 25 chairs are awarded to members in the Department of Psychiatry, with at least one in each of the teaching hospitals. These chairs put us on a solid base for scholarship. Not only do they emphasize the department's academic priorities but they protect the department from recessions (they account for about 30% of the department's $7 million annual budget). They also help us attract the best people and students to these programs. Significantly, they have connected academic psychiatry to some of the most altruistic citizens of our country: people who have become partners in fighting stigma and arguing for a fair share of dollars to this orphan field. We did very well in raising funds for the department, and despite the challenges along the way, we were second only to the large Department of Medicine in chairs that have been endowed in the faculty. The Clarke Foundation was a huge benefit to the university Psychiatry Department; because of this foundation and later CAMH's foundation, University of Toronto's Psychiatry has raised more external funds than any psychiatric group, anywhere.

During the 1990s, our university department emphasized several other issues, such as the role of women. We developed policies on harassment and boundary violations. We also improved the recognition and respect of teachers, including part-time faculty. The Faculty of Medicine switched to a new problem-based curriculum that had been so successful at McMaster, Calgary, and Harvard Medical School. Rather than traditional departmental teaching in lectures, this approach emphasized small-group, interdisciplinary, clinical problem-based learning. The psychiatry staff flourished with this new approach to teaching.

We increased our emphasis on developing teachers in those years. Teaching became another program unto itself, with an emphasis on how to develop someone as a teacher, and how to provide resources, rewards, and respect for teaching. Brian Hodges, my former resident, excelled as leader. Ivan Silver, an excellent geriatric psychiatrist at Sunnybrook, expanded continuing education and did a superb job in producing psychiatry leaders. Mark Hanson, a child and adolescent psychiatrist, improved undergraduate education. Jody Lofchy developed a summer institute for a subgroup of medical students to attract them to the field of psychiatry. The results have been outstanding in drawing people serious about a career in psychiatry to the University of Toronto.

There were disappointments too. Residents rebelled against the director of postgraduate education because they alleged they were treated unfairly. I listened carefully to the residents, but I dithered for months. I knew this director couldn't stay without the confidence of the residents' group, but I wanted to avoid a confrontation. Everyone suffered. In the end, I terminated his second term considerably early. Once he moved on, I appointed Allan Kaplan, a trusted junior colleague, and he established a very good, trusting relationship with the residents and the hospitals over the following decade.

Up North

The Clarke had long had a program on Baffin Island. I went there in the 1970s, and the program continues to this day; about 500 people were assessed in 2012. The University of Toronto's Faculty of Medicine had already developed a good program for medical care in Sioux Lookout, in northwestern Ontario, a medical service that included psychiatric care and was very active. But people in most parts of the province still didn't get the psychiatric treatment they needed, so they had to be referred to psychiatrists in a big city. This wasn't acceptable; people should have access to mental health care near their homes. So we as a department developed an outreach program, beginning in Kenora, Ontario. Under the leadership of Brian Hodges, we linked the five psychiatry teaching programs in Ontario with psychiatrists and residents travelling to many communities, including Baffin and Sioux Lookout. This has now created a large outreach program. By 2012, 40 psychiatrists and more than 70 residents from the University of Toronto spent about 300 days in 10 Ontario communities. About 2,000 patients are treated annually. These are people who would not have previously received treatment, or who would have had to travel to larger cities. The system is self-perpetuating, since new psychiatrists join the outreach program every year. A few years after the outreach program was established, the department took another step and began a program that sent psychiatrists to communities for a few months at a time. This is a temporary arrangement for communities lacking full-time psychiatrists, and both the community and the psychiatrist generally benefit; some psychiatrists even decide to stay on for several years. Finally, we added videoconferencing to the mix; patients did 4,165 sessions this way between 2005 and 2012. At first, staff were skeptical about videoconferences; surely they couldn't be as effective as a meeting in person. So we were pleasantly surprised at the results of an evaluation: the assessments and treatments were just as valuable and well-received by the patients and referring doctors as were face-to-face meetings. It's true that our staff didn't enjoy it as much as a regular office visit, but considering the size of Ontario, this is a hugely valuable service. I think that in this digital age, with so many electronic tools available, much long-distance therapy can be done.

• • •

In the late 1990s as I started to contemplate the end of my term as chair of psychiatry and CEO of the Clarke, I was feeling increasingly isolated. I had taken on the mantle of leadership, and although I thoroughly valued it, the role was unsettling. This is perfectly natural, as leadership involves an inner transformation, which may involve a shift in core identity and a significant change in relationships. I was spending more and more time alone, and my marriage was starting to fall apart. At that time I really appreciated the words of the great French poet Anatole France: "All changes, even the most longed for, have their melancholy; for what we leave behind us is a part of ourselves; we must die to one life before we can enter another."

For many years, Dorothy and I had a satisfying marriage as we raised three boys and carried on a busy life. We were much less connected by the mid-1990s when I became overwhelmingly busy with the merger of the hospitals that formed CAMH and was also teaching in Italy. We divorced in 2000 after 32 years of marriage. It is one of my life's real regrets that our marriage didn't endure.

Barbara Dorian had worked with me in 1979 as a resident and then later as a research fellow. After coming back from Stanford, she joined the staff at Toronto General. In 1994 she left Toronto General and joined the Mount Sinai group. When I was part of the search committee selecting a new chief of psychiatry at Women's College in 1996, we appointed Barbara to the position, and she and I again worked closely together. As my marriage ended, Barb and I developed a personal relationship, which eventually included her daughter Lindsay. This connection has been hugely rewarding for me personally and a wonderful support for my work.

As it turned out, Anatole France's eloquent words would sustain me in the challenging years ahead. I had been so focused on the demands of running the Clarke and the university Psychiatry Department that I didn't see clearly the profound changes occurring outside, in the community and in the political world. My world as a psychiatrist and as a leader in psychiatry was about to be rocked, in ways I could never expect.

CHAPTER 17

Who Do We Serve?

When I was chair of psychiatry, I often drove three kilometres west from my office at the Clarke to the Queen Street Mental Health Centre, on the site of the old asylum. In those days, the neighbourhood around the hospital was poor and depressing. I usually saw homeless people hanging out on the street. They were clearly ill, talking to themselves, begging for money, or wandering aimlessly with a grocery cart of their possessions, and I suspected that they were not able to access the treatment that could have helped them live more fulfilling lives.

These were people with the most serious psychiatric issues, the chronically ill living on the streets or in the woods, in slums or in jails. They were the sickest, from a mental health point of view, and yet our profession wasn't taking care of them. For the most part, we weren't interested in them.

It was a sign of a big and unacceptable gap. Scientists in the lab had made some astounding discoveries that could relieve the terror of hallucinations and the misery of depression. Evidence was starting to demonstrate the healing power of some of the talk therapies, such as cognitive behaviour therapy, and interpersonal and dynamic therapies. We were starting to see that, together, drugs and therapy could give people with depression, bulimia, and bipolar illness a full and rewarding life. But, somehow, we were not delivering this knowledge to the street, where some of the sickest patients were. It turned out, as a 2004 study later showed, that we were reaching only one-third of the people who needed psychiatric care. Two out of three patients would not or could not see a psychiatrist and get the drugs and therapy that could significantly improve their lives—this was as true of the 5% of the population with severe and persistent mental illness as it was for those with more mild forms of disability.[1] Over the last decade, the frequency of mental illness has remained constant, but large US studies show that the likelihood of being treated had increased from 20 to 33%, a significant gain that also demonstrates the huge unmet need, one that was readily apparent to me each time I ventured down to Queen Street.

The saddest thing was that this gap didn't just separate us from the very people we were supposed to treat; it fed the stigma that is so painful for people with mental illness. They were the outsiders—we were the insiders. Of all people, we should have reached out. And yet most of us, including me, didn't.

It took me a long time to appreciate the depth of this problem. At the outset, like academic physicians anywhere, I was focused on the goals of my research, solving one of the riddles that blocked our understanding of the chemistry of depression, or probing the mystery of anorexia nervosa. My office practice and the ward where I looked after patients were as busy as could be. My graduate students were curious and motivated. The residents were eager to learn the skills of the profession. Later, as a manager of psychiatrists, I tried to make connections between clinical care, research, and education, and between psychiatry in general hospitals and a specialist hospital like the Clarke. I tried to balance compassion and science at a time when our profession seemed to think that you had to choose one or the other. Only gradually did I come to realize that one of the biggest gaps was between us, the psychiatrists, and our own patients.

The problem emerged in the 1960s when mentally ill patients were dispatched from the asylums. In the 1960s and 1970s, Ontario closed 7,000 of the 11,000 psychiatric beds in provincial hospitals. By the time the wrecking ball demolished the grand old relic of Victoriana in the early 1970s, the resident population of the Queen Street mental hospital had dropped from a peak of 1,200 in the 1950s to just 400. There were valid reasons for this exodus from the mental hospital, such as the new drugs to relieve psychosis, as well as the furor over the soul-destroying features of institutional life. One of the big drivers, however, had nothing to do with the care of the patients and everything to do with money: the desire to spend less on the health of people with mental illness. As a result, there was no real investment in community programs to help mentally ill people live outside a hospital until the late 1970s, long after they had left the asylum. The funds that were reinvested into the community in the 1980s and 1990s were tiny relative to the need. The result was what I saw on the street—homeless patients, often cold and hungry, with nowhere to go and no one to care for them.

Other countries have acted decisively to improve services for psychiatric patients in the community.[2] In Ontario, the government's response was predictable: many well-written reports but little action.

The *Graham Report* in the late 1980s said we should focus on services for people with serious and persistent mental illness.[3] Ontario psychiatrists, Provincial District Health Councils chairman Robert Graham advised, should be treating the 3% of the population with severe impairment from their illness, rather than the 15% who were less impaired. (Impairment had previously been equated with diagnoses such as schizophrenia and bipolar illness, but that doesn't reveal how sick someone is. By the late 1980s impairment was thought to cross different diagnostic lines and referred to the degree to which the illness interferes with home life, work, and social skills, as well as activities of daily living.) The *Graham Report* proposed a plan for the development and implementation of a comprehensive community mental health system. There was never any real follow-through.

Five years later, another report, *Putting People First: The Reform of Mental Health Services in Ontario*, issued by the Ontario Ministry of Health, went further. It recommended that 60% of the government's spending on mental health should go to community services and 40% to hospital care. This would reverse over a 10-year period the traditional funding allocations, in my view a much-needed development. Over the next decade, psychiatric hospital beds were reduced from 58 beds per 100,000 people, to the targeted 30 beds through cuts to the 10 psychiatric hospitals directly operated by the Ministry of Health.

Meanwhile, Ontario acted slowly in the 1990s to develop effective and accessible services delivered in the community. Assertive community-treatment teams began to spring up. These multidisciplinary teams, composed like whole hospital teams, went out to the patients, instead of asking them to visit the hospital. This was mostly a good thing for patients, but the idea that people with schizophrenia were living in the community still scared many members of the public. Fear and prejudice prevented true integration, especially related to work and housing. There was too little support in the community for seriously ill people. Reducing the number of asylum beds was potentially such a positive development, but with no follow-through nor a network of community supports, many patients were worse off than in the days of the asylum.

I have been emphasizing the inadequate staff and lack of funding support for the community-treatment model. But this was complicated by other factors—some patients refused to come for treatment, or even to be labelled as ill. Others stopped their medications frequently, and most found that the communities did not welcome them. Some patients with schizophrenia had deficits in their capacity to plan for and follow a treatment routine. Without regular structure or supervision, mental illness spiralled them downward into behaviours or situations that ended in their living on the streets or in jails, and losing touch with their after-care clinicians.

The tragic result was that the gap between people with mental illness and the rest of society widened. Instead of caring for mentally ill citizens in the asylum, we left them on the street and impoverished, with too little help to manage even the basic necessities of life. Often, as noted, they ended up in jail, which is where they were before the asylums emerged in the mid-1800s to provide humane care for the mentally ill. As the gap between us and them widened, it was all too easy to fall for any number of stereotypes about people struggling with mental illness and to rationalize our own behaviour.

It didn't help that the media sensationalized every episode of violence involving people with psychosis. In 1995, a broadcaster and ex-hockey player, Brian Smith, was shot in a parking lot by a man with delusions that the radio was broadcasting messages into his head. To calm a frightened public, the Ontario government passed Bill 68, broadening the criteria under the Mental Health Act that enabled family members to commit a relative to a hospital. It also made it possible for the first time to force some patients (after repeated hospital admissions for psychosis) to take medication whenever they did not comply with the doctor's prescription after leaving hospital. These were Community Treatment Orders (CTOs). I spoke against the proposed new law initially, believing it infringed on civil liberties excessively. Most of us would agree that a severely delusional person who is about to cause harm should be detained in hospital, and when people don't comply with treatment and have potential to cause severe harm, it also makes sense to detain them. But it seemed excessive to order them to take their drugs when they weren't psychotic or threatening, just because of their potential to decompensate. I thought we could achieve this by different means, by the patient signing an advanced treatment directive when well, perhaps. CTOs have since been used carefully and rarely for people with multiple recurrences of psychosis after stopping medications and have been found to be useful in some settings but not others.[4]

Irrational fears about mental illness were firmly entrenched. According to a 1998 survey of nearly 3,000 people in Britain, over 70% believed that people with schizophrenia could be dangerous to others.[5] Nearly one-quarter thought that people suffering depression could be dangerous to others. These attitudes ignore the facts. Studies show that only about 4% of crime is related to mental illness. In fact, the mentally ill are more likely to be the victims of crime than those in the general population. Five times more crimes are committed against the mentally ill than the other way around. One Danish population study revealed that the mentally ill have a sixfold increase in the risk of being murdered; the highest risk occurred for those with substance abuse, personality disorders, and schizophrenia. They are more dangerous to themselves than they are to others: between 20 and 40% of people with schizophrenia make at least one suicide attempt.

What's more, people with serious and persistent mental illnesses die early. In Ontario, a man with schizophrenia has a life expectancy of 60 years, about 20 years less than those in the general population. One contribution to this problem is the medication we use to treat psychosis. The newer "atypical" antipsychotics, which have been heavily marketed by drug companies, are associated with severe weight gain and type 2 diabetes. These newer drugs do have an advantage, though: they are less likely to produce neurological side effects, and some patients find them more effective than previous drugs. Poor diet, lack of exercise, high rates of smoking, and lack of consistent medical care also contribute to early death.

In the British survey conducted for the Royal College of Psychiatrists, a substantial number of respondents blamed the mentally ill for their illness. One-third said that a person with an eating disorder caused her own condition; one-half felt an alcoholic could just pull himself together to be well. Fifteen percent of the population related mental illness to a lack of self-discipline and willpower, a number almost unchanged since an earlier British report in the mid-1990s.

In other surveys, respondents made it clear they feared the mentally ill, didn't respect them, and didn't want to socialize with them. In a survey that I later conducted in 2005 with Ed Adlaf and David Goldbloom, half of the respondents said they wouldn't want to live next to, or work next to, someone who has schizophrenia; one-quarter felt that way about a person with depression. An Austrian study in 2003 revealed that over half the population think that people who have been in a mental hospital are less intelligent and less trustworthy than the general public, and that the hospital stay was a sign of personal failure.[6]

Perhaps it is no surprise that physicians, including psychiatrists, share with the general public some of the stigmatizing views of people with mental illness. I saw this over and over again in the way that some mental health professionals treated the people under their care and even, by extension, in the way that I was treated by other physicians in my first years in practice. In 1998, when CAMH was formed, the organization's mental hospital treated many people with chronic schizophrenia. One day, I noticed the staff were covering the sofa in the common lounge with a blanket whenever they sat down. The reason: the staff thought that the patients with schizophrenia were unclean and could carry disease. Imagine the message this conveyed to the patients.

Another sad story is told in James FitzGerald's book about his family.[7] His grandfather, Dr. John Gerald FitzGerald, was a leading figure in Canadian medicine, a public-health expert who had a huge impact on the world. He later became dean of medicine at the University of Toronto. He experienced serious recurrent depressions but did not get adequate treatment, though he saw the leading psychiatrists of Toronto and Connecticut. He eventually killed himself in 1940 in Toronto General Hospital by slashing his femoral artery. The Medical Faculty, Toronto General, and his family hid his story for years, until his grandson, James, published it in 2010. Depression and suicide were cause for shame even among doctors, who seemingly can deal with illness and tragedy.

A patient I saw in a general hospital was admitted to an obstetrics unit. She was five months pregnant and abusing laxatives for weight loss. The nurses on this floor kept the door to her room shut and provided only minimal care in a hostile fashion, as they were so angry that she was "deliberately" hurting her unborn baby. Women with addictions particularly face difficulties obtaining care when pregnant. They are often viewed as irresponsible, immoral, and promiscuous by the very people they turn to for help. These attitudes greatly hinder a woman's ability to get treatment when she most needs help to get off drugs.

The discrimination against patients is patently illogical. Some caregivers think hearing voices because of depression is the person's fault, yet they would never accuse a person with hallucinations because of a brain tumour, an observable medical condition, of such a thing. Collectively, we display similar attitudes. As a society, we tolerate a health care system that houses people with addiction and mental illness in dilapidated buildings where conditions are worse than most prisons. We don't protest when there is not enough community treatment for people with mental illness—but we complain loudly if we wait too long for an MRI of our sore knee.

"Physicians are a reflection of their society when it comes to stigmatizing attitudes, but it's devastating when patients who need help encounter such attitudes," explained Dr. Manon Charbonneau, chair of the Canadian Psychiatric Association's 2011 Stigma and Discrimination Working Group.[8] Yet it happens. We are frightened by the strange behaviours or because these disorders affect our minds. Our minds represent our identities. We can be whole and ourselves if we have heart disease or cancer, but we fear the loss of our identity when our minds and personalities are altered. We fear the perceptions of the external world in a family with a mentally ill person, and in some cultures, the marriage prospects of other children are even affected.

Psychiatric Stigma toward the Mentally Ill

I have been a swimmer for more than 30 years, and one of CAMH's sites, at Queen Street, had a lovely pool that was open to staff from noon to 1 p.m., before it reopened to the patients for the afternoon. One day, when I was late to the pool, I finished my swim after one o'clock, and by the time I got out of the shower, I realized I was standing, nude, in the changing room with four or five male patients with varying degrees of psychosis. They were getting undressed and ready to swim. My response to this situation startled me. Without the costume of the CEO or of the physician, I felt ill at ease and was in a hurry to get dressed and get out.

I like to think that after 35 years I am comfortable and without prejudice toward those who are ill (and comfortable in dressing rooms). My response showed me otherwise, and it humbled me. It made me wonder about the subtle ways in which we all think and behave that perpetuate the very stigma we claim to be determined to eradicate. After this episode, I made it a point to swim late more often, until I was completely comfortable with my swimming buddies.

Many psychiatrists I know are compassionate and comfortable with mentally ill people. Psychiatrists as a group display more positive attitudes to the mentally ill than does the general public, according to a few European surveys. They are also more optimistic about recovery and far less concerned about violence. The same holds for residents in psychiatry in comparison to their medical colleagues.

But in other ways, psychiatrists contribute to the stigma—the experience of the mentally ill is that they often describe feeling patronized, punished, or demeaned by mental health professionals.[9] They complain that they are left out of decisions regarding their care, or not told of various treatment options, or spoken to like children. We sometimes use labels in a pejorative way—"hysteria" was such a term in the 1970s, only to be replaced by "borderline" in the 1990s.[10] Attitudes reflecting ignorance and fear develop early, often in medical school, and are directed to people who are seen as undeserving of treatment. Directing most of our treatment resources to less severe conditions may also reflect a type of stigma. Patients who have been hospitalized may have to wait a month to be seen in follow-up after discharge. In a Toronto study, only 44% of psychiatrists said they could see a new patient urgently within a week, compared with 60 to 80% of other specialists.[11] How could this be?

The number of psychiatrists is not the problem. Canada has sufficient psychiatrists: 13.2 per 100,000 people, far more than the number the World Health Organization says is reasonable (9.8 per 100,000)—although many of them are crowded into Toronto, which has 42 per 100,000, the highest concentration of psychiatrists in the country.

So what made it so difficult for a sick person to find a psychiatrist? Paul Kurdyak evaluated all office-based billings by Ontario's psychiatrists over a two-year period, from 2007 to 2009. Kurdyak found what we had been seeing decades earlier: more than half of the psychiatrists who graduated from the University of Toronto in the 1980s set up offices to deal with the worried

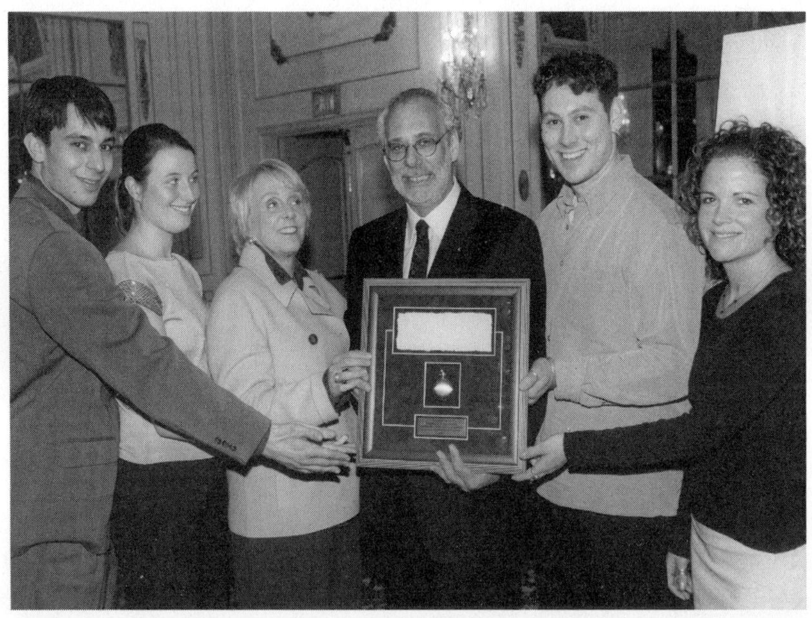

Honoured by the Schizophrenia Society of Canada, with Josh and Tiff Garfinkel, Barbara Dorian, and Steve and Leanne Garfinkel.

well—people who might have mild to moderate depression, anxiety, interpersonal problems, or personality challenges but who were not seriously ill.

It was nice work: the therapists enjoyed a steady income from people, often from professional or upper-income brackets, who came once or twice a week, sometimes for years. They worked regular office hours and didn't often have to respond to middle-of-the-night calls. This is not to say that these patients do not need treatment—most do. But many could be treated successfully with fewer visits, every two to four weeks, for example, or intermittently when problems recur. Yet they kept up their regular visits; they were the bread and butter of the private practitioners.

Pursuing an analytic or psychodynamic practice was certainly more lucrative and perhaps more readily rewarding than being a state employee in a mental hospital. There was little financial incentive to open up time for people with serious chronic illnesses like schizophrenia, which couldn't be cured by therapy alone, or even by a solo practitioner—a team effort was required to provide the necessary care.

All this therapy was being paid for by the Ontario government, and still the ample psychiatric care didn't help people who were mentally ill on the street or struggling with an active psychotic state. These people were left out in the dark. All the therapy for the moderately ill didn't even cut the hospitalization rate or reduce trips to the ER.

Even before these staggering reports were written, in the mid-1990s, it was clear that we were not taking care of the sickest members of our society.[12] I wanted to do something, but was it really my job? Some of my colleagues said no: our job, as university professors, was to educate doctors, psychiatrists, and other health care providers for the future, and to advance research and define new treatment for the future. It was not our role to decide who got the treatment: that was the job of government and our medical associations.

That was my position when I took over as chair of psychiatry in 1990. I was focused on my big goals of fusing science and compassion, bridging the gap between research and practice, and teaching multidimensional models of illness. But I would soon change.

A couple of years after I took over the Clarke, I was invited to the University of Toronto president's beautiful house in Rosedale to hear a speech by the new NDP minister of health, Ruth Grier. She was a real critic of the cozy world of the taxpayer-funded Toronto psychotherapist. Toronto's psychiatry, she complained, had performed poorly in meeting the province's needs, and office-based psychiatry was on its way out. I sat among other guests, smouldering with embarrassment. I couldn't respond because

I knew she was largely right. Office-based psychotherapy would disappear, deservedly so, if we didn't attend to the problems of the very ill.

I had come to understand this problem, and it was complicated. We were not doing enough to help our most severely ill patients. In fact, the care outside the hospital was so lacking that we were actually having to keep patients in hospital for longer than necessary. Despite all the bed reductions imposed on us, we were keeping people in hospital when they were ready for outpatient treatment. One key reason was that there was no decent place to send them. This was confirmed in a 1998 study of the inpatients at the Queen Street mental hospital that found that only 10% of the patients there needed that level of care, and another 45% needed some form of residential treatment. The remaining 45% could be better treated outside the hospital—in intensive community treatment (28%), community treatment (9%), or self-care (9%). This situation is a symptom of a huge problem in Ontario. We have so few resources for long-term care that we keep people in hospital beds (usually 12 to 20% of inpatients, depending on the setting), where they have a poor quality of life and block access for people who really need to be hospitalized.

While I was considering this problem, researchers asked patients what they felt they needed. Their answers were illuminating. Foremost they needed a job, skills training or education, and a connection to available services. Other needs identified in order of importance were income support, transportation, crisis management, counselling or therapy, and dental care. These kinds of studies, as well as those by more-vocal consumer groups, helped make us focus on the social determinants of health. If we really wanted to do something valuable for mentally ill people, these were the things to tackle. The job of helping mentally ill patients was about to get much larger.

By 1995, as my first term at the Clarke was ending, I was compelled to act. The men and women I saw on the street every day made me want to expand the goals for my profession and the university. This, I decided, was my responsibility: I had to find a way for my profession to care for the most vulnerable in our society.

I made my first step in 1995, while the NDP was still in power. The District Health Council of Toronto asked for advice on this issue. I chaired a group that made a number of suggestions in 1996. We agreed on the need to focus on the seriously ill, and the need for better access. Among other things, we suggested that new psychiatry graduates who wanted to practise in the city be required to provide service for the chronically ill. This could be as little as one day a month providing treatment in hospitals, community agencies, shelters, or jails. The remainder of the time they could attend to private practice and psychotherapy, but in the hospital they would be in touch with colleagues, attend rounds, have their work assessed, and contribute to caring for very ill people. A second recommendation was aimed at having physicians scrutinize their own practice patterns: if someone was seeing a patient in his or her office weekly or more often for over two years, without improvement, a second opinion by a colleague was warranted. I myself often request second opinions—we always learn, both the patient and me. This proposal also required the doctor and patient to clarify the goals of the further treatment, something that can get lost as therapy goes on.

After that proposal came out, I was invited by the Ontario Psychiatric Association to address the doctors at the Clarke to "explain" the proposal. The talk was on a Sunday, and I turned up in a tuxedo, as I was on my way to a wedding. The reception was frosty, to put it mildly. Clearly, the psychiatrists of Ontario didn't want change.

This was the mid-1990s and we were distancing ourselves from the very people we were supposed to help. Looking back, I suspect that the real issue was the ancient stigma against mentally ill people, the same stigma that has made its appearance in survey after survey. These psychiatrists obviously didn't want to deal with the people with the deepest mental health problems. They didn't want to see them on a regular basis. In this respect, I think the psychiatrists shared with other doctors and with the general public negative attitudes toward mental illness, even though they were the ones who were supposed to take care of them.

Strangely enough, it wasn't the socially minded NDP that finally shook psychiatrists out of their complacency. The impetus for change came from the 1995 election of the right-wing government of Conservative premier Mike Harris. Although the mental health of the men and women on the street was not the new government's primary concern, the Harris government would provoke a shakeup, and it would finally give us an opportunity to bring people who have been out in the cold into the heart of our mental health system.

CHAPTER 18
End of an Era

The news hit on August 13, 1996. The Clarke was going to close. According to a leaked provincial government report published in the *Toronto Star*, our hospital was to be merged with the Queen Street Mental Health Centre. The news sparked a furor at the Clarke.

It was a tumultuous time. The political climate in Ontario had been transformed since Mike Harris's Conservative government had swept to power in 1995, promising that the Common Sense Revolution would downsize government and restore the health of free enterprise. A radical change for Ontario was underway. For 42 consecutive years, the province had been governed by middle-of-the-road Tories, followed in 1985 by Liberals and then social democrats, who both favoured socially progressive legislation.

Now the new premier, Conservative Mike Harris, was leading a swing to the right: books had to be balanced, taxes could not be raised, more people had to get off welfare and back to work. While the Rae government thought doctors were too expensive—they were estimated to cost the public purse about $500,000 per physician (in compensation and diagnostic tests ordered)—the Harris government had a far more radical agenda. The Common Sense Revolution was a Darwinian exercise. It favoured the strong and denigrated the weak. Social programs would be cut or passed on to other levels of government, or costs returned to families who often could not afford them.

One of the government's first targets was health care. The health budget was 32% of the entire provincial budget, and hospitals accounted for 41% of it. The cost of health care was contributing to Ontario's $10 billion-plus deficit. There were many reasons for the escalating costs of health care—more elderly people, more expensive diagnostic tests, and more expensive medications, to name just a few. That didn't seem to matter. The focus was on inefficiencies in the health care system, and one way to deal with this was to merge hospitals, especially small ones like the Clarke.

The writing was on the wall. The year before the announcement, we had been hit by a surprise 8% budget cut, following four years of snipping. The Clarke had been shrunk to 88 beds, less than half the number it was in the 1970s, when I was working there as a resident. This was an impossible situation. As Ted Tremain, our board chair, explained, small didn't work for a hospital. We had to pay for cleaning and laundry just like any large hospital, but we had fewer resources to do it.

Tremain had urged me to think hard about the future: "You have an opportunity to do something significant, to do what's best for the people with mental illnesses, not what's best for Paul Garfinkel or the academic community," he said. I knew even then, a year before the *Toronto Star* article was published, that in the fiscally brutal climate of the Harris years, a merger might be the only way to guarantee the Clarke's survival.

With that in mind, I had already begun to strategize. The most obvious candidate for a merger was our neighbour, the Addiction Research Foundation, founded in 1949 to prevent and reduce harm from alcohol, tobacco, and other drug abuse. The ARF also operated a treatment centre for 4,000 addicts a year, with 530 staff and a budget roughly the same as the Clarke's. We shared a parking garage, and there were many reasons to share much more. We were both small, and getting sharp cuts from the Rae and then the Harris governments. Most important, we treated many of the same clients.

Many people with addictions have some form of mental illness, and people with mental illness frequently suffer from addictions. At least 50% of people with an addiction have a mental illness, and the overlap is even bigger in some groups. Of those attending a clinic for opiate abuse, for instance, 70% have a mental illness. Of those with an eating disorder, 40% have an addiction. When patients with schizophrenia leave hospital, their problems with addiction skyrocket. Violence connected to schizophrenia is related to two things: the person discontinuing his or her medications, and substance abuse.

Not only do mental illnesses and addictions co-occur, but researchers in both institutions were studying similar things, such as the role of neurotransmitters, the impact of early trauma and loss, and the influence of genetics. We know from autopsies that people who impulsively kill themselves have reduced levels of serotonin in their brains. Although the dopamine reward system plays a key role in the neurobiology of addiction, lowered serotonin occurs in some withdrawal states. The crossover between addiction and mental illness is substantial. Impulse control problems occur in addictions, bulimia, borderline personality, and chronic suicidality. Sexual abuse is three to four times as common in people with addictions, eating disorders, and depression than it is in the general population, according to our studies in Ontario in the 1990s. Couldn't we learn more if researchers collaborated, even if they worked across the street?

We shared an intellectual enterprise, but in the 1980s, the only thing we could agree on sharing was that parking garage. This reluctance to join forces has deep roots in the philosophical divide between addictions and psychiatry, which itself dates back some 70 years, to the founding of Alcoholics Anonymous. AA viewed addiction as a spiritual problem, not a medical one, and as a spiritual problem it could be addressed by a 12-step program, with support from the peer group and its appeal to a higher power. This approach has worked for many alcoholics and drug users, but its underlying belief system had helped create an unfortunate split with psychiatry. The addictions group resented that psychiatrists emphasized pathology—the causes, processes, development, and consequences—of the problem rather than the strengths of the individual. The use of medicines was seen as antithetical to the spiritual recovery model. Because of this split we learned little about addictions in medical school or during residency. We didn't teach the next generation of psychiatrists about addictions either. We assumed addictions were not our field, even though over half of our patients struggled with an addiction.

To my mind, a merger with the ARF, as difficult as it might be, made a lot of sense: it would be of great potential benefit to our patients, to the field of addictions, and mental health.

Early in 1996, before the new government announced its plans for Ontario's hospitals, we jointly asked for an external consulting group to advise on where the Clarke and the ARF could profitably link services. The group focused on the library and pharmacy (the ARF had 160 people on methadone daily); but rather than act, management from both sites decided to wait for a full external review of the ARF, scheduled for later that year.

While we were mulling over the merger issues, Harris was charging ahead, and he wasn't the kind to waste time. His government had set up the independent Health Services Restructuring Commission to study the province, region by region, and make decisions regarding the hospital requirements. This commission, at arm's length from government, had the power to issue directives—not suggestions—for the Clarke and also for every other hospital in the province.

This commission was set up to be removed from political considerations. The chair was Duncan Sinclair, a former dean of medicine at Queen's University. A veterinarian by training, Sinclair is one of the most straightforward men you could hope to meet. "We've got to do something dramatic; the government is out of money," he told the CBC after he was appointed. When he was asked why the government should target hospitals instead of other parts of the health care system, he said this: "Why do bank robbers rob banks? Because that's where the money is." He appointed as CEO of the restructuring commission Mark Rochon, a young, thoughtful, and experienced hospital executive who had once served as the Clarke's comptroller, and later served as an assistant deputy minister of health, so he knew the hospital system inside out.

In the spring of 1996, the Health Services Restructuring Commission began its work. In June, Andrea Baumann, dean of nursing at McMaster and the incoming chair of the Clarke board, and I were invited to appear and give our recommendations for the Clarke. We provided five possible candidates for Clarke partners: the ARF, Queen Street, and more than one general hospital. We favoured linking with the ARF and Queen Street, outlined why, and were invited for a further meeting in October. After this presentation we decided to hold meetings with representatives from the ARF and Queen Street to see if we could begin a process of merging the organizations.

By this time, the chances of merging with the ARF were even more remote. It had moved even further from the medical approach to addictions, placing less emphasis on treatment and more on health promotion and prevention. For instance, it had conducted good studies on government policies like the provincial RIDE program. This program, which stops drivers at random to see whether they are intoxicated, has saved countless lives. The ARF also worked on the science of selling alcohol, with arguments against selling alcohol at gas and convenient stores, and on limiting the hours that outlets are open. Since the late 1970s, the ARF had also provided Ontario with good data on use of drugs, alcohol, and other addictive substances in schools, through surveys done every two years.

The research coming from the ARF over the 1980s and 1990s was impressive and practical, and the organization commanded a great deal of respect internationally. At the same time, it was underappreciated in the province, and even at times resented by the government. The ARF had a fancy, plush bar in its basement for research on drinking behaviours, and to some government officials this was giving alcoholics alcohol at public expense. Besides the Clarke, the ARF was the only other hospital to suffer large extra budget cuts in 1994. As a result of both the cutbacks and its philosophical shift toward public policy, educational outreach, and prevention, the ARF had reduced its inpatient beds dramatically and some good doctors had left; it had difficulty retaining and then recruiting good medical personnel, including psychiatrists. The ARF didn't even want to be a hospital anymore; it had asked the government to declassify it as one.

Not surprisingly, our meetings with the ARF went nowhere, and it soon politely withdrew. Talks continued fruitfully with Queen Street. And as our meetings went on, I could see how a merger just might work.

Queen Street, a huge government-run hospital—also, however, a university teaching hospital since 1956—with 1,030 full-time, part-time, and medical staff, and an operating budget of $64 million, was by far the biggest player in Toronto's mental health network. It treated mainly chronically ill people with schizophrenia, and it seemed to be a slow-moving, cautious place. At this time, it had 436 beds, 736 admissions per year, and 2,000 outpatients, in six onsite and nine off-site outpatient programs. Upon its closure as an inpatient site in 1979, Lakeshore Psychiatric Hospital had its outpatient and support services integrated with the Queen Street Mental Health Centre. Queen Street had some real strengths. The hospital worked with 150 community-based agencies to help patients find housing, income support, rehabilitation, and training for jobs. The centre's research commitment was focused on such things as understanding housing issues for current and former psychiatric clients and the consequent shaping of public policy, which was nationally recognized. Very important to us, Queen Street was reaching out to the people in need in a way the Clarke was not.

Despite the breakdown of the talks with the ARF and the philosophical differences, our recommendation to the commission was to merge the Clarke, ARF, and Queen Street.

And that's when the news broke. The *Toronto Star* reported the closing of the Clarke when we had had no word of this—no report, no discussion. The leak was inopportune; I would have liked to send out a more positive message to staff about the merger but instead had to deal with all the anxiety and anger that comes with job insecurity.

I called a special meeting of all Clarke personnel: doctors, nurses, and maintenance and housekeeping staff packed into the auditorium. They were rattled. The Clarke was a tower of advanced research; the patients who walked into the emergency room came from all over the city, and the doctors were self-employed and strongly identified with the university. (The Clarke, as a fully affiliated teaching hospital of the University of Toronto, did not employ its physicians; the full-time and part-time psychiatrists were paid on a fee-for-service basis and were members of an academic financial partnership that pooled its income and shared expenses.) Queen Street, meanwhile, tended to the chronically ill, people who often looked dishevelled and confused as they hung around the institution. Queen Street was a depressing place, dingy, smelly, and poorly lit. The hospital was a ward of the state; its doctors were employees, the place was run by bureaucrats, and its unions were strong, having just completed a six-week strike. Queen Street, moreover, was a large institution. Would the Clarke disappear if we merged?

It was a very uncomfortable moment. I explained the situation as best I could to the anxious crowd: the Clarke was vulnerable, like many hospitals in Ontario, and the entire hospital network was being scrutinized by the new Ontario government to determine which hospitals should be closed or merged to save money, and also to create efficiencies. However, it was hard to offer much reassurance beyond the observation, based on my experience, that government personnel at the provincial and regional level seemed to respect the unique role of the institute.

No one was reassured. Some people suggested that I had a secret deal with the government to protect me if the Clarke merged with Queen Street. Maybe I'd even become the head of the merged institution if the Clarke closed. Some doctors were angry that the news had come as a surprise: Why did they have to read about it in the newspaper? Union representatives voiced their predictable outrage. A merger, if it happened, would inevitably disrupt the staff, and some of them might lose their jobs or be bumped to less desirable ones.

I heard the anger and pain in these comments, and I felt stung, but I realized that everyone, including me, was frightened by the prospect of change, especially when the province's aim was to cut the deficit, presumably by reducing the number of people on the government payroll. All I could say in that tense meeting and over the next few weeks was that we had to cover all possible options, and ultimately to do what was right for our patients, our staff, and the province.

By this time, the fall of 1996, I was convinced of the great potential in a partnership between Queen Street and the Clarke, but also including the ARF. The institution would have a synergy, forcing the Clarke researchers out of their concrete tower and learning to deal with the chronically ill patients who often had so little assistance. Queen Street could be removed from direct government control, recruit better staff, and begin to seek public support. It was chronically overcrowded and underappreciated, and the institution's expertise in treating hundreds of schizophrenic patients was not being spread effectively throughout the university network. This could all change. The ARF could provide its expertise in prevention, public education, and policy work, now applied to mental health.

Early in 1997, I was at a conference on eating disorders when I received a call at the hotel from Jean Simpson, the COO of the Clarke. I could hear the excitement in her voice. The commission had published its decision in a massive report. The upshot: the Clarke would merge with Queen Street, the ARF, and one other institution I hadn't even considered, the Donwood.

Founded in 1946 by Dr. Gordon Bell initially as a clinic in his home, the Donwood was Canada's first public hospital to deal specifically with the problems of addiction. With a staff of 120 and a budget of $7 million, the Donwood was designed to address the patient's physical, psychological, social, and spiritual well-being in a three-phase treatment over at least three years. Patients would begin by dealing with withdrawal and related medical problems, followed by four weeks of therapy, usually in groups. Finally, they would follow up with regular meetings to sustain the recovery. Patients would also be advised to join AA.

Simpson faxed over the commission's report—it was so weighty, it broke the fax machine, much to the displeasure of the hotel manager. But I couldn't wait to read the details. *We need this*, I thought. *If the Clarke is going to make it, we really need this.*

A few days later, I returned to Toronto to a dour scene. The staff at the Clarke, and at the three other institutions, were distressed. Some of the doctors at the Clarke were worried they would be turned into civil servants, just like their brethren over at Queen Street; others were just angry: Why were their worlds being turned upside down? Our nurses feared they would lose job seniority if they were swallowed by the Ontario Public Service Employees Union, the union representing Queen Street nurses (the Clarke's were members of the Ontario Nurses' Association, a union with different values and priorities). Researchers fretted that research money would be siphoned off for the care of the chronically ill. I could understand their concerns, though I suspected that beneath these complaints was an old-fashioned prejudice. They were about to gain a new responsibility for chronically ill patients who didn't always wash and take care of themselves. The ivory tower, in other words, didn't want to go out on the street.

But we had to make this work. The commission hadn't given us a suggestion; this was an order. We had no choice but to merge.

CHAPTER 19

Four Become One

The merger would be driven by a steering committee that was made up of three representatives of each organization: the CEO and two board members. Our first meeting was a Sunday retreat in the law office of Davies Ward Phillips & Vineberg, in downtown Toronto. This was the professional home of lawyer Stephen Sharp, board chair of our smallest partner, the Donwood. Articulate and charming, Sharp welcomed us into the comfortable boardroom. The key players were all there. Representing the ARF were its CEO, Perry Kendall; chair Bill Currie; and vice-chair, businessman Chris Gadula. A former schoolteacher, Currie had joined the Ontario Provincial Police and risen to the position of deputy commissioner. He was charming and well-spoken, and despite the ARF's earlier reservations, he seemed to accept that this merger had to work. The ARF was roughly the same size as the Clarke on a budget basis, each of us representing 20% of the combined budget. By far the biggest player in the room was Queen Street, with almost 50% of the combined budget and about 1,000 staff. Allison Stuart and two provincial government officials—an assistant deputy minister, Jessica Hill, and the director of mental health services, Dennis Helm—represented the interests of Queen Street on the steering committee. Stuart, the hospital administrator, had nursing training and a graduate degree in health administration from the University of Toronto. The smallest player by far was the Donwood, with less than 7% of the combined budget. It was represented by Sharp; physician David Korn, the CEO; and by another trustee and former addictions worker and policy expert, Pamela Fralick. The Clarke was represented by Andrea Baumann,

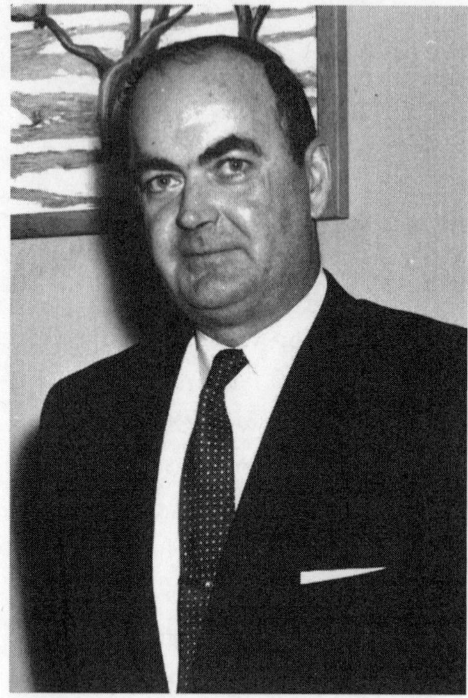

David Archibald was founding director of the Addiction Research Foundation from 1949 to 1976, and a former consultant with the World Health Organization and the United Nations. He was awarded a Membership in the Order of Canada for his service. Courtesy CAMH Archives.

the dean of nursing at McMaster and our board chair; the vice-chair David Weinberg, an architect by training but an expert in commercial real estate; and me.

The University of Toronto's dean of medicine, Arnie Aberman, also joined our committee because of the implications of a merger for teaching and research. Aberman is a prime strategist and negotiator. He speaks quickly, with thoughts crackling, and sometimes gets up in the middle of a meeting to walk around the room and talk one on one with people. He would phone you throughout the day, and it was common to get calls from him well into the night. Aberman's business and financial knowledge was highly unusual among academic physicians. He was never a researcher himself, but as dean of medicine he promoted the research enterprise and united a fractured faculty through the force of his personality and his relentless

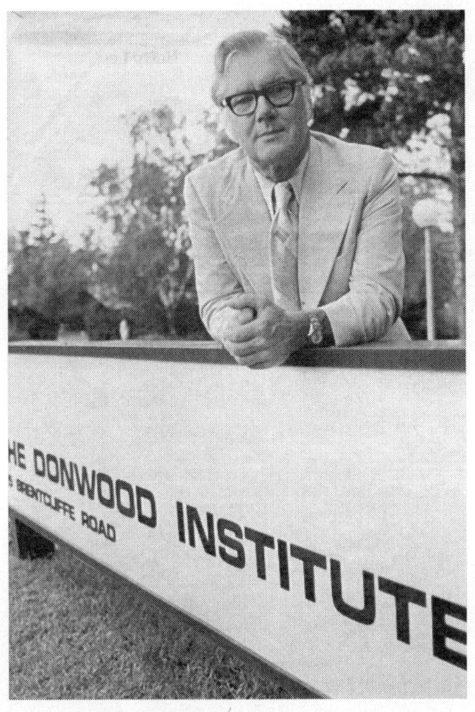

Gordon Bell founded the Donwood Institute in 1967, Canada's first public hospital for addiction treatment. In 1982, he was appointed an Officer of the Order of Canada for his pioneering work. Courtesy CAMH Archives.

communicating. These attributes turned out to be a real asset for our team. Aberman was later recognized for his exceptional service to Canadians by being awarded membership in the Order of Canada.

We wanted to keep the steering committee small, so we decided not to include representatives of the labour unions or consumer groups; they would get their chance to give input when we held public consultations.

In the comfort of the Davies law office and, I suspect, with thoughtful preparation, Sharp on the first day of meetings put forth two important suggestions: First, all four partners should be considered equal as we make decisions for the future of the merged organization. And second, we shouldn't vote; decisions should be made by consensus. It might take longer to make decisions, but we would then be more comfortable with each other and the results. It was hard to argue with these suggestions. This meant that, to develop something different and progressive in the new corporation, we had to start with the first order of business: equality of founding partners regardless of their size. This meant accepting that the Donwood would have a disproportionately large say in our future.

In fact, by making the four organizations equal, it diluted the antagonism toward any one organization or person, which in some ways made what we were attempting easier: the feeling was that you always had to watch your back against the other three, so there never became one enemy. At times, the addictions groups would be together on issues. The Clarke and the ARF were roughly the same size, but we were bound to clash because we started out with very different positions on the issue of merging addictions with the medical side of mental health. On the other hand, the two academic organizations, the Clarke and ARF, could be united to protect the role of scholarship. One thing was immediately clear on that first day: the Donwood represented a model of compassionate treatment and could be a significant partner in my goal to balance science and care. From what I could see in Sharp's boardroom that day, that would work out just fine.

I went home after the first Sunday meeting scared but excited. Suddenly, the seed of a merged institution had developed a life of its own. The process would not be in my control, and I had no way of imagining what the final outcome would be, but I knew this would be one amazing ride. Our main job was to develop strategies and plans for the creation of the new organization and advise the three boards and the Ministry of Health on the best way to proceed. In particular, we were supposed to determine the mission and vision of the new corporation, and its core values. We had to establish a governance structure and deal with the legal, human resources, and financial impact of the merger on the four institutions.

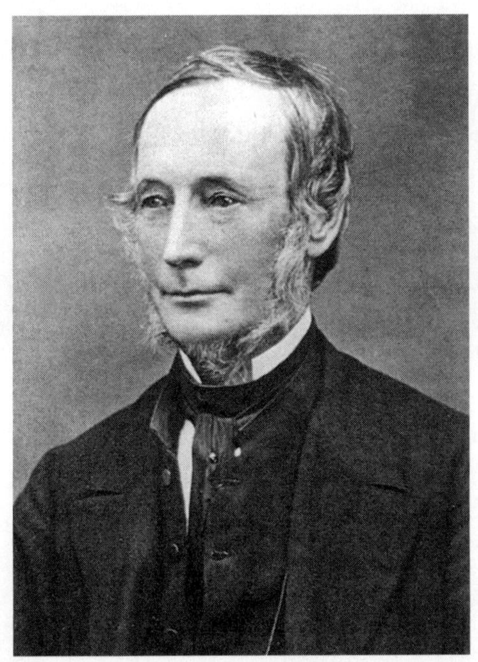

Joseph Workman was appointed medical superintendent of the Toronto Asylum in 1853. He was a progressive physician who followed the tenets of moral therapy. He fought hard against government interference, overcrowding, and underfunding. He devoted his life to mentally ill patients, and retired in 1875. Courtesy CAMH Archives.

I could see a huge opportunity. A merger was not necessarily a bad thing. Mergers provide unique opportunities to transform disparate parts into a single new organization that is radically different from what came before, to do something beyond merely reducing costs. There are opportunities to recalibrate organizational cultures, set new strategic directions, and reengineer major processes. To accomplish these goals in a successful merger takes considerable time, at least 5 to 10 years.

We met every Friday morning, from 7 a.m. to 10 a.m., for 34 weeks. Our first move was to hire the facilitators Graham Scott and Maureen Quigley, who both had experience in this type of work. They had been involved in the earlier merger discussions between the Clarke and Queen Street, so they knew two of the players. This had advantages and disadvantages. The Donwood and ARF groups were worried that this might give us a strategic advantage. We had already worked on our collective mission and vision during our earlier merger discussions and had even held public consultations late in 1996. Several members, including me, resented the idea that we were now going to start all over again. The process really tested my patience. When a couple of the steering committee members complained that we were moving too fast, I jumped on them: "If you're anxious, try meditation, or a walk in the woods, or valium, but don't hold us up!" I had a tendency to blow from time to time when frustrated, and this was one of those times. It was not my finest moment.

The facilitators created a roadmap for where we needed to go. They were also the focus of displaced anger; it was much easier to get angry at them than at someone who might be your board chair in six months. We all at various times were hard on Scott and Quigley.

At the beginning, everyone felt they were losing something, even when we were all convinced of the overall benefits of the merger, and we had to deal with this sense of loss. Meanwhile, the staff, patients, and their families, as well as health care providers in the community, were getting increasingly anxious; because of the information vacuum, rumours started to spread. Would the Clarke researchers eat up Queen Street funds, causing even more neglect of the chronically ill? Would money from the Clarke and the two addiction facilities go to Queen Street? Would addictions be medicalized? Would everyone suffer further budget cuts?

In the year leading up to the formal amalgamation, the atmosphere was consistently one of mistrust and fear. Who had a minuscule advantage in some imagined race to the finish? Who had promised what to whom? Who was saying one thing publicly yet being misleading in private conversations? Those were the questions we struggled with on an interpersonal level. Then there were the bigger issues: How badly would the addictions field be treated

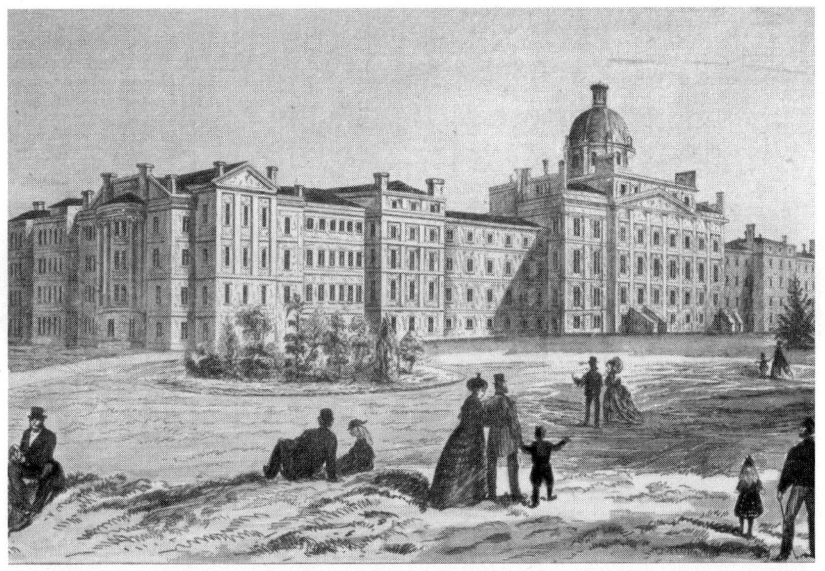

The Asylum in 1870. Courtesy Canadian Illustrated News.

over time? What about neglect of the chronically ill? Would the academic work all become "biomedical"? Behind all of this we were also worried about our personal fates. For the CEOs it was simple: Who would be part of the new organization? Who would get the job as CEO? Who could they tolerate? Who could they not? There were many moments of posturing in front of the people who would likely form the core of the new board.

We all knew, however, we had to move forward; there was no other choice. The chairs of all three boards and the government sent a clear message that the amalgamation was to proceed because it was going to be valuable for the province as a whole, regardless of who among us was affected. This was a powerful message to the four CEOs in the room, all of whom had so much personally at stake. The university also came in with decisive support for the merger. This prevented university faculty from mounting a resistance movement. The Ontario government had sent high-powered officials, Jessica Hill and Dennis Helm, to our committee as a sign of its support. They made it clear that the government was completely behind the merger process and especially the divestment of the Queen Street hospital. This merger would be the first of the 10 directly run hospitals to be divested by government. The Ontario government would no longer be in the business of directly running hospitals.

We knew we were in choppy waters because the cultures of the four institutions were so different, so we decided to avoid the issue that was bound to cause the most conflict: our mission and vision. We side-stepped the issue and at the time I felt that we had deflected it, unwisely, to the future board to decide. In retrospect, I think if we had started with this, it would have bogged us down for a long time. This decision also made the new board responsible for work on what was appropriately at its core.

Instead, we set to work on the practical issues. How would the staffs be melded? How would we deal with the unions? What were the budget issues? The composition of the new board was a big question. This can be a really thorny issue when hospitals come together. We decided that a board of 16 to 20 individuals would be the preferred size. Each of the four founding partners would have three members, in keeping with the philosophy of our steering committee. To bring in new views, we also decided to allocate four positions to members selected from the community at large. In addition, there were four ex-officio members: the vice-provost of the university, the CEO, the physician-in-chief, and the president of the Medical Staff Association.

The facilitators, along with the Donwood and Queen Street groups, suggested that at least half the board be people with direct experience of a mental illness or addiction—either former patients or their family members. This would be a significant change from

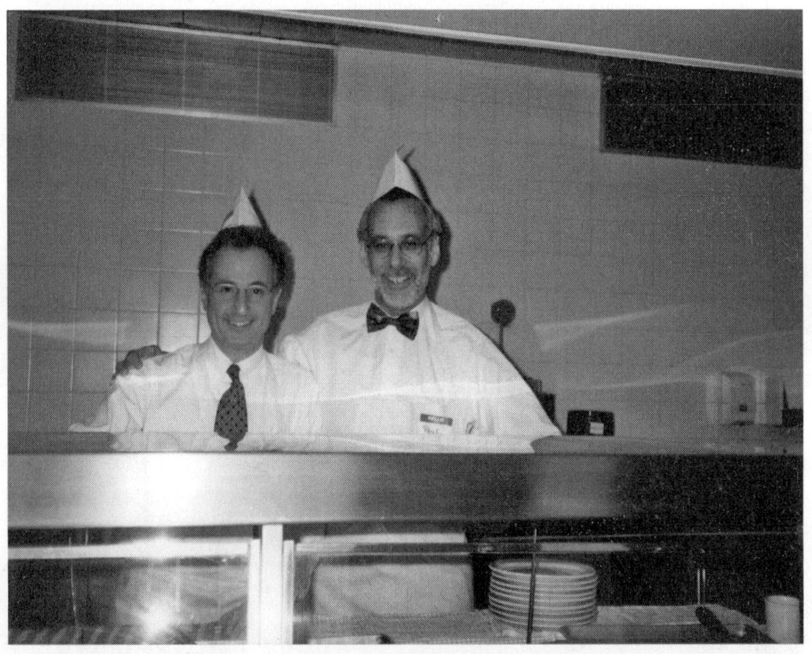

Serving at a United Way breakfast with David Goldbloom in 1994.

other hospital boards in the city, which had a more corporate feel. But who better to speak to the issues than people with lived experience? To some of us, this idea felt somewhat intimidating, but we eventually decided that 30% of the board should be people with these lived experiences. We also decided to have representation from regions outside the Greater Toronto Area, since the new organization was to be a provincial resource. Both decisions proved to work well. Members would be elected for three-year terms, renewable to a maximum of nine years. Members would be recommended by a nominating committee based on required competencies.

A nominating committee, chaired by Ted Tremain, was formed with representatives from all four founding partners, including past board members not involved in the merger. They polled the existing board members of the founding partners and constructed a slate of candidates for the new board. As well, advertisements were placed in local newspapers for the four new community representatives. In all, 88 applications were received.

To ensure board renewal, we adopted the form of an electoral college. This model allows for many stakeholders to have a vote on the nominations slate put forward by the nominating committee. There would be 70 members voting on new board members: 14 representing clients; 7 from families; 12 from community mental health and addictions agencies; 6 from public health; 5 from social service agencies; 10 from agencies representing addictions, mental health, seniors, and youth; 4 from the District Health Councils; and 4 each from the academic community, and from unionized and nonunionized employees. The staff and public loved the idea, but I was uncertain. I thought the process would be too cumbersome and might inject a partisan bias to the new board. But the model has ultimately proved to be enormously successful, as board members are carefully vetted by the stakeholder group and chosen according to the current need. The 70 members meet several times each year and provide excellent advice, especially those at the local level. The members are, and were, great ambassadors for CAMH, as the new organization would eventually come to be called, and, if anything, have prevented a partisan makeup of the board.[1]

One important issue in the merger concerned the medical staff. Each of the four institutions had very different approaches to working with its physicians. The two addictions facilities employed few physicians and were proud of having evolved to a less medical framework. Queen Street employed or had on contract about 30 full-time psychiatrists and many part-time general practitioners and psychiatrists. These physicians were members of a province-wide association, the Ontario Physicians and Dentists in Public Service (OPDPS), which had formed about a decade earlier and was perceived to have been effective in improving salary and benefits for the doctors in the 10 provincial psychiatric hospitals. Since the Clarke was a fully affiliated teaching hospital of the University of Toronto, it didn't employ its physicians. Instead, the approximately 60 full-time and 100 part-time psychiatrists belonged, as mentioned earlier, to an academic financial partnership that pooled its income and shared expenses. This partnership provided significant incentives for the academic enterprise in keeping with the university's principles regarding physician compensation.

The physician leaders of the four organizations—the chiefs of staff, as well as the presidents of the medical staff associations—established a group to develop medical staff bylaws and to examine the financial issues. This group readily came together to develop a unifying set of bylaws for a single medical advisory committee and a single medical staff association but appropriately deferred the partnership discussions until months after the merger had been completed. This was too volatile an issue to be resolved before the merger was complete. The unification meant the OPDPS would no longer represent doctors at Queen Street or anywhere else in the new organization. Not surprisingly, several of the Queen Street psychiatrists resigned as a result.

In mental health and addictions settings, the interdisciplinary team is far more important than it has been in an acute-care general hospital, and the steering committee, the physicians, and the leaders of the professional disciplines wanted the new organization to reflect this fact. So we made two important decisions. First, the leaders of the larger professional disciplines, including nursing, social work, and psychology, would be voting members of the Medical Advisory Committee, with one exception: only physicians would vote on the process of physician credentialing and oversight. Second, a new Clinical Practice Council representing all professional disciplines and interdisciplinary activities would be created.

We managed to solve many of the practical problems of merging organizations but there was one looming issue, the divide between addictions and mental health. The Donwood and ARF teams, ever vigilant about the potential for the medicalization of addictions, tried to fence off addictions from the rest of the mental health institution, as if it were a distinct society. They made one demand after another—a separate CEO for addictions, a separate allocation of money, and on and on. I was opposed and believed that we should seize the opportunity to create something new, something that would finally bridge the addictions and mental health gap that had been such a problem in the past. This was no time to fence off addictions. But between them, the two addictions facilities had 50% of the votes. In other words, they had the power to hold things up. Over time, however, they were able to respond to the argument that the board had to oversee the proper use of all resources and that this would enable a single CEO to bring the groups as closely together as was desirable.

The whole process was intensely frustrating. At one time or other we all felt like victims in this process, and we all wondered whether it was worth continuing the process ourselves. I kept telling myself that I had done well taking my views this far, and could easily bow out and let others do what they know, while I returned to what I knew: academic psychiatry. What did I have to gain from all of this? I had tenure and, as chair of psychiatry, I had one of the best jobs in the country, at least for two more years. The frustration made me consider removing myself from the process by saying I was not going to be a candidate for CEO and would just remain in my university role. But somehow I couldn't let go. Clearly, I am competitive and a big part of me wanted to stay in the game. There was potential for an exciting new enterprise, and I wanted to be part of it.

The CAMH experience shows that sometimes it's good to have no choice. In a new era of constraint, it was suddenly clear that we weren't going to fix the business by focusing on the small things and hoping the future would take care of itself. When the Health Services Restructuring Commission directed the merger, the game became about strategy and vision. Could we turn this disruption into an opportunity to make a difference for our field?

The steering committee and later the board rose to the challenge and clarified our vision: the understanding and care for people with mental illness and substance abuse should be on par with that for other types of human pain and suffering. Now the vision was clear, and it was both inspiring and inclusive to all involved. It was focused and easily communicated. People could see it, feel it, and know that it was right.

Conventional change literature suggests that fear is a necessary and even desirable motivator, particularly in a situation like ours where people didn't know each other and feared what "the other" represented. Fear may provide one initial spark for action, but aspiration is a far more important motivator. It is important to focus on a future that makes us all proud. We, both the patients and the caregivers, were the underdogs. Historically, our field had been disadvantaged and our patients on the whole had suffered as a result. All of the participants in the new enterprise—addictions and mental health, and the academy and community—could identify with this bigger goal. Our vision was to gain parity with other areas of health care, and to do so, we knew we would have to strive for excellence in each area of pursuit: clinical care, teaching and health promotion, research, public awareness, and fundraising.

This would be a formidable challenge for the organization's first CEO.

CHAPTER 20
From Belief to Reality

The search for the CEO of the merged organization began in the middle of this frenetic year of merger discussions. It was an international search, and seven or eight candidates were interviewed before they came to me. As for my competition on the steering committee, two key CEOs were out of the game. David Korn, the head of Donwood, had taken a buyout several months earlier. Allison Stuart decided not to compete for the role.

My comments to the search committee involved the same core themes as when I went to Toronto General and to the university/Clarke: we needed a mix of top science and caring for patients, especially for the chronically ill, who have been stigmatized for so long. Quality counts—we had to do all our work well. We had to respect the multidimensional nature of illness, so we needed a range of talent and skills. We needed to learn from one another. Team work was becoming increasingly important in all of health care.

In October I received the offer. I would start as head of the newly merged Addiction and Mental Health Services Corporation (later, the Centre for Addiction and Mental Health) in January. I was genuinely excited by this challenge and by what we could achieve. Yet I knew that the process was going to hurt many good people, including numerous close colleagues and friends who were feeling anxious and who might not have a role in the new organization. As CEO I would have to make decisions that would affect careers, and I felt guilty knowing some very capable colleagues would have to be let go. Then there would be an additional sense of guilt and shame if I felt I let down my own institute. What's more, I now had to deal with former rivals in a collegial way; we were now to be partners. Dealing with these conflicting feelings, I felt lonely and isolated. I couldn't share my concerns with other people inside the organization, or even with colleagues on the outside.

All eyes were on me as I selected my new team in the fall of 1997. To allay concerns about bias, I invited a board member, often Bill Currie, the former chairman of the ARF, to participate in each of the 16 search committees.

The plan was to have a competition initially to select internal candidates, and to recruit externally only if we couldn't find a suitable internal person. I had learned from my experiences at the beginning of the decade; rather than looking for "superstars," we wanted to find excellent people with shared values and competencies. There would be panels at each search, led by a professional recruiter and with formal questions based on the necessary competencies. The first two hires were obvious. Jean Simpson would be COO, and David Goldbloom would be physician-in-chief. Both had the perfect mix of experience, excellence, and ability to work with the team. Franco Vaccarino, a scientist who worked on pleasure systems and dopamine in the brain and had excellent interpersonal skills, was appointed vice-president of Research. The latter caused some resentment among those ARF people who thought there was an equally good scientist from their side of the house. Although the first selections were former Clarke people, others quickly joined the team: Clive Chamberlain, the outstanding physician-in-chief from Queen Street took over as a vice-president of Clinical Programs, and the ARF's CEO, Perry Kendall joined us for a few months before going to Vancouver to be the medical health officer. Other ARF people also joined us. Patrick Smith, the talented American psychologist, became a vice-president of Clinical Programs. Caroline Nutter took on responsibility for our provincial role; Peter Coleridge led the marketing and communications function; and Mariana

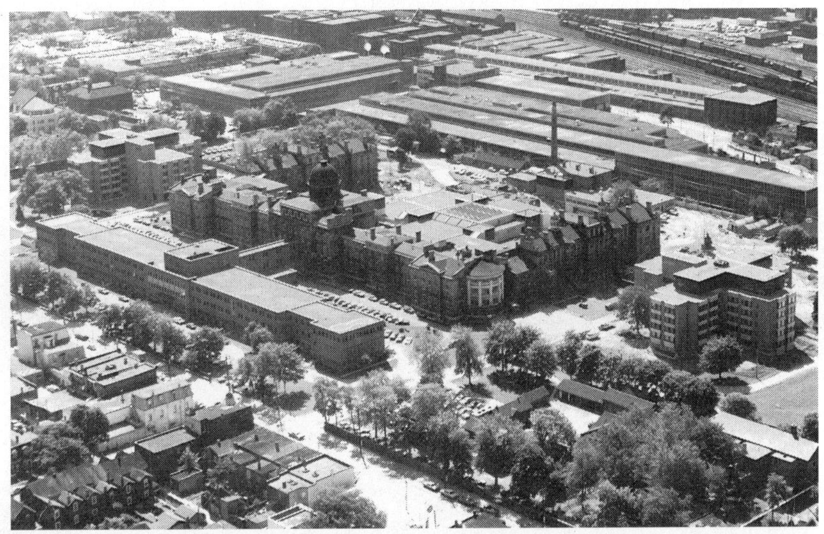

An aerial view of the Queen Street asylum in 1972, with the administration building that was added in 1956 in front of the old building. Courtesy CAMH Archives.

Catz, Information Management. Susan McGrail, who had earlier been at ARF, was selected to be head of the health disciplines and after a year moved on to government and, later, to run the Bellwood's addictions programs. Mike Prociw, an accountant from Donwood, was appointed to the head of finance.

We went to external people for some key roles. Georgie Beale from Montreal, who had newly completed a PhD, took over as vice-president of Nursing, and Rhoda Beecher came from Toronto Hydro to be executive director of Human Resources. Soon after, Dev Chopra, a very capable manager, joined us to oversee the finance, HR, IT, and building part of the operation. Jean Trimnell, a former nurse, became a leader/manager of several clinical programs. Shortly after, we recruited Elisabeth Stroback and David Cunic, who ably managed the physical redevelopment. Peter Catford ably took on the information management function when

The Asylum Evolves, 1846-1979

Over the following century, the asylum complex underwent building and landscaping changes in response to an expanding population of patients, financial constraints, changing psychiatric approaches, and urban growth pressures.

1879 to late 1970s
Massey Manufacturing Co., later Massey Harris and Massey Ferguson, farm implements' manufacturing

1972
Paul Christie Community Centre is completed.

1972
The first two of four Active Treatment Units are completed.

1956
A new administration and central clinic building opens, serving many uses until 2009. A walkway connecting the new Administration Building is punched into the front of the old asylum. This is the beginning of the end for the old building, which will be demolished in 1976.

1979 to 2009
The Joseph Workman Auditorium serves as a theatre and lecture hall for CAMH and the community.

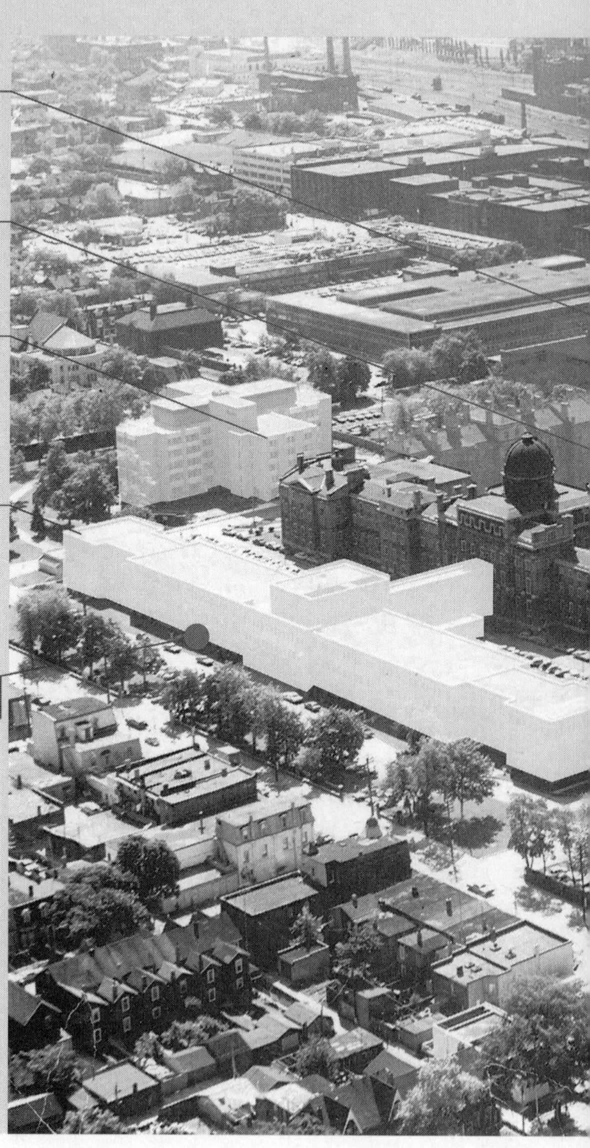

Aerial view of the Queen Street Mental Health Centre complex, 1972
CAMH Archives

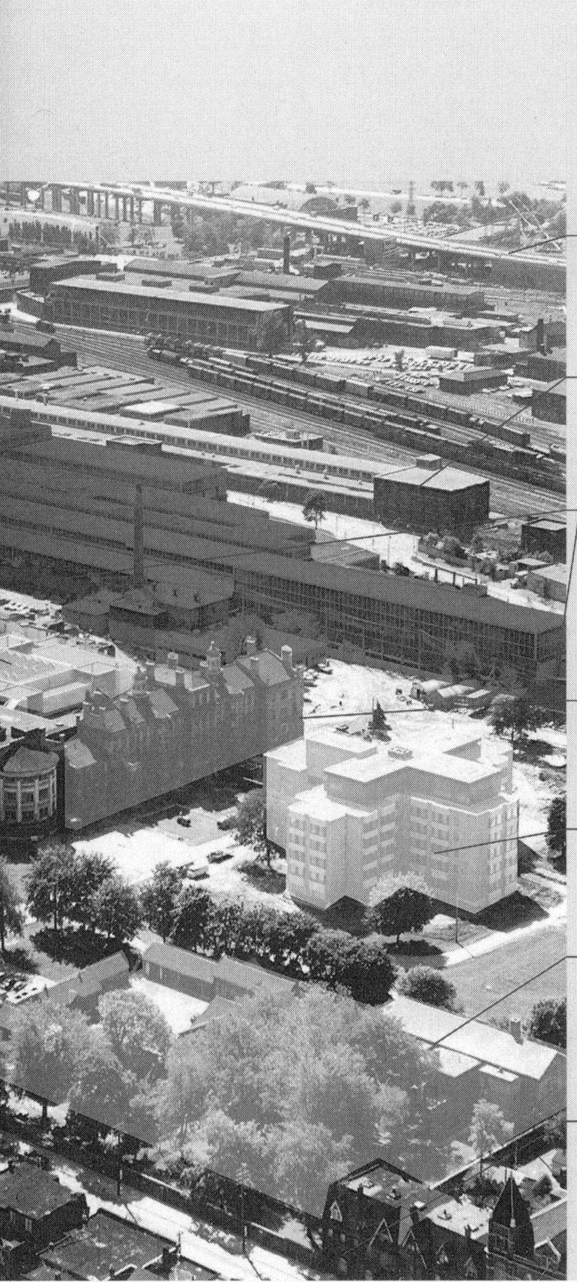

Gardiner Expressway

1888–1889
After the sale of 24 acres to developers in 1888– 1889, the original lot shrinks by almost half. No longer on the city's rural outskirts, the complex is now part of a fully urban and industrial landscape.

1889
Two brick workshops are added for use by staff and patients working in skilled trades. These are in existence today, designated as heritage structures, together with the surviving boundary walls, under the *Ontario Heritage Act.*

1866-1869
East and west wings are added to the main building to ease severe overcrowding.

1972
The first two of four Active Treatment Units are completed.

1870
Farm buildings are erected for agricultural purposes until 1912, when they serve as storage and utility areas. They are demolished in the late 1970s.

1861
By 1861, the entire property is enclosed with masonry walls. Parts of the east, west and south brick walls still stand as designated heritage structures under the *Ontario Heritage Act.*

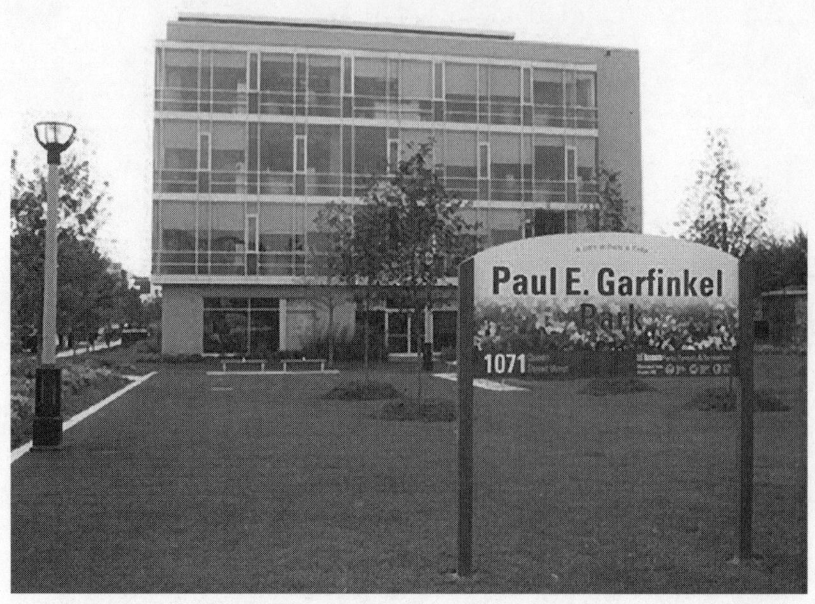

The City of Toronto named Paul E. Garfinkel Park in 2009. Courtesy CAMH Archives.

Mariana Catz left. Gail Czukar, a lawyer with government experience, and Joanne Campbell, an outstanding advocate for social causes, became instrumental in connecting CAMH to a broad community—they had a significant role in seeing CAMH change its nature relative to other providers and to our clients.

Then I made my first big mistake as CAMH CEO: I knew I had to leave the Clarke site to signify this was a new enterprise, and to avoid the appearance of bias toward my former institution, so I moved my office next door to the ARF building. (Really, I should have moved to Queen Street, where many of our staff and patients were located.) My new office was down the hall from Bill Currie, the former chairman of ARF who was now the chair of the CAMH board. He became the chair because of his experience and having come from the addictions world, whereas I came from the mental health world. This was a way of splitting up the power, a good idea in theory. Then the trouble began. Currie had an executive assistant who was always poking around, which irritated me. It was clear that Currie wanted to involve himself in management and saw me much like a vice-president, which I could never accept. He would complain that management was inappropriately seizing control of the organization. I would counter with: "We are trying to manage the organization and we will be led by the board's vision, values, strategy, and goals; we will consult with you and the board—but we have to make management decisions." It was a head-on power struggle.

Bill was soon appointed by the mayor to a task force on homelessness, and he used his position to push over and over again for more direct involvement on homelessness by CAMH. This direction was fine with me, considering how the homeless often suffer from addictions and mental illness, but we couldn't agree on how to make the work fit into our overall strategy.

Currie had allies on the board—Pat Capponi, an author and advocate for mental health and social change, as well as Nora McCabe, a vocal supporter of care for the chronically ill. They were constantly opposing what they saw as excessive spending by researchers at the cost of humane care for the afflicted. In many respects, they were on the side of the angels, protecting the disadvantaged. But the new organization had a mandate to balance the provision of care with the discoveries of science. One flashpoint was the food. When we proposed contracting out the management of the food services to an external company, believing that efficiencies could be realized by using a private company, they became furious. Once, I told the board that the performance in the different clinical services was uneven; to make my point, I said I wouldn't want a family member to be treated in some of our services. This was quickly reported to Andy Barrie, a former board member of the Clarke and a radio host for the CBC, which quickly aired the story. I was infuriated. Currie and I tried to work things out but never could. After one particularly stormy meeting in April 2000 I was extremely distressed and realized that one of us had to go. Currie resigned, and so did his allies on the board, Capponi and McCabe. Soon after, Capponi and McCabe were voicing in public, on the radio and in print, about our usurping clinical funds for the academic agenda.

I was downcast. I felt that this discord had nothing to do with the role of research versus care. It was all about governance, about who was managing the show versus who was governing. I also felt frustrated by not being able to speak out in public. Four days later, however, the board held a day-long retreat, and each member was forced to examine how difficult the past two years had been and how important it was to pull together. The organization's future was at stake. The openness proved a real turning point—the group really coalesced. The board appointed Pamela Fralick as chair. There couldn't have been a better appointment. Pamela, originally appointed to represent the Donwood, had once worked in the addictions field. She is by nature collaborative and direct and interested in bringing out the best in others, including some previously silent board members and managers. Pamela was sensitive and perceptive. "You feel like a pound puppy," she told me when we met. "You're unloved, unwanted, and harshly criticized." She was completely right. But after she took over, the board perceptibly changed. We all pulled together, and with support from the board, my team and I were invigorated and worked doubly hard.

It was a difficult period, but one thing helped: from day one, we knew we had to actively manage the transition. A new organization was being formed, and we were very aware of the need to invest resources in dealing with the endings, as well as the new

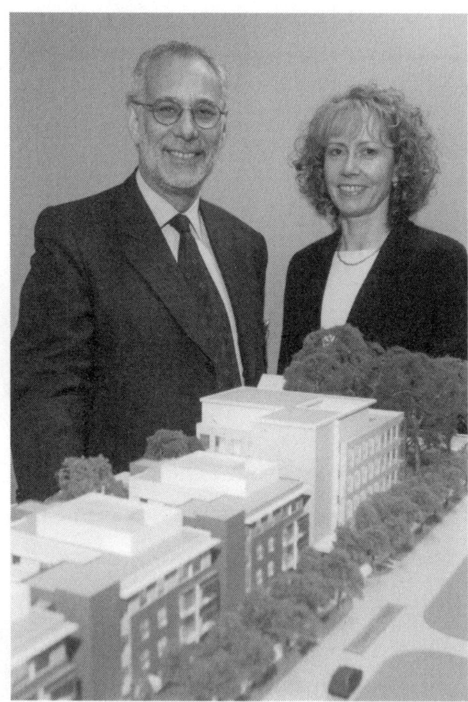

Paul Garfinkel with Pam Fralick, second board chair, and model of the redevelopment. Fralick led the board of CAMH through a difficult period, ultimately leaving it much stronger. She later became CEO of the Canadian Cancer Society. Courtesy CAMH Archives.

beginnings. The literature suggests most mergers are undermanaged; we did not want CAMH to end up in that position.

A big challenge in any merger is to integrate the different organizations on the ground, not just on paper; that is, to bring people together to create a new culture. Some organizations give this daunting task to a single individual, or even to an outside consultant, but we didn't think that was a good idea. We decided to embed the accountability for leading the planning and implementation of the integration in the Senior Management Group. Senior managers, meeting weekly, cochaired six major task forces on the key aspects of the integration: communications, culture, human resources, operational and clinical performance indicators, program management implementation, and transition support strategies.

We wanted to ensure the planning process was grounded in a strong conceptual model, and so used a theoretical frame from William Bridges as ours.[1] Bridges has emphasized the difference between change, which is external, and transition, which is internal, and encompasses the psychological changes we experience as we go through the process. This model emphasizes that transition starts with an ending—we were all leaving something behind. We repeatedly acknowledged that people had lost something important and that many of us could expect to experience Elisabeth Kübler-Ross's stages of grief. We never denied people their feelings, but provided support by explaining the gains.

We formally marked the endings. Hernando Cortés, the 16th-century Spanish explorer who led an expedition that caused the fall of the Aztec Empire, burned his ships when his men were in Mexico, to signal there was no going back. In order to have new beginnings, we had endings with appropriate symbols—ceremonies to close the old organizations and some programs, digging up the old time capsule, and recognizing the specific people who had brought us this far. We were always careful to put the new organization within the context of our honourable histories (when it came time to name the new streets on the grounds, for example, we honoured the Donwood's Gordon Bell, Queen Street's Joseph Workman, and the university's Aldwyn Stokes). Endings have been shown to demonstrate continuity with what really matters. According to Bridges's model, as you begin to let go, you enter a neutral zone. During this time, anxiety is heightened, people feel isolated, old problems reemerge, and there are many who want to go back to the old ways. People become concerned about the leaders, and there is usually a longing for definitive answers. This is the moment for real leadership, with a vision that reminds people how united they are and how their values are aligned. We quickly focused on five short-term goals that would give the process a

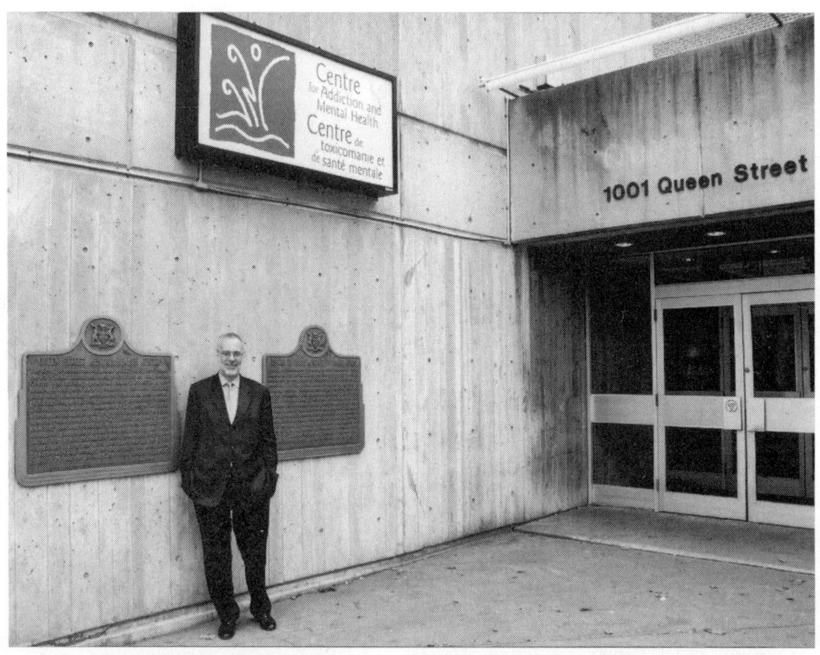

Outside the main entrance to Queen Street in 2000.

transparent structure: (1) efficiencies, such as in the administrative areas and bed consolidations; (2) synergies, such as in prevention, information management, distance learning and care; and fighting stigma; (3) anticipating areas of future increased need—adolescence, gambling addiction (Ontario had recently introduced legalized gambling); law, and mental health and dementias; (4) hot topics, such as concurrent disorders in older adolescents; and (5) what no one else would do: care for the chronically disadvantaged with schizophrenia and severe bipolar illness.

It was really helpful to tell everyone in the new CAMH network about these five main themes in the first year of the merger. Then staff could begin to consider the concrete benefits of the massive integration. Queen Street, for instance, had only 40 computers and 10 email addresses at the time of the merger. Now it

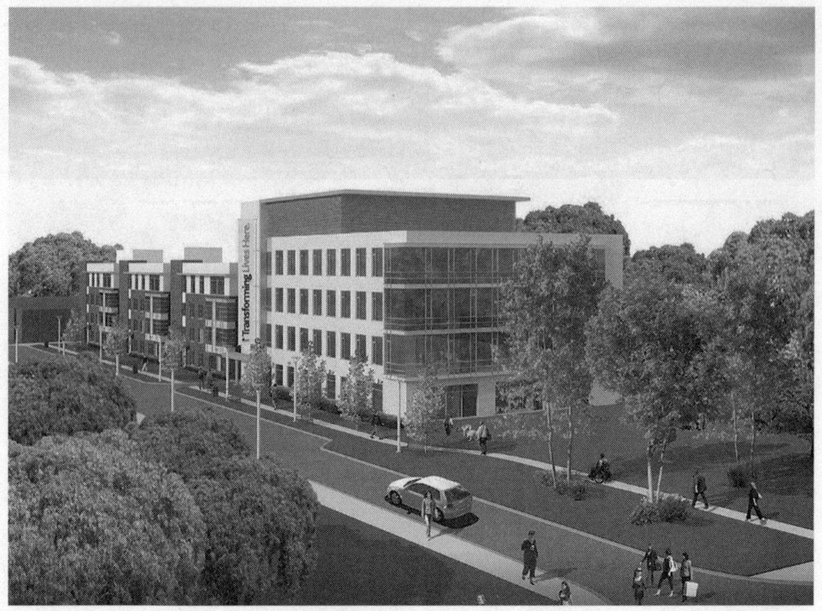

Sketch of the first four buildings of the new Queen Street site, which were opened in 2008. Courtesy CAMH Archives.

could discard an inferior information system and benefit from the ARF's excellence in this area. They could see us say forcefully that a humanitarian society doesn't run away from its most disadvantaged citizens, and that adolescents could be treated for concurrent disorders in Ontario. Staff were reassured by promises that administrative savings could be used for new clinical programs. We developed indicators to monitor and evaluate the implementation of the postmerger integration. To be accountable, we promised to disclose all details as they became available.

We also worked on the symbols of the new organization—name, logo, colour, and letterhead—by engaging our staff as often as possible. These decisions were not easy. We had trouble agreeing on a name for our new organization, so we compromised. We came up with something bland that displeased everyone equally: CAMH,

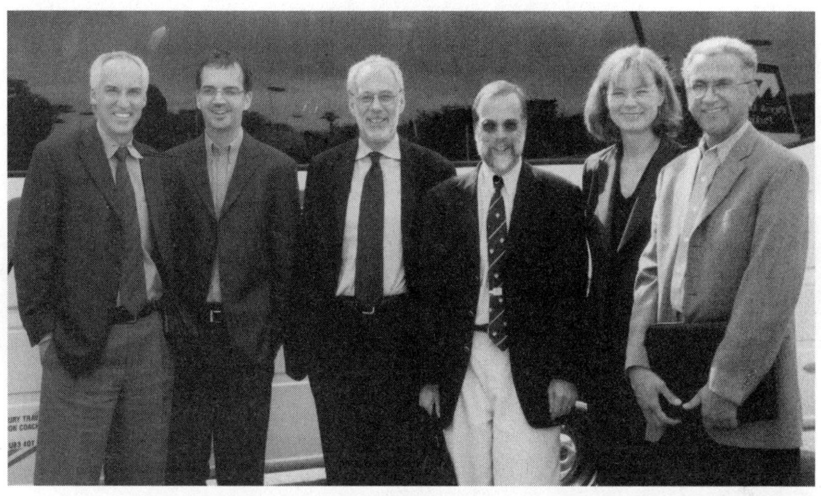

A CAMH group visited Birmingham and London in 2002 (left to right): Franco Vaccarino (vice president, research), Trevor Young (physician in chief), Paul Garfinkel, Steve Lurie (board member), Elisabeth Stroback (property development), and Dev Chopra (executive vice president, administration).

the Centre for Addiction and Mental Health. (The name could have been worse: the previous contender was the Addiction and Mental Health Services Corporation.) Even after the name was in place, it meant nothing to people. After five or so years, I was thrilled when cab drivers knew what I meant when I said I wanted to go to CAMH.

There could never be enough communication. We had a weekly internal newsletter, and an anonymous transition telephone hotline. What appeared to be most needed and wanted were more opportunities for face-to-face, two-way communication. So we took a number of steps: regular breakfasts with me, and with Jean Simpson, were instituted for small groups of staff, and the issues raised in these discussions addressed in the newsletter; regular forums for the middle managers were organized; all-staff meetings at each of the four sites were held; and senior managers

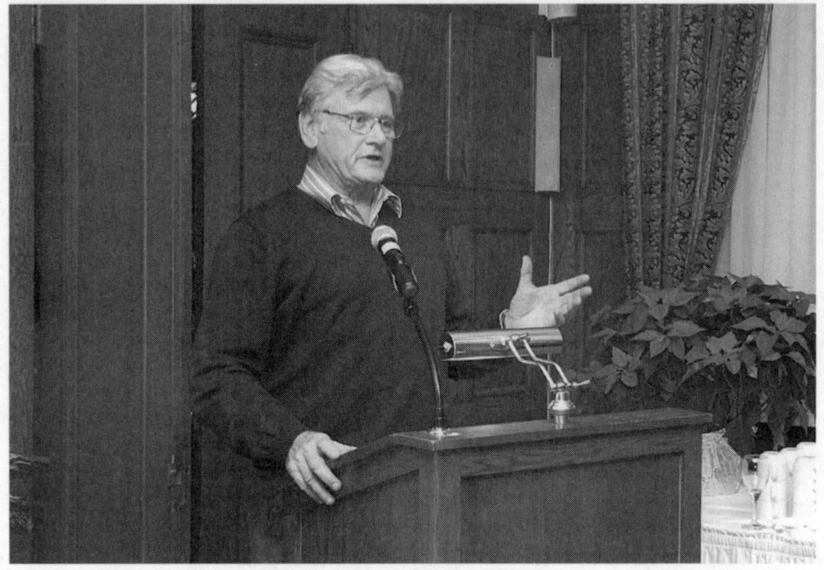

Clive Chamberlain, formerly psychiatrist in chief at Queen Street and then vice president of Clinical Programs at CAMH. Courtesy University of Toronto Department of Psychiatry.

were provided with overhead materials to inform their staff about important new developments.

We had a vision, to put mental illness at the same level as other medical conditions. But vision doesn't mean anything unless it's aligned with action, values, and behaviours. For the first few years, we received a lot of criticism, particularly that we had these excellent aspirations but were not living them. Staff accused us of not improving treatment quickly enough, or of emphasizing our international programs rather than improving health close to home. It took a couple of difficult years to bring people onside. Ultimately, the staff got it. In survey after survey and in accreditations, it was gratifying to see that our staff appreciated what CAMH stood for, why we were unique, and how we were going to succeed. They made fun of my descriptions "it's a win-win-win-win circumstance" and "we were handed a gift" and "research education, health promotion, and care are mutually enhancing" because they heard them so often, but they knew what these descriptions meant and agreed with what we were about.

Making the vision real took time. We invited patient and family representatives to a Patient Care Committee meeting of the board of trustees to discuss issues affecting patients. At the first meeting, we were questioned quite harshly about the eight patient deaths at the Queen Street site over the previous year. We explained the causes of the deaths, but our critics wanted to know where the bodies were buried. The rumour was that Queen Street had somehow hidden the bodies on hospital grounds. We were astounded by this, but we also saw this as an opportunity to build transparency, and hopefully trust. We developed a complaints office and publicized it widely; the clients then developed their own Empowerment Council and Client Bill of Rights with our support. Client representatives were on all the important committees, and they were compensated for their time. They taught us that, when we do surveys of patients, we get different results depending on whether another patient or a staff member interviews the patient. We turned to client interviewers. Later, the clients took over a business, a café and catering business, and made it financially successful as well as a source of employment for clients. (In 2013, they took on the catering for the entire organization.) An art gallery (later named the Jean Simpson Studio) was opened with artists in residence and opportunities for clients to sell or rent their art. We formed a collaboration with a local community college, George Brown, and special courses were set up to train assistant chefs and masonry workers. When we negotiated employment contracts for our redevelopment, we insisted that a certain percentage of the workers would be our clients. Later a thoughtful philanthropist, Sandra Rotman paired CAMH with the Rotman School of Management at the University of Toronto to provide mentoring and funding to clients who wanted to open small businesses. Over time we also started to hire peer counsellors. All of these initiatives demonstrated our values. They took time to evolve but were very successful.

On one occasion maybe too successful. We did have a governance model that required clients and family members to be on the board itself. We took this seriously and called for nominations from clients and from clients' representatives. One application came in from a man in our Medium Secure Forensic Unit. He had been in various institutions for lengthy times for arson, including attempting to burn down hospitals. We were seriously considering him for the board when a question arose: Is this appropriate? Joanne Campbell, then our outstanding vice-president of Communications and Community Relationships, said, "How would it look in tomorrow's *Star* if we turned him down—we're committed to clients." A wise board member, Herb Solway, a lawyer who had seen it all, remarked, "Just think how it will look in the *Star* if you put a psychopathic arsonist on the board!" The debate died immediately.

Facing a challenge that looks overwhelming at the outset can sometimes produce wonderful results. The CAMH merger was one of those times. Despite the early tensions, the vision for the new organization was coming together beautifully. Addictions and mental health were finally beginning to be acknowledged as significant and deserving of the same kind of money and public interest that heart disease or cancer receive. This was nothing short of phenomenal. Mental health was finally getting closer to the funding it deserved (though not the community sector). The budget CAMH received from government had far more than doubled. Research funding had quadrupled, and funding from philanthropy had reached heights none of us could have ever imagined. Recruiting excellent staff became a pleasure. It was much easier to recruit top people to CAMH than it had been to the Clarke. As our reputation developed, we could hire clinician-scientists such as Benoit Mulsant, Bruce Pollock, and Rohan Ganguli from Pittsburgh, Kwame McKenzie from the United Kingdom, and Tony George from Yale, all respected for their science but thoughtful caregivers as well.

In order to be considered like the other specialty fields, we had to strive to be excellent in all endeavours. Like our colleagues in the best general, pediatric, and cancer hospitals down the street, our clinical care had to be excellent, as did our work in research and teaching, public education, fundraising, and health promotion. What's more, we were starting to integrate the different streams of knowledge by actively bringing together research, teaching, and care, which was delivering benefits to all three. And finally, we were now on a path to bring together mental health and addictions: consultations were readily available across the programs; teaching and rounds were shared more often. People were learning from one another—some staff crossed over to work in other programs, learning new skills and bringing others to their teams.

We still lagged behind on one goal, though. The merger had not been able to deliver any real benefits to the rehabilitation and reintegration of chronically mentally ill people, who had been stigmatized for such a long time. We had to find a way to reach out to the sickest patients, and to accomplish this, we had to look west, to the former asylum on Queen Street.

CHAPTER 21

The Asylum as Urban Village: There Is No Plan B

A year after CAMH began life, we were, from a geographic point of view, everywhere. We had four main sites in Toronto, as well as 10 satellites scattered throughout the city, from the lush ravines of northern Toronto to the hardscrabble west end, where the old asylum had been built. We also had 30 regional offices spread across the province that were supposed to promote health, educate the public, and do community-development work. Yet, after the effort to merge four organizations, we had not come together in an actual physical way.

We needed a single hub, where the experts in addiction could mingle every day with experts in schizophrenia and mood disorders, as well as with the patients themselves. We couldn't afford to remain in our ivory tower—or a concrete tower, in the case of the Clarke. We had to find a place where we could reach out to the community to keep relevant and engaged. We needed a hub where researchers and the people who actually treat mental health problems could work together to become better scientists, teachers, and clinicians serving the public.

But where? The Clarke and the ARF were out. Municipal zoning rules wouldn't allow us to expand. What's more, building on the Clarke site could send the wrong message, that the CAMH merger was actually a takeover by the Clarke. Besides, these buildings were in a densely populated area of shops, restaurants, and clubs; there was no greenery or place of respite. The Donwood sat in a beautiful ravine setting, but it was too far north to be accessed by the patients in Toronto's west end and it was far from our university partners.

That left Queen Street, in the southwestern part of the city. Its drab concrete buildings housed over 300 patients, mostly people with schizophrenia, people with developmental handicaps and psychosis, or elderly patients with schizophrenia or dementia. There were also 70 forensic patients, mostly with schizophrenia, sent there by the courts.

To my eyes, it symbolized the pain and isolation that mentally ill people have suffered for so long. It was a miserable place. Its giant concrete and cinderblock buildings were reminiscent of Eastern European Communist-era architecture. Dull, cramped, and undignified, disrespectful of the needs of individuals, they hardly inspired hope or respected personal space. Patients had to line up in the halls for a quick shower in the morning. The lighting was bad, the corridors were too narrow, and some of the tiny rooms smelled of urine. Outside wasn't much better. The buildings were completed in the early 1970s and were called Units 1, 2, 3, and 4—not in geographical order but according to the order they were built, which confused most people when they tried to navigate their way around the site. There wasn't even proper signage. The 11-hectare site was mostly paved over with parking lots; prostitutes and drug dealers took over the few green areas on most nights.[1]

How would I attract the best clinicians in the world to work in a place like that? How would I persuade the staff at the other facilities to move out there? The entire place, both staff and patients, seemed to be operating in slow motion. It was a world away from the quick pace of the university hospitals I knew so well. However, as I thought about Queen Street and what it represented, I decided it was exactly what we needed. It was actually the ideal place to function as the heart of our new CAMH enterprise. It would signify a fresh start to a long troubled history.

The psychological history of the Queen Street was decidedly mixed, as Toronto psychiatrist Dr. Nicole Koziel showed in her 2009 paper "Psychiatric Spaces: The History of Therapeutic Design." When it opened on January 26, 1850, the Provincial Lunatic Asylum, as it was then called, was the largest and most modern public, nonmilitary building in Canada. It had central heating, hot and cold running water, and indoor washrooms.[2]

The architect, John George Howard, designed the original, Victorian building to fit the most advanced and humane treatment for mental illness at the time. "Moral treatment," popularized by British physician John Connolly at the Hanwell Asylum in the early 1840s, recommended that every patient be treated kindly.[3] Their health would improve in an ideal environment with plenty of fresh air and greenery. As Koziel tells us, patients were classified by symptoms and were only to mix with those of the same diagnostic class and gender, in a soothing and dignified environment. Patients who were classified as curable were allowed more time with staff and meaningful work within the asylum.

The architect tried to follow the guidelines of Thomas Kirkbride, the leading mid-19th-century American expert on asylum construction. He built an extensive system of staircases to separate different classes of patients. Gardens and farmlands were designed for therapeutic work, and the asylum was located just outside the city limits, three miles west of the noise, the smoke, and the smells of Toronto. Howard did have to bend to directives from government officials on the size, though—the asylum would have 500 beds, twice Kirkbride's recommended number.

It started out well, Koziel continues. Dr. Joseph Workman, the asylum's medical superintendent for 22 years, from 1853 to 1875, implemented a program of kindness, quality food, exercise, fresh air, and good medical care. He installed a library, chaplaincy services, and occupational therapy. He also introduced group work, outpatient care, and a halfway house. He and his successor, Dr. Daniel Clark, discouraged straightjackets and other physical restraints.

The building itself was a problem. Workman struggled with chronic problems afflicting the ventilation, sewage disposal, and heating systems. Meanwhile, government officials pressured Workman to get physically able patients to produce as much of their own food as possible. As a result, he had to divert energy to crop rotation, soil type, and inventories of farm animals and equipment.

By 1875 "moral treatment" was over; the institution got more and more overcrowded.[4] Thus began a vicious cycle. Patients were not cured; funding was cut back. Conditions worsened. Then came the "treatments," such as chemicals to induce convulsions. Tales of these treatments, along with the intimidating and alienating nature of the building, increased the intense fear of the asylum. The fear spread to the supper table—children were told to "finish your dinner or we'll send you to 999" (the asylum's street number). People would hold their breaths on the Queen streetcar when it rumbled past, lest they catch whatever afflicted the patients inside that looming building.

In 1964 the Ministry of Health announced quietly that the old asylum building, with its several wings, would be replaced. Staff and patients had hated the old building: with high ceilings, it was extremely noisy, and large floor cleaners, streetcars to the north, and a railroad to the south all made the background noise more intense.[5]

By the early 1970s, the provincial government of the time was eager to demolish it. Hardly anyone in public life disagreed, apart from the province's and city's heritage preservation agencies and well-known architect Jack Diamond, who wanted to restore the once-great Victorian building. So it was demolished, and when the new mental hospital opened on January 30, 1979, at a new address, 1001 Queen Street West, Ontario health minister Dennis Timbrell said it would not be like the "lunatic asylums of old."

Nonetheless, the campus was still an island, cut off from the city. Most of the wall around it had been torn down, allowing mentally ill patients to wander outside into the neighbourhood. But few outsiders came in. It was as if an invisible barrier separated mentally ill people from the community. A century of segregation, reinforced by the asylum's Victoriana architecture and concrete blocks, had magnified ancient suspicions of mental illness.[6]

So the idea of putting a modern academic health institution on the grounds of a 19th-century asylum was somehow rather perfect. With one bold step we could begin to create a new world of acceptance for people with mental illness. Queen Street also had significant practical advantages. It sat on almost 11 hectares of land in what was then a down-and-out part of town. The Ontario Realty Corporation (a provincial Crown corporation), which owned the property, was trying to divest some of its properties. It might sell the site. Of course, we had no money, but we could dream.

The board of CAMH and the executives quickly agreed with the plan—at least that our hub should be on the asylum grounds. We had to start at the beginning: What did we need? What did the patients need? What did the system need? We started to consider the implications of the deinstitutionalization of mentally ill people. The asylum was built to house people who were ill when all that could be provided was custodial care. Now new drugs and treatments were allowing mentally ill people to live outside the hospital. This fact would have a profound influence on how we designed the buildings on the Queen Street site. It wasn't just a question of how we would manage mentally ill patients on the inside. What counted just as much was how we would care for them on the outside.

Mental Health in the Community

Research and evidence pointed toward a new model of care. Reintegration to the community, when safety and security permit, was not only desirable from a humane standpoint but would lead to a better quality of life. The focus now was on recovery and emphasizing people's strengths and their ability to reach goals. We heard this message loud and clear from those who had experienced mental illness. They wanted paid employment, supportive housing, and other broad social supports that went beyond a narrow clinical view of "medical care." All of this would affect the architectural choices we were about to make for the new CAMH. It obviously could not be an old-style mental hospital; it needed to be open to the patients and connected to the community so that patients could get care regardless of where they were living.

To learn more about how advanced mental health systems handle these challenges, members of the senior management team flew to London to see how the Maudsley Hospital was dealing with the discharge of mentally ill patients; we then went on to Birmingham, another progressive place. We were encouraged to see that they were managing seriously ill patients outside the traditional institution, caring for the kind of patients who were still struggling with delusions that the moon would collide with the earth, for instance. It was thrilling to see. People were living in pleasant small townhouses, with doors that opened to the street. They had access to a nurse 24 hours a day, and they saw their doctor and did cognitive or other counselling or training on a regular basis. They were reassured they could have a quality of life whether they continued to believe their delusions or not. Some people were employed part time, or worked in supported environments. These facilities were, in other words, treating the sickest patients outside the hospital, and the model was successful.

What I saw was just a small part of an aggressive push to help people live outside psychiatric hospitals.[7] By 2000 the United Kingdom had closed 90 of its 120 psychiatric hospitals and moved the bulk of its long-stay psychiatric patients to group homes and community care. The government invested 700 million pounds to improve mental health services, the money focused on mental health promotion, primary care, access to services, service effectiveness, help for caregivers, and reducing suicide. This capped a decade of activity that successfully transferred long-stay patients to community settings. (Nevertheless, there were still significant problems to be solved in the United Kingdom, such as national shortages of psychiatrists and nurses, and the low priority of care for elderly people and children.)

To get a more detailed picture of the possibilities, we studied another international leader in mental health, New Zealand. In 1997 New Zealand set a straightforward goal: to decrease the problems related to mental illnesses, and to increase the health of and reduce the impact of mental disorders on patients, caregivers, and the community. New Zealand launched a national plan to ensure that the 3% of adults and the 5% of children and youth with severe mental disorders receive timely mental health services, to develop services for the 17% of adults with mild to moderate mental disorders, and to create assertive community-treatment teams for seriously ill people in the community. It also targeted more and better services for Maori. New Zealand is now a world leader in the mental health field.

While England and New Zealand were acting decisively to help mentally ill people live productive lives outside the hospital, Ontario was lagging behind. When we sent patients out of the hospital, we did develop community-based support—some housing and supported employment—but not enough. There is only so much you could do when Ontario devotes only 7% of its health care budget to mental illness—far below the 10 to 11% spent by New Zealand and the United Kingdom.

I saw what this underfunding meant in practice when some community activists took me on a tour of the west part of town, where many of our clients were living. They took me to a hotel where we sent discharged patients. It was filthy; street workers and drug dealers were hanging out in the dirty, dimly lit halls. It made me sick. Was this where we were sending vulnerable people to recover from a stay in a mental hospital? I was appalled.

My travels and research had shown me that deinstitutionalization could work if there was an investment in mental health services. It would take money to develop the community care that would allow mentally ill people to live decent lives outside the hospital. We calculated that $800 million extra per year would be required for Ontario to match New Zealand's system. It was a lot of money, but the potential benefits were enormous—patients could have a good quality of life; be productive; and if they stayed healthy, there would be financial savings for both the social service and justice systems. It would be the right thing to do.

We judge a civil society by the way it deals with its most disadvantaged members. But we had to be realistic. Ontario's financial picture was part of the landscape. We knew what we needed: expert care both inside and outside the institution. Now how should we start? Could we build a facility that would bring us closer to our ultimate vision?

Sharing the Vision

The consultation phase of the project started on a dour note. The staff were mostly suspicious and anxious about the new organization and even more so about the plan to merge the four hospitals on the Queen Street site. They worried any move would disrupt their daily networks—where they retrieved the medical records, who they spoke to in HR, who their colleagues would be at the lunch table, and so on. Some were in denial; most busy clinicians didn't believe it would happen. Many seemed to indicate they would come onside only when the funding and plans were finalized. Researchers thought that they would lose out, with money siphoned from research to this new enterprise. The neighbours were worried too. Back in the late 1990s, the site at the old asylum was on a desolate stretch. MOCCA, the Museum of Contemporary Canadian Art, had not yet set up on the north side of the street; nor had the other galleries, shops, and restaurants. But even by then, Trinity Bellwoods, the community northeast of the asylum, was evolving as the housing market warmed up and younger, well-salaried urban professionals renovated old Victorian houses and moved into lofts in converted factories, alongside the traditional residents, the artists, and the working-class immigrant families. People from the neighbourhood saw the site of the old asylum as a dangerous place where prostitutes and drug dealers were allowed to ply their trade, with insufficient attention from the local police. The senior management team responsible for the planning needed a process to bring people onside with the plan to integrate CAMH on the Queen Street site and to get their views on what form the new development would take.

At this point, we hired an outstanding team led by Frank Lewinberg, of Urban Strategies, to undertake government and community relations. Urban Strategies proposed that we seek input from people inside the organization, and outside, including the neighbours. We would start out in an unusual way for a large organization. We would ask people what they thought without taking a position ourselves. We would seek their opinions without trying to lead the process in any particular direction.

Many workshops were organized, and those invited to participate included representatives of staff at all levels, partner organizations from across the city, the university, families of clients, other caregivers, CAMH board members, the Ministry of Health, the City of Toronto staff and politicians, and, of course, CAMH clients and neighbours. We listened. Most people concurred with the integrative model. They wanted the heart of the organization on the Queen Street site, and they did not want it to be an isolated campus or asylum but a complex, accessible from the street and surrounded by greenery.

We held focus groups to tackle specific issues like the relationship between the site and the neighbourhood. We engaged people in many ways. We even had a competition to decide how the remnants of the wall that once surrounded the property would be featured in the new setting. Over 125 artists applied their imaginations, and their suggestions were featured at City Hall.

Step by step a vision emerged. This vision transformed the model of physical space for a mental health care facility from a large institution isolated on a large site to an "urban village," a real neighbourhood—a mix of buildings with different uses and activities, integrated into the surrounding community. We were not seeking a purpose-built facility that looked or felt like an institution. The goal was to "disappear the institution" and thereby reduce the stigma associated with it.

The vision that came out of the meetings had three parts. First, we would create a hub on the Queen Street site for the CAMH organization. It would be designed to encourage collaboration among the people involved in client care, prevention, education, and research. The new hub would be linked to a network of community-based programs in satellite locations. Placing related programs as well as education and research facilities at the hub would establish it as a multipurpose health care, education, and research village. (Not all research could be located at the hub, though. The PET, cyclotron, and animal labs could not be readily moved and would remain at College Street, close to the university.)

Second, we would design the new Queen Street site as a village linking with the surrounding urban landscape. The institutional stigma related to the old Queen Street asylum was to be replaced with an accessible community setting for client care. The hub was to be designed with a pattern of buildings, streets, sidewalks, and green spaces fully open to the surrounding neighbourhood. The goal was to create a safe, comfortable, and welcoming place. We planned for a mix of CAMH and non-CAMH buildings (CAMH needed only about half of the space on the site), including stores and small businesses providing supportive employment, university and research centres, restaurants and cafés, and galleries. People seeking help would arrive at office-type buildings rather than at an imposing institutional facade.

Third, we would respect the landscape on the Queen Street site. We were influenced by the strong community concern that the existing openness of the property would be compromised if many more buildings were added. The existing landscape was a significant resource. It was to be maintained and improved to create a high-quality, client-centred, and health-promoting environment. The landscape features were to have many functions, including private healing spaces for patients; public open spaces and activity areas to integrate with the surrounding community, and attractive public amenities along the streets and sidewalks.

The architects we chose came from a group that called itself C3, made up of Montgomery Sisam (Terry Montgomery and Alice Liang), KPMB (Bruce Kuwabara), and Kearns Mancini (Jonathan Kearns). They were all taken with the project and were a pleasure to deal with, since they understood our vision so completely.

Once we had the vision clear in our minds, we presented it to the CAMH board for adoption as policy. It was an exciting moment. We emphasized what a great change the plan represented, how exciting it was for the community, and how we had to engage both government and private supporters in this once-in-a-lifetime opportunity. Most of the board members were enthusiastic, but several felt overwhelmed by the magnitude of the project. One board member said that it all sounded terrific but "What is our Plan B if we fail to get the necessary supports?" I was surprised by the question. It never occurred to me that people wouldn't rally around such a progressive plan. While I was struggling to respond, Jamie Anderson, the Royal Bank of Canada's vice-chair who was our board chair, responded for us all: "There is no Plan B."

We forged ahead with program planning. There would be 10 clinical programs, including mood and anxiety disorders; schizophrenia; addictions; women's mental health; child, youth, and family; geriatrics; developmental disorders; and forensic psychiatry. A ninth program was designed to support chronically ill people in their transition from the hospital with regard to quality-of-life issues, particularly housing, work, income, and social support. The final program, a consultation assessment and triage program, would triage patients to the appropriate level of care and provide acute treatment for people in crisis. Within each clinical program, careful study determined how much hospital, ambulatory, and day programming would be required.

The geriatrics program required about 35% growth, and a new focus on clients with long-standing psychiatric disorders and on support for nursing-home communities. Twelve new beds were created for young people with serious, concurrent disorders—mental illness with substance abuse. Addictions moved its existing 47 beds to homelike alternate milieu settings, with one floor for

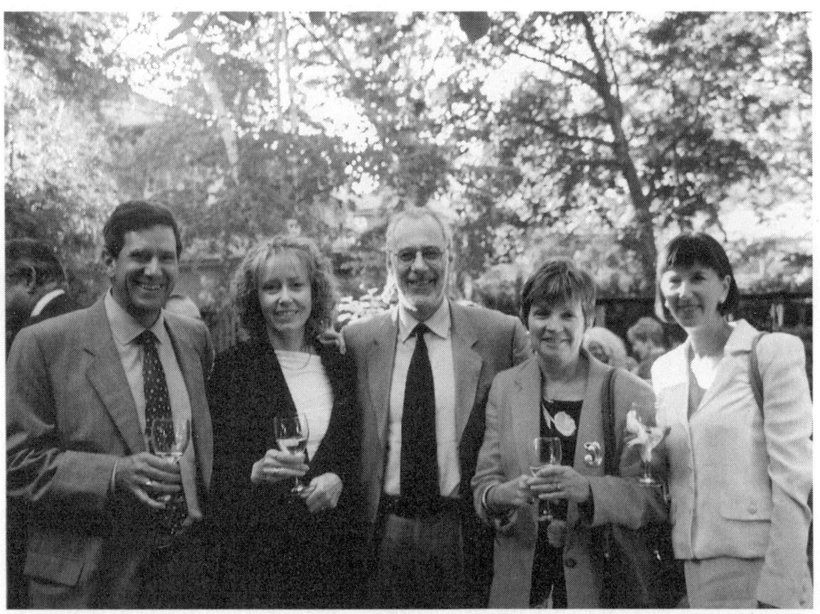

Paul and Jean Simpson celebrating the opening of the first new buildings in 2008 with board members Jamie Anderson and Pam Fralick, and (extreme right) Jan Stewart.

a medical withdrawal unit. These settings are similar to a neighbourhood walk-up apartment building, with single bedrooms and private bathrooms for each person. They have private spaces to read and relax, and general living spaces, including kitchen, dining and living rooms, and television and computer rooms, just like an ordinary home and very unlike a traditional hospital.

Many people with chronic schizophrenia do not require long-term treatment in a hospital, so we transferred more of the chronic care to the alternate milieu setting and eventually were able to have many clients off-site. We formed partnerships with landlords to give chronically ill people a home and social support. By 2010 some 60 long-stay patients were discharged to community settings. We also had negotiated for new community housing in a building on our property that is rented out to various businesses. We were

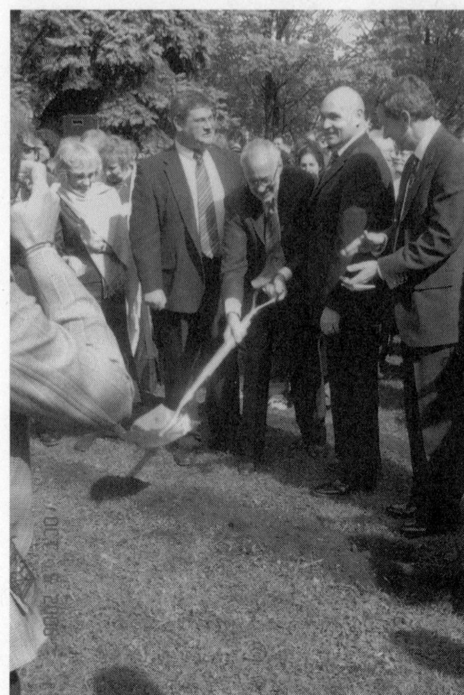

Breaking ground for the first new buildings with cabinet minsters David Kaplan and George Smitherman, and board chair Jamie Anderson. Courtesy CAMH Archives.

able to obtain about 170 community-supported apartments, a portion of which were allocated to our clients.

We could not overlook the forensic population. These are the mentally ill people who have broken the law. Sometimes the infringement is minor. About 85% of the forensic population are people with schizophrenia, and often they have been unable to access the regular mental health system. The forensic program is growing in CAMH; beds have increased from 70 in 1998 to 155 in 2012. I am pleased that people who were languishing in our jails have been appropriately directed to mental health care. Yet I fear we may be recreating the old asylums with forensic patients who are kept for long periods in institutionalized settings, not because they needed to be but because of public fears and a lack of programs in the community.

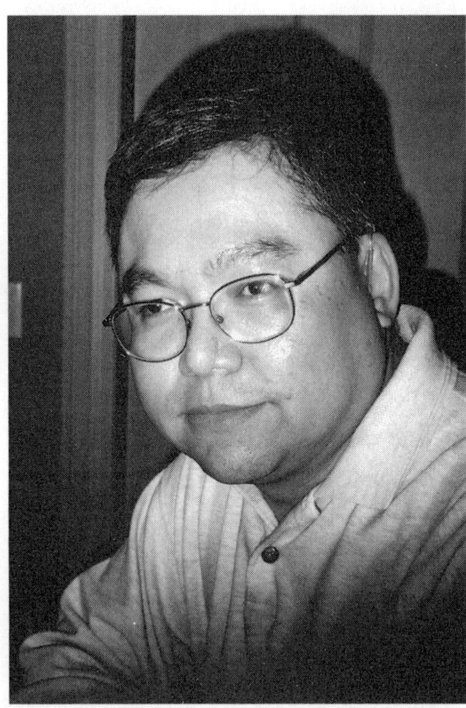

Clarke Institute and CAMH board member Raymond Cheng, a strong advocate of progressive care for the mentally ill.

A forensic program is necessary in our current world, but to function well it must have proper resources. We were faced with a terrible example of what happens when systems fail. In 1996, a woman was placed in one of the general forensic units (at the time, there were no gender-specific sites), where she was raped and later died in childbirth. It took us eight years after forming CAMH to get funding for a female forensic unit.

• • •

The next step was to transform the vision into a master plan for the Queen Street site development.[8] At this point, the vision was in the form of a narrative that everyone could understand. Now a more specialized design and real estate development process was required. So we established a working group comprising CAMH senior management and three real estate developers to advise CAMH on the practicability and feasibility of the master plan as it evolved. So, for example, this group repeatedly considered concerns about the value of new roads within the property, eventually concluding that permitting roads met the goal of making the hospital true to life in the city. Ultimately, it was agreed that all the surrounding streets to the north would be extended southward into the property as new public streets, much like any street in the neighbourhood and thus accessible to everyone. There would also be two new east-west streets, one an extension into the property westward of an existing street, the other a new street. Thus, the Queen Street property would be divided into a series of blocks, each of which could contain a number of separate buildings, again much like any other part of the city. Two blocks were to be dedicated as public parks, encompassing existing mature trees, and a further three areas of land would be reserved as permanent open spaces for the use of the adjacent buildings, again reflecting the location of mature trees.[9]

The master plan also went through a long public process, including the neighbourhood community, which was invited to a series of open houses and presentations. As a result of these consultations, when the master plan went through the city's approval process, it was unanimously approved by City Council with the full support of the community.

Throughout the process of developing the master plan, we were fully involved with the provincial and city governments. Mike Harris's Conservative government was surprisingly helpful. I say "surprisingly" because when I first met Harris, when he was Opposition leader in 1993, I wasn't impressed. He was a former golf pro who seemed to have little interest in people who were sick or poor. He wanted to shrink government, and I was worried

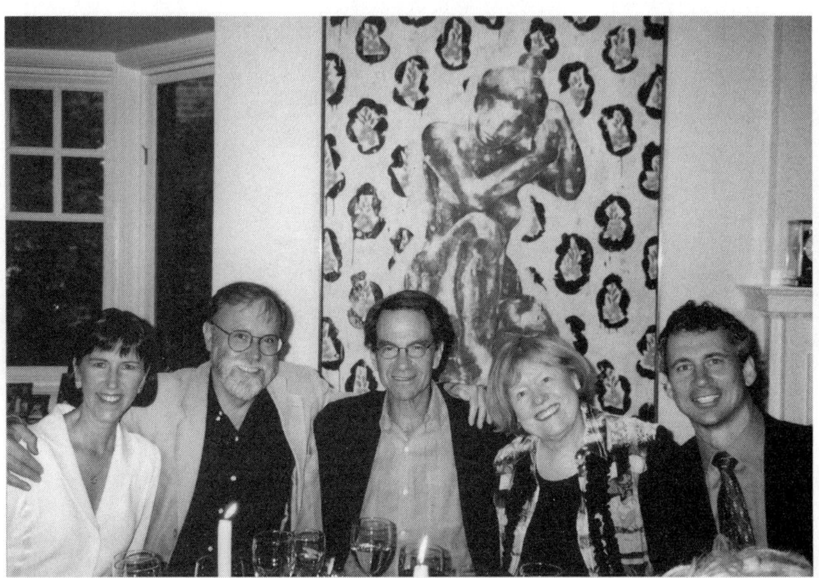

Vice president, nursing, Georgie Beale (second from the right) flanked by CAMH board members Jan Stewart, Dan Burns, Herb Solway, and Greg Rogers. Burns became chair for the CAMH board in 2009.

that mental health would be one of the first items on the chopping block. But when he became premier, Harris acted decisively in ways that would eventually help CAMH. His line of thinking was straightforward: Ontario has too many hospitals, so let's give an independent body, at arm's length from the government, the power to decide which ones should be shut down and which ones should merge. Then let's sell the property. The Ontario government divested the Queen Street hospital and gave the four institutions that merged into CAMH the money to buy the land. They also helped by giving us the money to harmonize the labour contracts among the four institutions. We got a real boost from Harris's health ministers, Elizabeth Witmer and Tony Clement, both of whom supported us from the start. The Conservatives were strong backers of the CAMH vision. They helped us with costs for the

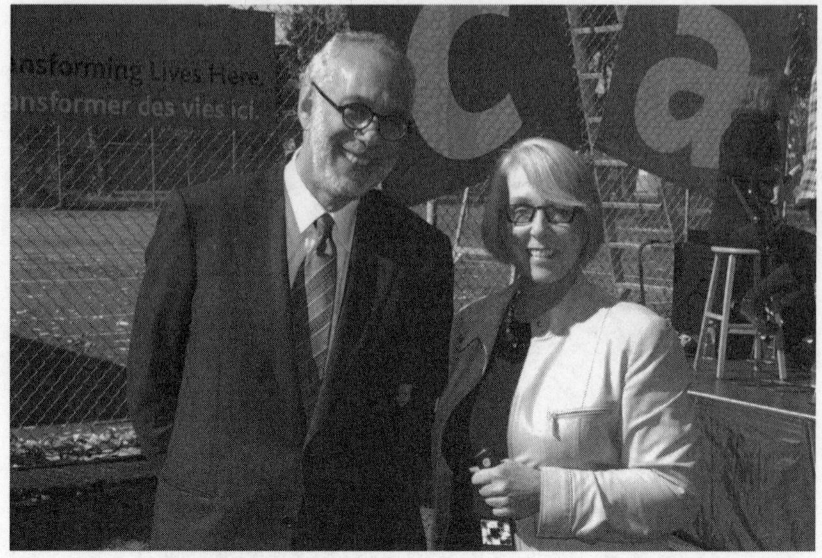

With Barbara at the site of the construction of the new CAMH buildings. Courtesy CAMH Archives.

original planning processes and liked our approach. I still have a letter from Minister Clement dated August 2003, stating that the ministry intended to have us proceed with the redevelopment. Two months after I received this letter, the Conservatives lost the election to a Liberal government.

Premier Dalton McGuinty was very much interested in this project, but his government slowed down the process. Things ground to a halt while McGuinty and his health minister, George Smitherman, pondered the financing of all capital projects. After a couple of years, the Liberals introduced capital project financing, a variation on public-private partnership (P3) financing that had become popular in Britain. This involved selecting and then working with a consortium of private business to design, build, finance, and maintain the buildings for 30 years before turning them over to CAMH. Although there would be a premium to be paid to private business for carrying the risks of cost overruns and delays, we felt that this was the only way to get the job done.

To keep our entire clinical programming going during the construction, we proposed that the project be built in three phases extending over about 12 years. In hindsight, the timeline probably should have been collapsed to half that. The first phase consisted of four small apartment-like buildings to house the alternate milieu beds for mood disorders and addictions patients, and a large ambulatory building for the addictions outpatient programming. The provincial government paid for these relatively inexpensive buildings directly with a capital grant of $40 million. But the next two phases were of far greater magnitude and required the P3 approach. If we wanted to build, we would have to raise a significant portion of the money ourselves.

The Foundation Leads

We had an unlikely advantage in that only one of the original hospitals, the Clarke Institute of Psychiatry, had an active foundation. After the formal merger, the Clarke Foundation board began a process of redefining its role to support the priorities of the new organization; it rewrote its bylaws to reflect this, changed its name, and accepted new board members who could relate to the broader mandate. A capital campaign had been planned for the year prior to the merger. Support for this campaign was reworked to reflect the addictions as well as the mental health issues, and the campaign, chaired by former federal finance minister Michael Wilson, raised $11 million between 1998 and 2000. We were euphoric.

But the redevelopment project four years later required a very different level of private commitment. One of our foundation board members, Pamela Fralick, who did an excellent job as our second board chair, suggested, in response to a question, that we target $100 million. Everyone laughed. It sounded like a joke. But amazingly, over the next seven years, we raised an unprecedented $108 million to provide CAMH's share of the building project; two years later, the foundation had raised about $160 million.

This capital campaign was led by an outstanding team from Toronto's financial and business sectors: Jamie Anderson, Michael McCain, and Tom Milroy. These three capable individuals and the Foundation Presidents Mary Deacon and Darrell Gregersen were supported by countless volunteers and staff. After a few years we had received very large family and corporate donations. The Labatt, Beamish, McCain, Ward, Godsoe, Fidani, and Younger families donated funds for named new buildings or wings, an extraordinary phenomenon for a mental health and addictions facility in Canada. We held dinners to honour people who had recovered from, or learned to cope with, serious illness. These dinners often attracted close to 1000 people, many of whom were thought leaders in Toronto's business community. An important effect of taking our message out to the business community was to educate them in problems in the workplace that had previously been ignored. Many corporations began to take mental illness and addiction seriously in their work settings. George Cope of Bell Canada, for example, insisted Bell's managers be trained in recognizing and dealing with these problems.

This achievement is a tribute to the spectacular support from donors and volunteers who recognized that mental health and addictions should be treated like any of the other medical conditions receiving broad public support. Forming a partnership with these community leaders became one of the most significant parts of the CAMH experience. Surprisingly to us at the time, the Foundation's board as well as the board of CAMH itself came to be seen as highly desirable places for volunteers to serve.

In the end, we hoped the transformation would extend beyond the services we provide and the environment in which we provide them. For mental illness and addictions to truly achieve parity in both care and compassion with physical illnesses, we must all reconsider our assumptions; a new physical environment for CAMH was unquestionably necessary but not sufficient. New buildings and new models of care are just part of the story of hope for people with mental illness and addictions. Our goal wasn't just to do a better job of delivering care to the people who needed it. Our goal was much bigger: to end the isolation of mentally ill patients and begin to wipe out the stigma against mental illness once and for all.

Research shows that three things act to overcome stigma: protest, education, and contact. All of us within CAMH, and the outstanding community leaders who rallied around CAMH, did all three. We launched campaigns to raise awareness of the cause, the stigma, and the organization. An advertising campaign, appearing in bus shelters, on radio, and in newspapers, emphasized recovery. We held events to recognize people who had successfully battled mental illness or addiction, to "unmask" these illnesses. Courageous people spoke up. Ron Ellis, a star player on the last hockey team that won the Stanley Cup for Toronto in 1967, described overcoming depression as a far more powerful achievement than winning the hockey trophy. Michael Wilson, Canada's outstanding finance minister under Prime Minister Brian Mulroney and later ambassador to the United States, spoke about the effects of stigma and how it contributed to the suicide of his son Cameron.

We spoke out whenever people were demeaning in reference to the mentally ill. When Jim Carrey made a movie about mental illness that was denigrating, we were part of the protest. We spoke in schools and in workplaces; we educated doctors. We wrote position papers to influence thought leaders in government and the media. We supported Workman Arts, an art collective founded by a creative nurse, Lisa Brown, at Queen Street in the late 1980s. This patient group put on plays, art shows, and a wonderful movie festival, Rendezvous with Madness. I don't think any of us were naive—it takes years to alter attitudes and behaviours—but we believed that we had set the right path.

Protest and education are important, but nothing is more significant than contact; when people rub shoulders with those who have had a mental illness, they can no longer dehumanize them and discrimination fades. This is why we encouraged patients to develop work skills; to become peer counsellors, masonry workers, and chefs, and to run the coffee shop. The more we live and work together, the more we fight discrimination.

By acting on many fronts, both physical and psychological, we created a new place and a new way of being on the site of the old asylum. Instead of a relic of Victoriana designed to shield the mentally ill and the citizenry from each other, we created an urban neighbourhood with buildings that were ordinary by design. When you walk down the street, you would never know what was inside. This was the dawn of a new era for mental illness. An era in which we all belong.

CHAPTER 22
DSM Dysfunction

Psychiatrists today face a major problem: the scientific revolution that has provided us with so many powerful tools to treat mental illness has in some ways diminished us as a caring profession. Take the business of diagnosis. As we've seen, psychoanalysis and its obscure language were banished from the DSM, the diagnostic manual, when its authors started classifying mental illness by symptoms in 1980.

This change has had a profound effect on the treatment of mental illness. The DSM has become the bible for insurers, managed health care providers, and the courts. They rely on it to decide whether treatment is funded or not. In many ways, the DSM has been a useful advance. It has helped the practice of psychiatry by enhancing the reliability of diagnosis and has allowed physicians to talk to each other, knowing they are discussing the same thing.

But it has also influenced psychiatry in less positive ways. The checklist approach downgrades psychological understanding, and a new generation of psychiatrists are diagnosing by formula rather than sitting with patients to understand their problems in the context of their life and psychological makeup. To me, this is a major issue. It is a loss for our profession and a loss for our patients. A diagnosis is just the beginning and can never substitute for a deep understanding of the person.

The DSM has always been controversial and has other limitations.[1] For one thing, the line it draws between sick and not sick is arbitrary. I could see that problem when I was working on the DSM committee for eating disorders. The rule was that a female had to lose her menstrual period to qualify as an anorexic. However, my colleagues and I were able to show, through a large Ontario population study, that young women who lose weight because of a terror of fatness demonstrate the same degree of impairment in their lives whether or not they've lost their menstrual periods. (This criterion has since been changed.) A criterion for bulimia nervosa was bingeing and vomiting twice a week. This too was arbitrary: people who vomit once a week can otherwise be just as ill as those vomiting more often. In focusing on reliability, the DSM created problems with qualification. If you don't meet the criteria for a disorder according to the DSM, you might not qualify for funded treatment despite serious impairment.

Further difficulty arises when the DSM turns a normal experience into a medical issue. Depression is a good example. According to the DSM, one must have five of nine symptoms lasting for just over two weeks in order to qualify for this diagnosis. Yet this set of criteria blends in with many normal mood states and inflates the frequency of clinical depression in any population. When Gordon Parker and his colleagues in Australia conducted a community-based study using DSM criteria, they found that by the time people were aged 40, an astounding 79% had met criteria for clinical depression at some point in their lifetime.[2] How reasonable is the two-week duration? All we have to consider is our own responses to significant loss or setback—most people feel down for a couple of weeks. Moreover, evidence shows that mild states like this frequently remit rapidly.[3] A six-week minimum would be far more appropriate for a clinically significant diagnosis.

In DSM-5, published in May 2013, the scope of depression was significantly expanded to include people who feel sad for several months after losing a loved one; previously, bereavement had been excluded unless extremely prolonged and severe.[4] The science behind the DSM-5's decision to eliminate the bereavement exclusion is this: there are no clinical studies showing that major depressive syndromes shortly after the death of a loved one differ markedly from other depressions that happen spontaneously. Apparently, the committee wanted to make sure the bereaved got the treatment they need, to reduce suffering and prevent suicide, though suicide among the bereaved is extremely rare, much less than in the general population. The inclusion of bereavement in this way raises troubling questions: Are we turning a normal human emotion into a medical problem? Will this increase the use of antidepressants? Is there any evidence that the antidepressant medicines will work for what is an expectable human response to a major loss?

It is impossible to say with any accuracy when normal grief ends and depression begins, but we can say that when the experience is prolonged (over a year) and severe, it requires treatment. However, by linking grief with pathology, we are creating a situation where normal emotion is seen as abnormal. Grief has a useful function for human beings: it permits us to pay respect to the lost person while enabling us to withdraw and recover from the loss.

Medicalizing the worried well could drain resources from the seriously mentally ill to people who might have modest symptoms and no real impairment in their lives. It might also lead to unnecessary drug prescriptions. When family doctors can spend only 6 to 10 minutes with patients, they will be inclined to prescribe medications. According to Allen Francis, an emeritus professor from Duke University who headed the previous revision of the DSM, expanding diagnostic criteria is a "bonanza" for drug companies. Frances has commented that the DSM originally had the goal of establishing a common language for the discipline but now is regularly misused as a guide to specific treatments.

Are the DSM committees being influenced by pharmaceutical companies to make decisions that will ultimately lead to more drug sales? DSM committee members in the last iteration

(DSM-5) were allowed to earn consulting fees from drug companies, although David Kupfer, the chair of DSM-5, limited the amounts individual members can earn to $10,000 per year, and limited stock holdings to less than $50,000. However, I don't believe that individual committee members have been swayed by the drug companies and their consulting fees. Rather, they are influenced by a bias: they see more and more problems as medical conditions requiring treatment, not as variants of natural experiences, behaviours, and feelings. This bias toward medications has been growing for the past 30 years.

Social anxiety disorder is another example of shifting boundaries regarding normal variants of behaviour. Social anxiety was inserted as a disorder in DSM-IV in 1994. Critics claim that the normal and at times useful quality of shyness is being pathologized. On the other hand, a case can be made regarding extreme shyness that causes distress and impairs quality of life. If one panics at the thought of going out, or is unable to speak in a group, for example, treatment is valuable. The only way to get treatment in many countries is to have a diagnosis. Creating social anxiety disorder permits many people who suffer to get help, but it may also change how we view variations in temperament and certain personality characteristics.

In fairness, the DSM committee sometimes resists the temptation to make new diagnoses. Recently, one of the committees considered a new diagnosis: attenuated psychosis disorder, also known as psychosis risk syndrome. This was supposed to describe young adults who have suffered subtle symptoms such as hearing barely audible sounds or whispers in their heads, or perceiving objects as frightening or threatening. Some of these people might be at risk for full-blown psychoses, and for them, earlier treatment may be valuable.

But many others captured by this category would never become ill. A study conducted by investigators at Brown University, in Providence, Rhode Island, showed that among a large sample of psychiatric outpatients, all of the patients who would qualify for the so-called psychosis risk syndrome met criteria for another DSM disorder. So why have the new diagnosis, especially when it might result in the unnecessary prescription of powerful drugs to someone who doesn't need them? The proposed disorder was sent back for further study, wisely in my opinion.[5]

While pulling back on some new conditions, others were added in the latest version, including binge eating disorder (in DSM-IV, this was included but only as a topic for further study; it is now fully in the text); excoriation disorder, characterized by repetitive and compulsive picking of the skin, resulting in tissue damage; as well as hoarding disorder, in which sufferers have persistent difficulty discarding possessions regardless of their value. The DSM keeps casting a wider net, by expanding the criteria for different disorders. This identifies many more in the population as having a diagnosis than previously.

ADHD provides us with a good example of how the criteria changed and further inflated already high prevalence rates. ADHD, already far more diagnosed in the United States than in the United Kingdom, will now only have to have an age of onset of 12 rather than 7, thus increasing prevalence further.[6] Similarly, Joel Paris at McGill has described a group of our colleagues as "bipolar imperialists," people who are ever expanding the spectrum of bipolar disorder so that more people can be treated with medications. But the DSM-5 committee wisely held the line at not shrinking the minimal length of a hypomanic episode from four days to two. DSM-5 has also made some changes that in my opinion have improved the diagnostic criteria—for autism, for example.[7]

Over and over we hear that the rationale for expanding the pool of people who are diagnosed as having a disorder is to permit people to obtain needed treatment. But perhaps we should be more concerned about diverting extremely limited resources to less severe problems when we expand the definition of a disorder. The DSM can also complicate things for the researcher because the categorization lumps too many different people into one camp. Proper clinical trials are next to impossible if many different types of problems become mixed. DSM diagnoses are devised by a group of experts sitting around a table utilizing symptom clusters to create diagnostic categories. Committees are invariably forced to make compromises that also influence the final outcome of clusters and categories. The symptom clusters are descriptions of the way people commonly suffer but do not reflect the underlying causation or process of illness.

For example, DSM bundles all depressive disorders in the same category. For almost 100 years, researchers and clinicians have argued over whether there's a difference between an endogenous depression, which seems to arise unprovoked from within, and a reactive depression, which occurs in response to the external world. The current DSM supports the idea of depression as a homogeneous disorder, as described by Edward Mapother and Aubrey Lewis, the leaders of the Institute of Psychiatry in the 1930s. They correctly claimed that most depressions have some initial precipitant or stressor, however subtle—a blow to one's self-worth or a conflict with a family member or loss of a loved pet, for example. Despite how it starts, however, there's no clear line between the symptoms of an internal depression and one provoked by something meaningful outside (losing a pet may mean a great deal to one person and much less to a second). What's more, as David Kupfer of the University of Pittsburgh has shown (and as I mentioned earlier), most depressions after the first episode require less and less stress to provoke an episode. Somehow the brain changes so that one becomes vulnerable to a recurrence with more modest life difficulty.

Depressive states may also be considered from another perspective: depression may occur along a continuum of severity, with severe forms getting locked in, and because of changes in brain circuitry, becoming self-perpetuating. This severe group falls into what was once known as melancholia. These patients have more physical symptoms, particular energy disturbances such as psychomotor agitation or retardation, in addition to the alterations in mood and affect.

These differences are relevant. The severe-melancholia group respond to SSRI and tricyclic antidepressants and to ECT, whereas less severe states may not respond to biological interventions. People with bipolar depression are different in another way. Antidepressants without mood stabilizers may worsen their condition. People with psychotic depression often require an antipsychotic medicine as well as an antidepressant, or perhaps ECT.[8]

The largest category of depressed people consists of those who are depressed because of a combination of life experiences and personality factors. Personality characteristics such as severe self-criticism, or extreme shyness and anxiety and especially rejection sensitivity, are vulnerability factors, with recurrent life stressors. Patients in this group are much more responsive to specific psychotherapies, such as cognitive behaviour therapy or interpersonal or psychodynamic therapy. They seem to be less responsive to antidepressant medication. A careful understanding of the patient and his or her symptoms is necessary to determine an appropriate therapy for depression. The DSM, in grouping all depressions under one headline, can easily mislead a doctor into prescribing the wrong treatment.

Broad classifications can also interfere with the evaluation of drug efficacy. There has been a great deal of criticism stemming from the fact that the newer antidepressants appear no better than a placebo in many studies. This is a fascinating finding, since the older studies showed large differences between the people who took the drug and those given a placebo. The critics are not addressing that the new studies include people with minimal symptoms who still meet the DSM-IV criteria, whereas the old studies were based on a much stricter definition of depressive illness.

As stated, the DSM has never been free of bias. Since 1980 it was anti-psychoanalysis and pro-medical. In developing the new versions of the DSM, social beliefs of committee members can matter as much, or more, than the scientific evidence. When DSM-IV was being developed, I served on the committee (of four psychiatrists and one psychologist) to revise the criteria for eating disorders. We met in Washington, DC, every few months over three years and had lively discussions on, for example, whether a diagnosis of bulimia nervosa required one, two, or three binge episodes a week. We were asked to, whenever possible, use research evidence to support the diagnostic criteria. Most of our work focused on small changes to the criteria, but there was one large area of new development. Some colleagues, especially Robert Spitzer, wanted to include a new diagnosis, binge eating disorder, to include people who binge but don't purge. But there was little research data on this subject—Spitzer felt that the DSM could be used to stimulate research. On the other hand, the new head of the DSM, Allen Francis, thought that the field would be enhanced as a profession if current evidence drove any diagnostic changes.

This is an interesting debate because it illuminates how DSM criteria evolve. An anthropologist from a nearby university (Lucille Parkinson McCarthy, from the University of Maryland) asked if she could sit in on our committee meetings. We agreed and quickly forgot about her presence as we entered into our debates. She later wrote a paper about her observations: we repeatedly would use the research base but often had underlying strong beliefs based on clinical experiences or other factors that we attempted to dismiss.[9] McCarthy emphasized the social and political forces on our minds, sometimes acknowledged and often beneath the surface—concerns about the stigmatization of some obese people; economic concerns regarding insurance companies' willingness to pay for the large number of people who would seek treatment; and even concerns about the public impression of psychiatry so rapidly expanding its patient base—would this be seen as trivializing and self-serving? But the entire tilt of DSM since 1980 has had a self-serving quality: DSM-III made psychiatry more medical at a time of competition from other mental health providers, making psychiatry more prestigious and adding a uniqueness to the profession.

The members of the DSM committee were hesitant to include the new diagnosis, so even though all of us knew this group of people existed from clinical experience, we all thought the data should drive the decision. Spitzer pushed hard—he brought forward epidemiological studies, studies of comorbidity, and analyses of the way the proposed criteria worked together. He persuaded the group to have the new diagnosis in the manual. Nineteen years later, in DSM-5 the definition is being expanded. Instead of two times a week for six months, patients can be diagnosed if they binge eat once a week for three months. It is not yet clear how many more people will be seen as having a disorder with this change.

One can see into the future by looking at today's HMOs (health maintenance organizations) in the United States. In many of those settings, the psychiatrist's job has become about changing or initiating medications. This is how organizational jobs are defined, and this is what trainees learn and see for their future. Huge money from pharmaceutical companies is driving this trend. Pharmaceutical research funds contribute to academic credentials and advancement for young researchers. Academic departments have far fewer positions for those who are primarily clinician-teachers or psychotherapy researchers. The paradox is that many still choose psychiatry because it promises more personal and closer relationships with patients and a better understanding of the human condition than any other field of medicine.

David Brooks, the excellent *New York Times* columnist, has described the problem of the DSM well: "The recent editions of this manual exude an impressive aura of scientific authority. They treat mental diseases like diseases of the heart and liver. They leave the impression that you should go to your psychiatrist because she has a vast body of technical knowledge that will allow her to solve your problems. With their austere neutrality, they leave a distinct impression: Psychiatrists are methodically treating symptoms, not people. Psychiatrists are not heroes of science. They are heroes of uncertainty, using improvisation, knowledge and artistry to improve people's lives."

Brooks is right when he goes on to say, "The best psychiatrists are not coming up with abstract rules that homogenize treatments. They are combining an awareness of common patterns with an acute attention to the specific circumstances of a unique human being. They certainly are not inventing new diseases in order to medicalize the moderate ailments of the worried well."[10]

Recognizing this, the people who developed the DSM put in a qualifier. They caution us against taking too literally the sharp boundaries between disorders and between illness and the normal difficulties of life. The problem, as New York psychiatrist Sally Satel has commented, is that key public institutions often disregard these caveats—they treat the DSM as the literal truth. Equally important, the teaching of psychiatry is distorted by the DSM. The next generation is learning to diagnose psychiatric illness using the checklist in the manual. In doing so, they're losing a huge part of our knowledge and skills.

Despite all the controversies over the DSM, the checklist approach to psychiatry has helped us make more reliable diagnoses. But it comes with a price. It is impossible to treat suffering individuals without understanding personal history, symbolic meaning, conflict, ambivalence, social context, and the primacy of existential concerns. This is particularly true when dealing with the impact on humans of violence and poverty, which contribute to current levels of depression and other psychiatric disorders. Sadly, some psychiatrists today don't want to know. They are so fixed on categorizing the symptoms they observe and then choosing an appropriate drug that they don't search for the deeper meaning of their patients' problems. The diagnosis becomes the end in itself—and the treatment with medication follows.

I believe this is regrettable, both for patients and for our profession. Accurate diagnosis is obviously important, but we as psychiatrists have to move beyond the DSM to preserve our unique capacity to develop a deep understanding of individuals and the mechanisms, both biological and psychological, that underlie their suffering. If we persist on this course of defining our field primarily by checklists of symptoms and making drug treatments the primary answer to human troubles, what will we be?

CHAPTER 23

Psychotherapy: The New Evidence

In the last 20 years, just as psychiatrists were running away from the talk therapies, particularly psychodynamically based ones, there's been a growing body of scientific evidence that shows talk therapies work. In fact, there is overwhelming evidence that nondrug therapies can be a powerful way to handle psychiatric conditions if we specifically define which therapies for which types of problems. Psychiatrists today have a wide array of treatments beyond medications to offer individual patients. There is a huge opportunity for psychiatrists, presuming we take it.

Talk therapies are making a comeback in a scientific age because the evidence shows they are effective for specific problems. Cognitive behaviour therapy (CBT), developed in Philadelphia by Aaron Beck and his colleagues, including Brian Shaw, who came to the Clarke in the 1980s, examines the types of distorted thinking that may affect emotions and behaviour.[1] Patients are helped by examining misguided thoughts and learning to challenge them. CBT has been proven to help people with depression, some anxiety disorders, and even bulimia. More than 70 clinical trials of CBT for unipolar depression leave no doubt that it's effective—better than placebo and equal to medications for mild to moderate depressions. CBT also reduces the rate of relapse as well as or better than medications. It is useful for the eating disorders and addictions when modified for the specific problem. It is now being adapted for use as an aid to treatments for schizophrenia and bipolar illness. Research has also shown that behaviour therapies are of value in specific circumstances, such as desensitization to phobias or for compulsions.

Another treatment for depression, interpersonal therapy, evaluates the patient's relations with other people from a psychodynamic perspective. It was first developed as a control condition in a trial of new antidepressants by Gerald Klerman of Boston and Eugene Paykel of London. When the surprising results began to show the treatment was beneficial, it was refined by Klerman and Myrna Weissman and their colleagues, in the New Haven–Boston Collaborative Depression Research Project for the treatment of moderately depressed patients. By the late 1980s, there was evidence for its real effectiveness, especially for depression in the context of acute relational problems, losses, and transitions.[2] Another form of psychotherapy, supportive psychotherapy, is useful particularly when combined with medication and rehabilitation. It aids the patient in developing a greater understanding of his or her current situation, defining alternatives and fostering adaptive coping and resilience. Supportive therapy helps to buttress the individual's self-esteem, encourages expression of feelings, and works to instil a sense of hope.

More recently, Marsha Linehan of the University of Washington developed dialectical behaviour therapy (DBT), a treatment she wished she had received when she was ill as an adolescent.[3] Originally used for suicidal adolescents with borderline personality disorder, DBT has been adapted for substance abuse and eating disorders. Linehan hypothesized that people with borderline personality disorders struggle to experience and integrate the dialectic, the opposing views. Self-destructive urges are commonly part of borderline syndromes. Suicidal behaviour, according to Linehan, is both harmful and maladaptive but may serve a useful purpose, perhaps to release emotion, or to alter feelings, or to convey distress. Thus, there is a need for both self-acceptance (Linehan calls this radical self-acceptance), and change, the latter for parts of the self that can be altered. Acknowledging that behaviour makes some sense as a relief from suffering is important in providing validation for the person (they are not "just bad"). Although validation and acceptance of the self are important, modifying maladaptive behaviour is also critical. Linehan showed that entrenched behaviours can change, and when they do, can alter the person's emotional state (the opposite of what many people had intuitively thought). As part of treatment, people are taught "action opposite to emotion": when they feel an emotion is inappropriate, they are to act in a manner opposing that emotion. These interventions diminish impulsiveness and help people tolerate distressing "bad" feelings. Mindfulness has been an important part of this treatment, and has been since pursued for its own benefits.

Mindfulness-based stress reduction was first developed by Jon Kabat-Zinn at the University of Massachusetts Medical School in the late 1970s from experiences in the application of Buddhist meditation techniques.[4] A core goal of mindfulness meditation is to develop an ability to experience thoughts as purely mental events that can be allowed to pass through the mind without generating feelings or reactions. The focus is not to change "aberrant" thoughts but to learn to experience them as internal phenomena separated from the self. Mindfulness meditation has been shown to be effective in preventing relapse once a patient has recovered from depression. Mindfulness-based cognitive therapy (MBCT) was specifically developed by Zindel Segal and his colleagues to reduce the number of relapses in patients with recurrent major depression.[5] Mindfulness is also useful for people in recovery from substance abuse.

• • •

After hundreds of studies, we now know that psychotherapy is effective for most people. One meta-analysis found that "the average person who receives therapy is better off at the end of it than 80% of the persons who do not."[6] Another more recent meta-analysis of more than 50 controlled studies of adolescents and children, comparing evidenced-based therapies (such as CBT or family therapy) with general support, found a large benefit to the evidence-based therapies.[7]

The real issue, then, was not whether psychotherapy worked. The question was what kind of psychotherapy was useful for what sort of disorders, and when to apply it with other forms of treatment. Those decisions, I believe, should be based as much as possible on the evidence a priori and not on the theoretical biases of the individual psychiatrist.

Clinicians may not be changing their practices in response to psychotherapy research data. In the 1999 study I did with Christine Dunbar, Mike Bagby, and Barbara Dorian of Ontario psychiatrists, we found, that 40% of the physicians had altered their theoretical orientation—the belief system that guides understanding of a person—over the course of their careers. The majority did not. Whether they had incorporated these new therapies into their treatments is not clear from our study, but anecdotally it appeared that most had not. Psychiatrists can use different therapies in their practice even if they specialize in one area. It is possible to learn the skills of another approach to better tailor treatment to the individual patient, or at least to recognize when an alternative intervention would be effective.

Dynamic psychotherapy is a powerful treatment, but it is not useful for all conditions. Those with chronic depression or certain personality disorders can benefit from this treatment, but those with severe depression, OCD, or psychosis generally do not. Combining dynamic therapy with medications can enhance the results for conditions such as moderate depression and bulimia.

Psychologist Allan Abbas of Dalhousie University, in Nova Scotia, published a meta-analysis of more than 20 studies of the effectiveness of psychodynamic treatments that lasted for fewer than 40 sessions.[8] These included almost 1,500 people suffering from depression, anxiety, or stress-related problems. The analysis demonstrated a very large beneficial effect from the dynamic therapies. Equally important was the finding that when people were followed up over the first year after therapy had ended, the positive effect had continued to grow. Psychodynamic therapy may set in motion processes that lead to further psychological growth and maturity.

Although there is strong evidence that talk therapy is effective in some cases, we don't know exactly how it works. (This is also true for many new medications that are introduced generally in medical practice.) Is it the therapist's interpretations (the formulations of the meaning of feelings and behaviour) that leads the patient to new insight and benefits, or something else? There is strong evidence that trust, faith, hope, consistent concern, and attention are important for the success of therapy. In studies where patients and therapists fill out notes after each session over one and a half years, it had been demonstrated that intellectual insights were not the only thing that produced change. Emotional interventions were considered to be most powerful, according to both therapists and patients. Other studies comparing CBT and dynamic therapy have shown that CBT is most helpful when therapists have incorporated components of dynamic therapy—exploring recurrent themes, emotions, and fantasies, as well as defences and relationship patterns.[9] The precise mechanisms that produce change may not be clear, but this doesn't undermine the strong case for the effectiveness of talk therapy.

Too many clinicians ignore the evidence for psychotherapy and rely too heavily on prescribing medications. This is a symptom of a major problem afflicting our profession. We have swung too far in the direction of prescribing drugs for mental illness and even for problems that are a normal part of the human condition. We have traded the hours of therapy, and the search for meaning in a person's life, for the checklist diagnosis and the quick prescription.

This is hardly what we signed up for when we became psychiatrists and committed ourselves to helping people with mental illness. If we really want to serve our patients, we need to deploy the full scope of treatments to relieve pain, and intervene to help them live more fulfilling lives. Psychotherapies, as we have seen, have been proven effective for some people. Decent housing and jobs are essential to recovery. Above all, we need to treat our patients as complex individuals, not as one-dimensional figures. We need to devise layered treatments addressing their biological, psychological, and social needs.

Unlike other professionals working in the mental health field, psychiatrists potentially have the training and ability to integrate the complex and powerful interactions between biological and psychological makeup and experience. Ideally, we can balance the science of the brain with the art of managing the mind to produce innovations in treatment that merge these aspects in tailored and specific ways.

For psychiatry to be a strong profession, it must have a conceptual centre. The domain of the psychiatrist is the mind and the personal consciousness of the patient.[10] We study the physical brain as an index of the mind. We study behaviour as an index of the person's makeup. Psychiatrists should aim to understand the person, and why disorders of thinking, feeling, or behaving have evolved as they have in that person. The problems may involve some changes in the person's brain that impact thinking, memory, perception, and mood; aspects of temperament such as genetics, attachment, or intelligence; life experiences like loss, separation, abuse, or trauma; and the broader context, such as family, relationships, and work.[11] Only when all these factors have been considered does the ideal psychiatrist determine the necessary interventions. Many mental health workers can provide good psychotherapies, and many general practitioners and internists can learn to be capable psychopharmacologists. Psychiatrists should provide a unique understanding, integrating medical knowledge, neuroscience, psychological models of the mind, and social determinants of behaviour.

Our domain is the interface of mind, brain, and body. We have to evaluate and integrate information, from the molecular, to the neurochemical, to the intrapsychic (within the mind), to the interpersonal, to the systemic, to the sociocultural. The territory is the broad science of human behaviour, including psychology, anthropology, and sociology, as well as the complex activities of the central nervous system. Our tools range from our capacity for empathic listening to sophisticated neuroimaging systems, such as PET scans and functional MRIs that show detailed pictures of brain functioning in health and disorder.

What an amazing time to enter the field of psychiatry. We now know how common the mental illnesses are. There is a real need for new, well-trained people in our field; jobs will be plentiful. As well, there is great variety in the type of work, and it is never boring. We are now able to draw understanding from complex fields to make psychiatric care and treatment comprehensible to patients and families, and to engage the public and our colleagues. We are becoming more able to battle the prejudice to our patients and the field, and we are advancing treatments dramatically. Someone entering the profession today will be certain to see remarkable increases in knowledge and continual therapeutic advances throughout their careers.

One of the distinguishing features of psychiatry is in the diversity of models we use to understand the human conditions. They provide us with a frame of reference to appraise a problem. Take a 12-year-old boy, James, who is afraid to go outdoors at his father's farm. He is afraid of horses, convinced they might kick or bite him. The traditional Freudian analyst might see the boy as gripped by an Oedipal fear, which in this case is a displacement of a fear of his father onto the horse. A more modern dynamic psychiatrist could highlight a problem in attachment, associated with anxiety in being separate from his mother and fears of abandonment that keep the boy indoors.

The behaviourist would focus the problem from a different point of view. Perhaps the little boy went outside a long time ago and a horse snapped at him. This caused anxiety that led to a fear, which has now generalized to all horses and places with horses. An interpersonal framework might focus on the issue of unresolved conflict between the father and son, and on the fear and avoidant behaviour as representing the boy's ambivalent struggle with anger and wishes for independence. The geneticist might evaluate the family to see whether any blood relatives were predisposed to high levels of anxiety. There could be an inborn defect in the brain's neurotransmitters and receptors that regulate anxiety. Ultimately, one may propose a dimensional model—the boy was born with a vulnerability to anxiety and stress, which is stimulated by certain circumstances that have a specific meaning to the boy and thereby influence his avoidant behaviour.

Six psychiatrists, six different but possibly overlapping explanations. Each one might be convinced that his or her model provides the complete and only answer to the mystery posed by the boy's fear of going outside and being with horses. In real life, though, one explanation rarely provides a full view of one person, let alone all people who present with suffering in a particular way. People are complex, and each individual's presentation is impacted by different life circumstances, temperament, and experiences, and psychiatrists' ability to vary and integrate the models of understanding enriches our experience of the clinical situation.

By using the model that best fits the situation, we can gain a more comprehensive understanding of the problem, which will lead to a more thoughtful and effective treatment plan. Ideally psychiatrists of the future will have the training and knowledge to use various models of the human psyche to improve the quality of life for our patients. This understanding will open the door to all kinds of strategies, from prescribing drugs, to interpreting unconscious motivation, to meditation and cognitive behaviour therapy, to helping the patient find a home and a job.

A Comfortable Home Is Good for Therapy

The traditional view of housing for people with addiction and mental illness has been that they should cut out drugs first, then get into treatment, then training, and then finally, find a place to live. In the early 1990s in New York City, psychologist Sam Tsemberis and researcher Ronda Eisenberg tried the opposite approach based on what homeless people told them.[12] They began providing the housing and rent supplements, and then individualized supports based on the person's need. After five years, 88% of the program's tenants remained housed, whereas only 47% of the residents in the city's residential treatment system remained housed. A large multisite Canadian study program called At Home/Chez Soi, run by the Mental Health Commission of Canada, with Paula Goering as the academic lead investigator, has shown not only better outcomes for the homeless who received housing as a first step in treatment but also significant monetary savings for the health care system.

A Job Is a Part of Good Treatment

A job is good therapy too. There has been a striking evolution from the old vocational rehab approach (think wicker baskets) to supported employment strategies, which provide job coaches, job development and training, transportation, individually tailored supervision, and support on the job. There is good evidence that these interventions are effective and promote confidence, self-esteem and well-being. According to a 2004 review by Indiana University psychology professor Gary Bond, 60% of patients enrolled in these programs found jobs, compared with 20% in other programs.[13]

Research demonstrates without a doubt how powerful work, income, housing, and social support are to recovery. Friends and family who develop mental illnesses need us more at those times than any other, and our very presence has a strong mitigating influence on their symptoms. The common social distancing that accompanies mental illness and addiction can be as devastating as the illness itself, if not more so. Human beings are social animals who need to connect and belong. Care, attention, and connection are even more important if we have an addiction to painkillers or a serious depression. We don't stop needing a comfortable and safe home because we have an alcohol problem or schizophrenia. In fact, how could we begin to recover without this essential security? Eugene Paykel and others have summarized the strong scientific evidence for social support playing a critical role in the outcome of mental illness.[14]

There is no doubt that effective treatments now exist for people with mental illnesses. These have been evaluated in many scientific trials, and the results are overwhelming, if only psychiatrists use this evidence for the benefit of reducing the suffering of their patients.

CHAPTER 24

What Makes a Good Psychiatrist?

It takes significant scope of human skill to be a first-rate psychiatrist today. A 2009 British study by Dinesh Bhugra and colleagues surveyed over 100 clinical tutors on the key characteristics of a good psychiatrist and member of the Royal College of Psychiatrists. The most valued characteristic was overall competency in diagnosis, management, and investigations (98%); followed by being a good communicator and listener (96.5%); the ability to make appropriate clinical decisions (97.3%); and bringing empathy, encouragement, and hope to patients and their families (83%). A critical self-awareness of emotional responses to clinical situations was also found to be important to 69%. Having a basic understanding of group dynamics was valued by 40%. The skill rated least important was the ability to appraise staff (13%).[1]

Clinical Judgment

The results of the Royal College survey of clinical tutors show that virtually all agree on the need for clinicians to have skills in diagnosis, management, and investigations, and an ability to make appropriate clinical decisions. What goes into these qualities? Kathryn Montgomery, a medical humanities professor at Northwestern University, has described medical thinking as neither an art nor a science in her 2006 book *How Doctors Think.*[2] Montgomery argues that, although physicians make use of science, medicine is not in itself a science but an interpretive practice that requires clinical judgment. These days, physicians' opinions are informed by knowledge that is based on science. The science base is critical and has led to innumerable advances in practice. But the general laws of science—certainty, reliability, dependability—have to be brought down to the specific person who is ill and facing the physician.

A physician takes the patient's history along with the presenting physical signs and symptoms and puts these together with clinical experience, that is, the lessons learned from others and from the basic and clinical scientific literature, in order to come to a clinical judgment. The essence of clinical judgment is knowing how to "particularize" to the individual person an observation that has been made on a population. As Oliver Wendell Holmes said, "The physician must generalize the disease and individualize the patient."[3] It also involves determining when the rules don't apply, or when a working diagnosis must be revised in light of new data. Whether we call this "practical reasoning," as Montgomery does, or the "art" of medical practice, as most of us do, it is central to becoming a capable clinician.

Flexibility

A good clinical psychiatrist needs to be flexible. Sometimes one has to be direct; at other times, it is important to allow patients to tell their stories in their own way. Sometimes it's valuable to hear the patient's fantasies; at other times, it is more effective to use an intellectual or cognitive approach. Sometimes common sense is what's needed. Although often underappreciated, it can be quite useful, particularly when guided by knowledge of the person's conflicts and strengths. Supportive psychotherapy is sometimes equated with talking to a kind neighbour but actually requires specific skill. This therapy takes into account the individual's personality and life history, adaptive and less adaptive coping mechanisms, and recent stressors to enable the person to gain a greater understanding of themselves and their current circumstances and options. The supportive therapist also works to instill hope and to enhance self-esteem and resilience.

Flexibility also means appreciating how psychiatric disorders do change over the years. For example, in Freud's time, hysteria, or conversion disorder, was a common diagnosis. Today these problems are called the somatic symptom disorders and dissociative disorders, and have separate categories in the DSM. The somatic symptom disorders are defined by disturbances in physical sensations or in motor functions, whereas dissociative disorders involve involuntary alterations in the sense of memory and identity. These specific disorders are rare now because they are thought to occur primarily in societies with strict social systems that prevent individuals from directly expressing feelings and emotions toward others. Such symptoms become an indirect means of communicating in less open cultures. In modern Western societies these types of syndromes are now very rare. However, other problems such as anorexia and bulimia have increased in my lifetime, in my view because of cultural shifts such as pressures for women to be thin and to perform to a certain standard.

Other psychiatric disorders that have increased are related to HIV infection (depression, delirium, dementia), as the infection has changed from a fatal to a chronic illness. Borderline personality disorder is typified by an intense inner pain and the attempts to express and manage it. Although we don't know if BPD has increased in recent decades, the associated behaviours (drug abuse, cutting, binge eating, gambling) used to reduce the emotional pain do vary in different circumstances. The frequency of problem gambling has, of course, increased greatly as governments have all scrambled for more revenues and made gambling legal and widely available.

Hope, Faith, Caring, and Support

Psychiatrists need to have a deep understanding of the physical brain, but we can never overlook a crucial component of therapy: giving a patient hope, faith, caring, and support. All physicians, including psychiatrists, should consider this an essential element of treatment. I think this was why the war veteran I met in Winnipeg when I was a medical student back in the 1960s regained his voice, at least for a short while. We gave him hope, attention, respect, and enthusiasm and encouraged him to face problems and master them. This faith helped him overcome the forces that were keeping him from speaking, though in his case only temporarily.

A generation ago, Johns Hopkins psychiatrist Jerome Frank studied patients who felt demoralized and hopeless because they were unable to bear their symptoms. Therapy offered hope, along with trust, feeling understood, being respected, and being encouraged to develop active coping strategies. Studies have demonstrated that these factors have as great an impact on outcome as the specific theory and technique.[4]

Empathy and Formulation

Sir William Osler had an elegant description of how doctors understand their patients: "It is as important to know what kind of a man has the disease as it is to know what kind of disease has the man." He went on: "There is a tendency among young men about hospitals to study the cases, not the patients, and in the interest they take in the disease lose sight of the individual. Strive against this."[5]

Psychiatrists, in other words, need to develop empathy. An empathic therapist accurately understands the subjective experience of the patient and is able to disentangle it from his or her own experience. Empathy is the ability to connect with another's internal world through understanding that person's situation, perspective, and feelings. A therapist may then communicate that understanding or act helpfully on that understanding.

"Empathy" is an often misunderstood word. Empathy means you appreciate the other person's point of view and you can understand how that person feels and views life. It doesn't mean you emotionally experience that person's pain or cry with him or her. It is sympathy when you join in the experiences and feelings of the other. This distinction is important. Empathic psychiatrists have an objective view of their patients' problems; they share their understanding but maintain an appropriate emotional distance. Sympathetic physicians may share emotions with their patients, but this can interfere with treatment if they give up the detached objectivity that leads to deeper understanding.

Empathy is significant in all kinds of medical care. A review of primary care physicians shows that health outcomes are related to the capacity for empathy.[6] "Greater physician empathy has been associated with fewer medical errors, better patient outcomes and more satisfied patients," according to Dr. Pauline Chen. "It also results in fewer malpractice claims and happier doctors."[7] The psychopharmacologist is better if she is empathic; the surgeon can avoid lawsuits if he communicates in an understanding way with patients and their families. In psychiatry, numerous studies have shown that empathy contributes largely to the outcome , as do the qualities of openness, nonpossessive warmth, and genuineness.[8]

Yet studies of medical students and residents show that the capacity for empathy decreases over the time of training, whereas cynicism increases.[9] Clearly something is wrong. Melanie Neuman's excellent review from Germany highlighted several factors contributing to this disturbing trend—the mistreatment of students by their superiors, the students' own vulnerability and lack of social support; the high workload and short length of hospital stay.[10] Critically important is the attitude of role models. Many teachers think empathy is too vague to teach, but the opposite is true. Empathy can be defined, and there are good methods to measure it. Although everyone starts out with different natural degrees of empathy, empathy can also be learned, and it should be embedded in the students' educational experiences with patients.[11,12,13]

The anthropologist T.M. Luhrmann believes people are wrong to think of empathy as a mystical quality. Empathy is part of human intuition, and some are born with a greater capacity for it than others, but clinicians can actively enhance their skill in empathic understanding.[14]

As a teacher, it is always tempting to work with the most empathic, gifted, and brilliant students, but often the most valuable clinical gains (for the population) come from helping the less naturally empathic move a step up the scale. Interviewing skills, with the right mix of empathy, rapport, and directed questioning, are crucial. Psychiatrists can improve by observing others and practising with feedback. The good psychiatrist also knows how to synthesize the material from the interview (and other sources) and communicate it succinctly and meaningfully to the patient, family, and referring doctor. Synthesizing or formulating the patient's story into a coherent and meaningful narrative is essential for the practice of psychiatry.

Formulation requires active empathic listening, and connecting and spending time with the other person. One can make a diagnosis in 10 minutes, but you cannot provide a synthesis of the causes and context in less than an hour; and often it takes two or three. The integration follows. Some students are able to grasp this concept quickly, and for others it is a painful learning process. I can always tell how naturally psychiatry comes to the young doctors by their formulations—have they "plugged in" all the material they've been taught is relevant, or do they construct a narrative that is unique and feels meaningful to the particular patient? The formulation should incorporate all predisposing factors in the biological, psychological, and social spheres; all the precipitating issues; and the various forces that sustain the disorder. A formulation should also include a comment on the patient's personality traits, core conflicts, for example, with identity, sexuality, aggression, or dependency, and on his or her relational world—parents, siblings, friends, teachers, romantic partners, and employers. A thorough formulation is invaluable for the understanding of complex and multidimensional human beings. Recently, psychiatric training has moved away from the detailed formulation to focus on diagnosis. I believe we weaken the profession when we no longer demand these skills of the graduating residents.

Humanity, Integrity, Ethics, and Values

Today's graduating physicians and psychiatrists need to care. In this era of highly technical, exceedingly specialized medicine, medical schools typically overlook this. So what should young professionals care about? Students should care about their education, particularly about getting a broad education that develops them as well-rounded citizens with a broad perspective on both their society and their profession. Unfortunately, the current environment of rigid premed preparation doesn't reward a broad education, which might include study of the classics, literature, and philosophy. Instead, students become experts at studying science in a hypercompetitive, narrow environment. They miss out on the experiences that could give them a broader and deeper view of humanity.

Physicians should also care about integrity. Consider one of the big issues in medicine today, patient safety. Our profession cannot deal with this issue until we create an environment in which we can openly discuss errors and how to prevent them. This does not exist. Only 54% of residents discussed their most significant mistake with their attending physician, according to a 1991 article in *JAMA*.[15] This review suggests that a great many young doctors would prefer to get through their residency training without embarrassment than use the medical educational process to prepare them to be better physicians.

Preparing students for this type of integrity is difficult when medical school culture is permissive of bullying. In a *New York Times* article in 2012, Dr. Pauline Chen described an outrageous bullying culture in medical schools.[16] Most students said they had been harassed, or told they were hopeless or the stupidest student, or threatened with poor grades. As many as 85% of students acknowledge this type of behaviour by teachers in their third year. Schools have been reluctant to come forward and recognize this problem. UCLA, however, instituted faculty-wide reforms, including policies to reduce abuse and promote prevention; created a gender- and power-abuse committee; and mandated lectures, workshops, and training sessions for students, residents, and faculty members alike. The university also set up an office to accept confidential reports, and to investigate and then address allegations of mistreatment. This program has had only modest results: 13 years later, over 50% of students still reported some form of bullying, indicating how long it takes to change an entrenched culture.

Our students also have to care about ethics and values. Patient autonomy and dignity are particularly important for those of us who work in mental institutions. A patient's judgment can be affected by the mental disorder, thereby altering the appropriate degree of autonomy, or freedom of action. The degree of autonomy may vary in different periods of illness. In some such periods, we may have to make decisions for the patient's benefit. Patients with cyclical illnesses, like bipolar disorder, may be able to specify, through an advanced directive, what treatments they would wish when they fall ill. In many circumstances, the mental illness does not compromise the patient's judgment or autonomy; here, the clinical team and those closest to the patient have to know when to defer to the patient's preference and when it is necessary to intervene. Appropriate decisions can only be made by fully knowing the person as well as the illness.

Ethical dilemmas face the clinician every day. When do you order someone to go into the hospital as an involuntary patient? When does someone have the capacity to provide consent? How do we maintain confidentiality, and when and where do we breach it? End-of-life decisions can be as vexing as in any part of medicine. I was once asked to provide a consultation on a woman in her late 30s, with a 20-year history of restricting anorexia nervosa (that is, with no purging). She was severely emaciated and was being kept alive by nasogastric feedings. She wanted the feedings to end. Her psychiatrist, although ambivalent, seemed in favour of her decision, but he recognized that this was an uncertain area. I felt that because of the severe starvation and its duration, this woman's cognitive functioning was impaired and that a substitute decision maker was required. The problem was that she had no family member or close friend to act in this role. We recommended on the side of caution—review the patient's wishes when she has had the starvation effects reduced through refeeding and weight restoration. Eight years later she is still alive. Life has more meaning to her, and she has satisfaction in volunteer work.

Respect and a nondiscriminatory attitude to all patients are values we must all care about and uphold. None of us should define people by their illnesses any more than we should define people by their job, their colour, their ethnicity, or their size. A person should not be labelled "a schizophrenic" any more than a person should be viewed as simply "a diabetic." Human beings are nuanced and layered, and respect requires that we never categorize or label people by a single feature. I learned this lesson well from a single incident over 40 years ago when I was a medical student. A classmate and I were running down the hall on our way to see a patient, and my classmate said to me, "Come on, Paul, let's go see the stroke in Room 4." A senior clinician stopped us in our tracks. "There is no stroke in room 4," he said. "Mr. Jones is in Room 4. Let me tell you about him … He is an elderly man who served his country bravely in war, came back, and married his high-school sweetheart; they had four children and now have 11 grandchildren. He has worked all his life for the post office and has volunteered extensively for his community. Now that he is close to 80, he has experienced a stroke, which he is handling with great dignity. There is no stroke in Room 4; Mr. Jones is in Room 4."

We live in a society where the value of respect has diminished and we quickly define people by superficial characteristics, like money, appearance, or power. Such superficiality can be deadly. I have spent much of the last 40 years trying to understand and help people with anorexia nervosa—self-starvation in the face of plenty. This illness is related to a definition of the self through a self-image defined by our culture. Young people strive for an impossible standard of thinness to enhance their self-esteem and are governed by beliefs about body size and shape rather than by the enduring values that lead to a full and rich life. Not coincidentally, in our current world these eating disorders have increased greatly in frequency and have significant morbidity and mortality.

The unique potential of psychiatry is our way of understanding people, both in a broad context and in the application of our medical and psychosocial knowledge to a particular person. But at a time when drugs are dominating psychiatry, our new graduates are becoming less skilled at the very thing that is distinct about being a psychiatrist. We should be able to work comfortably and knowledgeably across many domains of symptoms, disorders, personalities, and life circumstances. We cannot provide this unique perspective if the only frame is the functioning of the brain.

We owe it to our patients to take such a broad perspective of understanding. Psychiatrists need to be aware of new areas of medicine that could impinge on their field. We have to incorporate developments in related fields such as neuroscience, sociology, philosophy, cultural studies, and psychology. I have seen at least three patients in the last two years who have complained of depression and fatigue. I referred them to a sleep clinic; they came back with a diagnosis of sleep apnea. Once the sleep disorder was resolved, their depression and fatigue were greatly diminished.

We owe it to our patients to use the many different models and treatments that are effective and to respect them as unique individuals. The only valid question is whether they help the patient. All treatments must follow the same rules: they should mix science with caring, and must be evaluated in a scientific manner, following accepted methods of design. The hypotheses regarding cause or course of illness should be tested with a desire to disprove them. Biological reductionism, in overly simplifying the human condition, allows simple erroneous theories to become the new reality. People hold on to the conclusion that they have a chemical imbalance instead of facing complex life problems.

We have to acknowledge that we have only a poor understanding of the mechanisms of the brain. But that in no way means we should throw up our hands and say we're completely ignorant. We know many of the contributors to clinical states, such as trauma, abuse, poverty, neglect, loss, drugs, and genetic makeup. But we are just beginning to learn how these are linked to the brain and the final mechanisms of disorders. This science is in its infancy. We do know, however, many of the factors that protect us from illness, particularly the inner and external resources that we bring to deal with adversity. The strengths we have, and their role in preventing mental illness, is a fruitful area of research. The evolution of a model of recovery built on the principles of hope, empowerment, self-determination, and responsibility is an important shift away from biological reductionism and toward humanism in psychiatry.

Psychiatrists today occupy a crucial place in mental health care and must embrace the full scope of clinical care. We need to turn away from purely biological models and the checklist approach to treating mental illness that is dominating our time. It's creating a factory-type approach for treating human troubles. We need to be masters in the art of care, and to blend compassion with knowledge of the new science of the brain and its chemical interactions. I do hope that future physicians will be better than my generation at avoiding false dichotomies. For decades our profession has been fixated on the split between the art and science of care. Yet the split occurs only in the minds of those who imagine it. There is no choice between art and science; they complement each other. Science serves the art of caring.

CHAPTER 25

Restoring the Public Trust

When Gallup asks North Americans how they view different kinds of professionals, psychiatrists typically get low marks. On ratings of "honesty and ethical standards," psychiatrists are rated highly by only 41% of the population. We do better than bankers and HMO managers, but far worse than nurses (who received a high rating from 85% of the population), medical doctors (70%), and dentists (62%).

These attitudes appear to be in part stigma by association; discrimination against the mentally ill spills over to people who look after them.[1] This has even spread to nursing. Among nurses, psychiatric nursing is the least preferred specialty of 10 areas, according to a 2008 survey by Ashland University professor Margaret Halter. Psychiatric nurses were least likely to be described as skilled, logical, dynamic, and respected.[2]

As psychiatrists we ourselves have contributed to our poor public image. When psychiatrists espouse strange theories that make no common sense (like Canada's Brock Chisholm, the first director general of the World Health Organization, who spoke out against the so-called mind-crippling myth of Santa Claus in the mid-1940s), when they blame parents for all ills, or claim that therapy can save the world, people notice. When psychiatrists offer opinions on people they have never examined, others begin to wonder how in the world can we comment when our skill lies in the examination itself? When doctors describe patients by name at a cocktail party, how does this make people feel about the privacy of their most intimate feelings and thoughts? (One person has told me he would never go into psychotherapy because of this.)

Psychiatrists who view the clinical examination as purely a checklist of symptoms and then make no effort to understand the person behind the symptoms leave patients feeling frustrated. Worse, physicians who put a premium on their own research and see the patient primarily as a means to completing their studies leave patients feeling exploited. When practitioners become identified with one side in disputes, like the doctor who is known to be available to take the father's side in custody battles, it's a terrible blow to our credibility.

Our public image has improved somewhat over the last 35 years, according to the same Gallup data. I believe this is related to the ascendancy of biological psychiatry. Psychiatry's return to its foundation in medicine has helped our image and has made us more respectable in the eyes of the public. However, we still have a long way to go to earn the trust of the public.

When one looks at the relationship between physicians and the public, one finds a paradox: people love their individual practitioners, but they don't love the profession. They see their doctor as a healer who is concerned with the ethics of caring and the relationship he or she has with the patient. This has traditionally been the heart of the practice of medicine. The physician uses knowledge and skills to act in the best interests of the patient. The core values of the healer should be psychiatry's greatest asset, and here the public can be our ally. Patients do not wish individual decisions about their health to be made by either a corporation or the state, but rather in the context of a respectful, participatory relationship with their doctors.

So we live with the paradox: people have high expectations for their healers but a low opinion of the profession. This distinction between healer and professional was recognized over 40 years ago by the sociologist Elliott Friedson. Medicine, he said, has convinced the public that it is trustworthy because of its credo of ethical behaviour and the integrity of its body of knowledge.[3] This professed altruism conflicts with doctors' self-interest and professional aggrandizement. The Canadian government's move in 2004 to pour an extra $40 billion into health care over 10 years is a case in point. The bulk of the money didn't go to health care innovation, as was its purpose; most of it went to compensation for strongly organized groups, like doctors and nurses. Over the decade, doctors' compensation rose by 3.3% annually, whereas the average Canadian's compensation went up by just over 1%.[4]

This points to a fundamental problem: psychiatrists have effectively formed a social contract with government and with the people we serve. Society entrusts us with the important job of caring for the mental health of our citizens. In return, we have a duty to behave in a responsible way toward the citizens and the government. Are we fulfilling that social contract?

The idea of the social contract goes back to the seventeenth- and eighteenth-century writings of philosophers Thomas Hobbes, John Locke, and especially Jean-Jacques Rousseau, and was widely promoted in America by Thomas Jefferson. Originally, it was used to explain the nature of the relationship between the state and its citizens. It outlined a series of reciprocal rights and duties as being fundamental to this relationship. The essential characteristic of the social contract is the agreement. It can be between society and an individual, or it can be between society and an institution and its members.

Psychiatrists are a party to a social contract, one that grants us status and privilege but in return entails an obligation to serve the public good. Psychiatrists have tremendous advantages—a type of monopoly control, use of the professional title, and the ability to charge patients a fee.[5] In Canada this fee has been paid by the provinces' health budgets. Mental health professionals who are not medically trained cannot bill these public resources. In return, we have a responsibility to provide a high standard of care and improve care for future generations. To maintain standards, we regulate ourselves via a regulatory body that is supposed to act in the public interest.

The universities' faculties of medicine are entrusted with producing the next generation of practitioners, and with improving care for the future. I think they should do more: as Jock Murray, then dean of medicine at Dalhousie, put it two decades ago, they should be "academies in the community." This means, among other things, that universities should convey to the public the complexities of modern health care, the difficult challenges, and the need for advances in basic and clinical sciences where their immediate relevance to the social agenda may not be obvious. They should instill in students a commitment to care for the seriously mentally ill. Young doctors should be encouraged to work in psychiatric and general hospitals, to become valuable members of teams, and to provide care to smaller communities and within community care organizations. There should be a greater focus on the development of specialties in underserved areas of adolescent psychiatry, forensic psychiatry, and addictions. The public good requires that Canadian psychiatrists embrace a fundamental transformation of the health system and that we advocate passionately for the changes—patient-centred care, a shift to the community, and facing down discrimination and social inequities.

These are the responsibilities we accept as part of our social contract. To fulfill this contract we must face some important problems.

We Need to Fight Discrimination against the Mentally Ill and Accept the Humanity of Our Patients

Discrimination against the mentally ill is alive and well. As we have seen throughout this book, people are still afraid of human beings who seem so different from them, particularly people who have schizophrenia and other serious mental illnesses. The evidence suggests that these fears are irrational. In fact, the mentally ill have more to fear from others in their world than the public does from them. And yet, sadly, many people do not want to associate with people who are mentally ill. Many even believe they are responsible for their own illness.

None of us are immune to these stereotypes. Psychiatrists, like other physicians, absorb the attitudes of our society, including the stereotypes of people with mental illness and the prejudices against them. Although we may be less likely to believe some of these myths, we are, in some respects, no different from the general public. You can see the troubling signs: we sometimes use labelling in a pejorative manner—hysteria carried this tone in the 1970s, as did borderline personality disorder in the 1990s. Our patients with psychosis say their psychiatrists aren't interested in them as people.[6] Some psychiatrists blame anorexic girls for their disorder, or alcoholics for their addiction. The problem is even evident in private practice: some psychiatrists only want to see the worried well because they are "more interesting" than those with psychosis. These troubling signs suggest we can place ourselves at a distance from our patients in ways that may influence our attitudes toward care.

In Ontario in the early 1900s, the public used to gawk at mentally ill patients on Sundays after church. Psychiatrists did not speak out. In fact, they led the eugenics movement in Canada in the 1920s and encouraged the sterilization of the mentally ill. They found a way to rationalize this behaviour: it was supposed to be in the interest of public health. In fact, psychiatrists participated in dehumanizing their patients, and treated them as if they were lesser beings. As history would soon show, this kind of thinking was disastrous for the mentally ill, and for the world.

The most sickening example was in Nazi Germany, where physicians played a significant role in the Holocaust.[7] Physicians joined the Nazi Party in far greater numbers than other Germans (7% versus less than 1%). Psychiatrists screened people for mental illness, and over four years participated in the sterilization of 300,000 people. By 1940 the sterilization program gave way to mass murder of the mentally ill. Over five years, a significant number of psychiatrists played an active role in an appalling program to kill their own patients. About 200,000 mentally ill patients were gassed or shot, leaving the question of how physicians of all people could condone these grotesque and unconscionable acts. In an excellent article, Alessandra Colaianni explains that most doctors who participated in the Holocaust believed they were doing an unpleasant but morally appropriate and necessary job.[8] She suggests that numerous factors contributed to this state of mind: the rigid hierarchy and socialization that exists in medical training, the licence "to sin" in medicine (students and doctors are allowed to perform actions that, in other contexts, are taboo), the detachment that medicine teaches, and the very ambitious nature of many physicians who strive for success. These physicians also absorbed the Nazi ideal that Jews, gays, Gypsies, and those with disabilities were not fully human, and they viewed their actions as being for a greater good. Exterminations, then, became medical procedures; doctors signed off on these routinely.

The Nazi story is a terrifying one of psychiatry's misuse, and it should remind us of the ultimate danger of stereotyping mental illness. We of all people need to fight the stigma that still surrounds mental illness, and fully accept the humanity of our patients. At all times, we must remember the core values of our profession: relief of suffering, compassion, and healing.

We Need to Fix Our Relationship with the Drug Industry

Chasing pharmaceutical companies (and being chased by them) for dollars, for grants, and for speaking and consulting fees rightly plays poorly with the public, especially when we proclaim that the drug company money does not affect our thinking or our decisions.

The pharmaceutical industry is the major source of most new drugs effective in treating human disease and it will continue to be. The estimated cost of bringing a compound from the laboratory, through all phases of testing, to the bedside is from $700 million to $1 billion per new drug, far too high for any government to fund. Doctors, academic institutions, and government must collaborate with the pharmaceutical industry to make advances in drug therapies. But the boundaries need to be clearly defined and maintained.

It is important to keep in mind the differing goals. A pharmaceutical company's goal is to maximize value for shareholders; a doctor's primary interest is the ethics of care. Tom Beauchamp defined the ethics of care almost 15 years ago as meaning respect for the decision-making capacities of autonomous persons, the avoidance of harm, provision of benefits, and fairness in the distribution of benefits and risks.[9] The physician must be prepared to place the patient's interests above his or her own and, in exchange, to receive an appropriate form of compensation and a great deal of satisfaction and sense of purpose. Any encounter involving a physician with industry should have as its aim improving individual patient care or the care of the broader public.

However, some serious problems have arisen in the ongoing relationship between psychiatry and the drug companies, problems that raise the question of whether we are living up to the trust that the public has bestowed upon us as physicians.

When Doctors Accept Gifts and Money from Drug Companies

"There are few beliefs in current medical practice that are held with greater passion than physicians' confidence in their ability to resist the influence of the pharmaceutical industry on their professional behaviour," says BC general practitioner Robert Woollard.[10] A classic example is the findings of a 1995 study by Brian Hodges, who surveyed the attitudes and activities of postgraduate doctors at seven teaching hospitals affiliated with the University of Toronto. He found that house staff generally reported that they would not maintain the same level of contact with pharmaceutical representatives if they did not receive promotional gifts. At the same time, the more money and promotional perks a physician received, the more likely he or she was to rationalize that discussions with drug representatives did not affect prescribing. One-third of the group believed that discussions with representatives would have no impact on their prescribing practices, whereas one-half felt that receiving gifts would not influence treatment decisions.[11] However, there is significant evidence that pharmaceutical companies' funding of continuing medical education, "all expenses paid trips" to meetings, and drug detailing have significant impact on the prescribing patterns of physicians.

Many guidelines have been developed as a result. These generally emphasize that only gifts of no substantial value be accepted. But D.R. Waud, a Canadian physician who was a professor of pharmacology at the University of Massachusetts Medical School, presented a more rigorous standard in 1992, asking, "Can any physician really believe that patients would be happy to know that their doctors were taking bribes, no matter what size?"[12] In my view, physicians may engage constructively with informed representatives of industry but should never accept gifts from them, even gifts of little value.

Still, one would never advocate the total separation of the academic community from industry. Much is to be gained from collaboration. Industry employs many brilliant people doing excellent research and can apply large resources to discovery. Industry is also responsible for informing physicians about the benefits and risks of promising therapeutic discoveries.

A total ban might not even change a thing. McMaster University banned interactions between internal medicine residents and drug representatives in the early 1990s. Several years later, the impact of the ban was assessed. McMaster residents were compared with those at the University of Toronto, who were not prohibited from meeting drug reps.[13] A ban did not predict whether a physician would see drug reps in his or her office in later years. On follow-up, 88% of physicians reported that they had met with a pharmaceutical rep in their office in the past year, regardless of whether they were allowed to do so during their training. The ban had no effect on the frequency of such meetings, and it is even possible that McMaster trainees had not learned how to interact in a constructive manner with these pharmaceutical sales people.

It is more important to teach residents about the nature of these relationships. Fifteen years ago, we were not doing so well. A survey of Canadian psychiatry residents found that just 19% were aware of specific teaching in their program about the pharmaceutical industry and conflict of interest, and 27% thought industry had too much influence on their training.[14] Fortunately, the teaching programs have improved in the last decade; there is now more open debate about physician–drug company interactions and its effects on patient care.

When Drug Companies Fund Continuing Education

At continuing medical education (CME) meetings, industry often hosts lunches or dinners (often at the best restaurants) and has a speaker afterward; or it may pay for groups of doctors to attend specific industry-organized meetings or national or international medical conferences. These are all extremely seductive and inappropriate.

I believe that we as a profession need to tighten the area of CME and industry. It is important for a self-regulating profession such as medicine to reclaim continuing medical education. The ultimate decision on the organization, content, and choice of CME activities for physicians should be made by the physician-organizers. All funds from a commercial source should be in the form of an unrestricted educational grant payable to the institution or organization. Physicians can afford to pay for their own meals. In 2002, then American Psychiatric Association president Paul Appelbaum put it this way: "Are there any psychiatrists in America who can't afford to buy their own pens, notepads, and Frisbees, or to call home from the annual meeting on their own dime? What other than a feeding frenzy can explain the shopping bags crammed with giveaways …? I don't blame the companies for trying to foist this stuff on us; I blame us for taking it."[15]

When Industry Funds Research

Assuming appropriate regulation, rapid and effective translation of basic research to practical applications often requires collaboration between academic medicine and industry. Pharmaceutical companies have also become a significant source of funds for research. Here, academic physicians can be easily brought under the influence of large grants that provide both for the science and for the investigator. External funding has the potential to alter an organization's agenda, influence its policy positions, or weaken its credibility. Research funds from industry can be accepted when there is a clear acknowledgement of the relationship in all communications derived from the work. I believe that academic physicians should participate in such research only when they maintain the rights to define how the study will be conducted and communicated. It is difficult to understand why scholars would become involved in research that is not within their control, especially with regard to the use and publication of the data. When industry funds are received, care must be taken to ensure an accounting of how the funds are spent, with the accounting being both to the donor and to the institution.

Significant abuses of this have occurred in the past. Companies have had research papers ghostwritten, then recruited leading psychiatrists in order to add heft to them. It's a terrible practice.

In some instances, the reporting of research has been seriously biased. If you read the literature on antidepressants in scientific publications, you might conclude that 90% show that the drug is more effective than a placebo. However, if you examined all the studies in the field and not just those published in scientific journals, you'd find that only 55% show a benefit. This type of selective reporting is being corrected by new reporting requirements for clinical trials. There is now a mandatory registry with the National Institutes of Health of all studies to be undertaken and their results, as they become available, to be posted on the Internet. Health Canada is developing mandatory requirements for the registration of clinical trials. The World Health Organization has been pushing for clinical trial registration, and many countries are signing on.

A significant problem has been the hiring of top academics and researchers to be consultants or members of advisory boards and to speak out in favour of a company's drug. At times, these psychiatrists have been given slides made up by the company or encouraged on what to say. Other times, the drug company permits the speaker to provide his or her own views, knowing that just being associated with the "academic star" will be good marketing.

The hiring of academics by drug companies has been a hot subject in the United States, where Senator Chuck Grassley chaired a congressional committee on this issue. The committee uncovered some outrageous examples of underreporting of funds from drug companies. Dr. Melissa P. DelBello of the University of Cincinnati told university officials that she had earned about $100,000 from 2005 to 2007 from eight drug makers, but AstraZeneca alone paid her $238,000 during the period. Dr. Joseph Biederman, a well-known child psychiatrist at Harvard Medical School, has been calling on doctors to diagnose bipolar illness in even very young children. He has been advocating the use of powerful antipsychotic medicines to treat the disease, but much of his work has been funded by the drug company that makes the antipsychotic medicine. He has even had a clinic at Massachusetts General Hospital named for the drug company sponsor, Johnson & Johnson. According to the *New York Times*, Biederman's work has helped fuel a 40-fold increase from 1994 to 2003 in the diagnosis of bipolar disorder in children. To comply with the university's conflict-of-interest policies, Biederman was to report earnings from drug makers. He told the university he earned several hundred thousand dollars in consulting fees from 2000 to 2007, but Grassley's congressional committee found that in fact he had earned at least $1.6 million. Biederman, who was subsequently disciplined by the university for violating the conflict-of-interest policies, is not alone. Charles Nemeroff, a top academic and researcher at Emory University, did not disclose over $1.2 million of the $2.8 million he earned in consultancies from 2000 to 2007. He was eventually asked to step down as chair of the university department but remained a professor until he moved to a chair in Miami.[16]

Grassley sponsored legislation called the Physician Payment Sunshine Act, which requires drug and device companies to publicly list payments to doctors that exceed $500. Some states already require such disclosures. Canada does not.

I am not stating there should be a complete ban on these consulting arrangements, but the terms of the relationship should be completely defined. A written contract outlining the services is crucial. The purpose and objectives must be clearly defined at the outset; remuneration must be in the form of a reasonable honorarium. Travel and accommodation expenses should be reimbursed where warranted. Many such policies have been developed in the last decade, with a significant impact. However, there are always people who slide past the rules.

The National Institutes of Health has strict rules about conflicts of interest among grantees, but the member institutes rely on universities for oversight. So far, the findings suggest that universities are not able to police their faculties' conflicts of interest. Almost every major medical school and medical society is now reassessing its relationships with drug and device makers.

Psychiatrists lead all specialties in amounts of consulting fees from industry. It is unclear whether this is because our science base is slight or because the fee schedule makes psychiatrists among the lower-paid specialists, so they're tempted by the additional remuneration. Irrespective of the reason there is no justification for this behaviour.

When Industry Funds Hospitals

Many hospitals and universities require large fundraising efforts for research projects, for academic chairs, and for capital redevelopment. Companies, along with wealthy individuals, donate money for these kinds of projects. Should some companies not be permitted to give? When I was CEO at CAMH, we decided that the tobacco companies were off limits because tobacco smoke is so detrimental; it's the only substance that, if used as intended, kills 50% of its users. We did accept gifts from families who made their money in brewing beer or from distilleries. What about money from drug companies? Can this confer to the company some undue advantage? Would this allow a drug company to influence research?

This was the one area of fundraising and of dealing with industry that led to criticism of me and of CAMH, when we accepted a gift from Eli Lilly toward a training centre, a seminar room for students and young doctors. It was a psychiatrist in Wales who criticized us for accepting the donation: Did it give Eli Lilly undue influence over doctors at CAMH? Would it affect how they handle mental illness? It's an interesting question with no clear answer. Industry donors are in a special position to foster academic work and to determine what work is conducted. Over time, donors can tilt the field and influence what is studied, who gets hired and promoted in university faculties, who become the influential role models and teachers. They can influence the practice in the long run—what the next generation of practitioners knows and practices. Does Eli Lilly's name attached to a training centre give young doctors the impression that the academy or CAMH specifically believes that drugs are the answer to mental illness, and not meditation or therapy, which are proven to work for some kinds of problems? However, we had not received a major donation from a meditation centre or a yoga expert. So we were in a bind. We needed external funds to build our strength in psychiatry and enable us to help people with mental illness. If were to say no to Eli Lilly and to other drug companies, we would have a hard time achieving our aim at CAMH, that of putting mental health on a level playing field with other medical specialties. Every other medical field accepts such gifts. We were preoccupied with these questions soon after CAMH was formed, but on reflection I still think that the value of building mental health strength outweighs the branding value of a plaque on a seminar room door and that the mental health field should be like other medical disciplines. We should make sure the funds do not determine selection of people recruited (we never have) and that together with our students and the public we enter into healthy debates about branding and influence.

When Industry Influences Treatment

When there's money to be made, industry does a great job of pushing doctors to prescribe drugs "off label"—to people who were not in the original target market. Take the new generation of atypical antipsychotic drugs. They don't have the frequency of neurological side effects of the previous antipsychotics, but they can cause severe weight gain and expose people to the risk of diabetes. The original population for these atypical antipsychotic drugs was patients with schizophrenia and bipolar disorder, but there aren't huge numbers of them. The lifetime prevalence of schizophrenia is 1%, and bipolar disorder is just a little more common (1.5%). Drug companies have had a powerful economic incentive to explore other psychiatric uses and target populations for these medications.

Psychiatrist Richard Friedman has described this problem well in the *New York Times*.[17] The drug companies began dozens of clinical trials to test these drugs in depression, a common disorder. Sales skyrocketed—in 2011 antipsychotic drugs were prescribed to 3.1 million Americans at a cost of $18.2 billion, a 13% increase over the previous year, according to the market research firm IMS Health.

Now these drugs are being promoted heavily to treat various forms of anxiety, the most common psychiatric symptom, whether as part of depression or other disorders or on its own. Almost one in five psychiatric visits is related to anxiety. Family doctors and psychiatrists have begun prescribing the atypical antipsychotics as antianxiety agents and as sleeping pills. These drugs have not been studied in controlled trials for any anxiety disorder, and they have many more severe side effects than the readily tolerated benzodiazepines or behaviour therapies, meditation, exercise, or yoga.

I am not against off-label use of a drug—a physician's clinical judgment is critical, and research evidence is often limited for any newer compound. There is a problem, however, if industry claims of rapid benefit preclude sequential use of less toxic approaches to anxiety and insomnia.

When Drug Companies Pay for Diagnosis

The drug industry has not caused the shift to the modern diagnostic categories. It happened because of the rage at psychoanalysis, the lack of reliability of earlier categories, and psychiatry's desire to appear and feel more like the rest of medicine. But the drug industry has benefited from the development of the DSM and has profited greatly from each new version of the diagnostic manual and its proliferation of diagnoses.

The drug industry is a big funder of organized psychiatry. The DSM is owned by the American Psychiatric Association, and in a typical year the drug industry accounts for about 30% of the association's multimillion-dollar budget, including large sums for advertising in journals and exhibiting at conferences, and sponsoring symposia, fellowships, and meetings.

Until recently, the drug industry paid large sums in consulting fees to most of the doctors on the DSM committees. This was a conflict of interest because the experts on the committee were in a position to widen the diagnostic categories. Although the DSM deals with diagnosis, not treatment, this would be an inducement to many doctors to prescribe drugs for problems that had not been considered medical disorders before. This would therefore expand the market for a drug. In the most recent round, the overseers of DSM-5 said that doctors on the panels could earn no more than $10,000 a year in consulting fees from the drug industry. One might say there is still a conflict of interest. But ruling out consulting fees to people on the DSM committees entirely would mean many fine researchers would not participate in the formulation of diagnoses, which is so important for our field. It would also separate the drug industry, which employs many top-rated researchers, from academic psychiatrists.

The answer to this dilemma is transparency. It should be made clear online where a researcher's money is coming from. Up to now, the universities have not been effective at tracking consulting fees, and in medical journals, the fees are disclosed only in the fine print. But in today's wired world, we can count on the community, armed with the powerful tools of the Internet, to make sure everyone knows how a researcher is funded.

The drug industry's influence on our profession is a huge problem. Although there have been some wonderful new drugs that have provided significant help to people I see regularly, the undue influence of pharmaceutical companies has been a significant negative force for the field. The drug companies have turned from what was a more noble industry to one that has to drive profits even when good new drugs are not forthcoming. In doing so they are contributing to the loss of professionalism, which our field will have to fight to regain.

We Need to Make Sure the Sickest People Receive Treatment

The publicly funded health care systems in Canada pay for intensive psychotherapy, mainly to treat people with mild to moderate mood disorders and personality disorders. But what about the people with severe disorders? Despite the presence of a publicly funded system, the most severely ill often do not receive the care they need. Private practitioners in particular have focused on the more "rewarding" treatment of the less seriously ill. It's true that our society and institutions recognize that we should give priority to the most seriously ill. Academic medical centres and physicians are now beginning to realize that their duty to society, their social contract, includes a duty to care for people with severe chronic disorders—more so than in the 1980s, but this way of thinking gained ground extremely slowly in Ontario. If we continue to widen the diagnostic net and provide unlimited psychotherapies primarily for mildly ill people, we will not have the resources to give the sickest in society the attention they need.

We have a long way to go. According to current community surveys, 26.2% of the adult population in our society suffers from some form of mental illness within any one-year period.[18] At least two-thirds of these individuals who require care don't receive any. This latter figure represents an improvement—over the last decade when the frequency of these disorders was steady, the percentage of people receiving care increased from 20 to 33%. Despite mental disorders being widespread in the population, the main burden of illness is concentrated in a much smaller proportion: about 5.5% are classified as severe, often when there are co-occurring conditions (about 45% of patients have more than one disorder) or serious illnesses such as schizophrenia and bipolar disorder. This group requires much more help than is generally available.

We as a society and as a profession need to address this problem. The academy has already taken a valuable first step by emphasizing more training in the care of psychosis during residency. Government has started to add financial incentives. But that's not enough. I still believe that to get a licence to practise, psychiatrists should be required to devote a part of their time to work with seriously ill people or in underserviced community settings, as the District Health Council of Toronto suggested 20 years ago.

We need to do more. As psychiatrists we need to consider how to deal with the growing demand for mental health care.[19] A large part of the solution may be in collaboration with other mental health professionals. We need to share the job with colleagues in other professions and rethink how we, with our specialized training, can be most fruitfully useful. We should be part of interdisciplinary teams with other professionals, like nurses, psychologists, and occupational therapists. Psychotherapy can be practised effectively by professionals from many disciplines as long as high standards are met, with clear training requirements, self-regulation, and accountability.

This does not mean psychiatrists should stop practising psychotherapy. But we have to consider our unique skills—the ability to apply medical knowledge to the diagnosis of behavioural disorders, order appropriate medical tests and procedures, evaluate the interactions of psychiatric illnesses with other medical disorders, and deal with the complexities involved in prescribing medications. Psychiatrists can increase their efficacy by using their skills to inform other groups, especially primary care providers and other mental health care providers.

More and more primary care is occurring through family health teams. This "shared care" involves the psychiatrist in both educating the primary care team about mental disorders and providing a system of formal and informal consultation to assist in the diagnosis and management of patients with chronic mental illnesses, as well as those with acute conditions such as anxiety disorders and depressions. Medical illnesses in which anxiety, depression, or personality disorder contribute to the severity of suffering may also be more readily managed in this model. Often, these illnesses can be successfully treated by the primary care team, with the psychiatrist as consultant. People with severe chronic mental illnesses may benefit from a mental health team. Such a team could take advantage of the unique skills of psychiatrists, psychologists, social workers, counsellors, case managers, and groups specializing in job-skills training and lifestyle interventions. Nothing in either of these models prohibits the psychiatrist members from spending part of their time delivering direct psychotherapy and pharmacological care to individual patients. In this way, psychiatrists may utilize their skills for maximum benefit as consultants and teachers, and as clinicians.

All of health care, including psychiatry, is evolving away from an individual enterprise to a team endeavour. Solo medical practices are gradually disappearing, and multidisciplinary teams are being developed. As described, these teams have the capacity to provide better care presuming the members work together, communicate with one another, and develop an atmosphere of mutual trust and respect. The Royal College of Physicians and Surgeons of Canada recognized the need for new skills required for specialists in the 21st century when it developed the important CanMEDS guidelines (2005).[20] These are competencies now expected of graduating specialists. The competencies of the medical expert remain at the centre for each specialty, but with six others—scholar, professional, manager, collaborator, communicator, and health advocate, in addition. The requirements of the CanMEDS guidelines are influencing the education of the next generation of psychiatrists in Canada. However, judging from my experience, further progress is needed in the areas of collaboration and management.

We Need to Contribute to Developing a System of Treatment for the Seriously Ill

Treating seriously ill people is a complicated challenge. Some patients lack awareness that they are ill—they deny the illness as soon as they are out of hospital. Some have delusions that they are being persecuted by the authorities or the hospital team. Some lack family supports to keep them connected to care. Some patients had a difficult time with the side effects of medication and stop treatment. For many, the fear of being labelled mentally ill outweighs the potential benefit of seeking help. Substance abuse also contributes to the fall-off from treatment, as can issues beyond the underlying mental condition. Poverty undermines treatment if patients can't afford a bus ticket, or if they are living in miserable conditions and become too worn down to make the effort. Income has a profound influence on patients' well-being and their response to illness.

Mental illness is so complex and multifaceted that the only way to meet this challenge is by creating a system of care, tailored to each region and population. It can be done, as progressive countries such as New Zealand and United Kingdom have shown, if the system has some essential ingredients.

Clear Policy

Many reports outline the deficiencies of the psychiatric system and what's needed to fix it, but the recommendations have not been implemented. What is needed now is clear policy designed for action, addressing the following points:

- This is where we will selectively place public funds.
- These are the areas where psychiatrists and other providers need to be trained.
- This is where we need to coordinate our efforts.
- This is where we will emphasize prevention and research.

Australia developed a policy framework for mental health in 1992 that addressed these issues. New Zealand developed and began implementing its framework in 1997, and the United Kingdom, in 1999. Now, at last, Canada has introduced a clear policy.

It came in 2012 from the Mental Health Commission of Canada after extensive consultation. The commission stressed the need for thinking "in terms of different 'levels' or 'tiers' to the system. Such an approach permits a focus both on the settings where services are located and on the level of intensity of service. At the lower tiers, the focus is on providing less intensive and less expensive services to large numbers of people. At this level services should be available in most communities, and can include population-wide mental health promotion and prevention initiatives. They may also include low-intensity community-based supports for people with milder mental disorders, school-based prevention programs and primary care screening for depression. While there is variation across the country, services at the upper tiers will often be available on a regional basis and can involve longer term, facility-based services" (forensic specialty programs, specialized treatments for eating disorders or borderline personality disorder, for instance).[21]

Incentives

To induce psychiatrists to spend more time with the seriously ill, we need a carrot and a stick. I proposed the stick two decades ago—young psychiatrists should be required to spend a portion of their time tending to the people who are most in need. I still think this is valuable, but I would also now add a carrot—financial incentives to make it worthwhile for psychiatrists to treat seriously ill people who may have difficulties in attending appointments regularly and who may require a high level of social service organization and support.

New Technology

In its 2012 report, the Mental Health Commission of Canada describes the use of new technology well: "There are tremendous possibilities for new technology in promoting mental health and preventing mental health problems. Technology makes collaboration easier and can be a remarkable tool for supporting self-management, especially for younger people, who use the Internet in every aspect of their lives. E-health offers new opportunities for interaction and engagement between people who need services and providers."[22]

Evidence from various parts of medical care supports the value of follow-up contact by phone or by text message for everything from medication adherence to diet and exercise. Such services are relatively inexpensive to provide and deliver large benefits relative to cost. "Electronic health records, telemedicine, Internet-based screening and treatment, videoconferencing, and online training are all tools that can enhance collaboration, access, and skills. Although telephone help lines have been a mainstay of community crisis services for decades, new forms of phone-based services are now helping people deal with moderate depression and anxiety, and aiding in the prevention and identification of mental health problems and illnesses in childhood."[23]

Publish Results

We in Canada do not collect enough data, and even when we do, we rarely share it. We should publicize results—the money spent on mental health, the patients served, and the outcomes. Then we can establish benchmarks to help us improve results. Australia collects and disseminates data that makes it possible to monitor critical elements, such as quality of life, satisfaction with services, and how people with lived experience are involved in making decisions at all levels. We should know how our money is spent.

Prevention, Social Inclusion, and the Needs of Special Populations

New Zealand has focused on improving the health status of Maori, Pacific people, and immigrants; Scotland, Australia, and the United Kingdom have all focused on having people with mental illness fully connected to society. Italy and the United Kingdom have set up supportive housing to replace institutional living. In Canada, we face a major gap in the delivery of adequate mental health service to First Nations. Although the Mental Health Commission of Canada underlined this problem in its 2012 report, we have a long way to go before First Nations will see genuine change.

Peer Support

Peer support works because people who have experience with mental health problems can support, encourage, and give hope to people facing similar situations. Peer support can be offered at peer-run organizations, workplaces, schools, and health care settings—wherever people need it. It can help reduce hospitalizations, reduce distress, and improve social support and quality of life. CAMH did introduce this type of peer counselling in 2010, but this was fully a decade later than in countries such as New Zealand.

Public Money

Looking at the changes in the mental health system over the last 15 years, we can see slow but significant progress. Still, we don't spend nearly enough to help people with mental illness manage their condition. Medications, for example, are covered by public insurance when people are in hospital, but when they are discharged, they have to pay for themselves, unless they are eligible for public funding through disability support. Medications are expensive, so many people stop their drugs and end up back in hospital, at public expense.

Society's understanding and care for people with mental illness and substance abuse needs to be put on a par with other types of human pain and suffering. These disorders account for 14% of human disability but receive about 7% of funding. This is far below the 10 to 11% of public-health spending devoted to mental health in countries such as New Zealand and the United Kingdom, two countries that have reformed mental health with significant new funds.[24] In Canada, on the other hand, mental health funding has declined slightly in proportion to health spending since 1989, and the targets for community mental health spending relative to institutional spending have never been reached. We should raise mental health funding to at least 9% of health funding. This would be intelligent public policy: the beneficiaries would have a good quality of life and be productive, while society would save money on the social and justice systems. In addition, concerns about equity and social justice could be addressed: a civil society is judged by the way it deals with its most disadvantaged members.

Accountability

Therapy can now be tested and evaluated to see if it works, and patients ought to know what the evidence says: the more the broad public knows about hospital groups and individual doctor's outcomes, the better. This kind of accountability keeps us on the evidence and striving to improve. Recent studies show that certain types of therapy work well on certain types of people, but not others. So, for example, dialectical behaviour therapy has been proven effective for borderline personality disorder. Cognitive behaviour therapy is very useful for depression and anxiety disorder; CBT and family therapy may be combined with medication for people with schizophrenia. We now know from the research that the silent, withholding therapist is not all that effective. We also know that too much self-disclosure is also not useful, and that short-term therapies can be very beneficial.

However, many clinical psychiatrists either don't trust the evidence or don't keep up to date. We need to create an effective dialogue between investigators and practitioners. At a time of evidence-based care, we have to be more accountable to our patients, and to the public. In other words, we have to demonstrate the effectiveness and the cost-effectiveness of the care we provide.

Some psychiatrists are not prepared for this. They feel misunderstood and retreat into a siege mentality, defending their usual practice. When psychiatrists run away from these debates, the results are often terrible. Take ECT, for example, which has stirred up a negative public furor. There is ample evidence that ECT is one of the most effective treatments we have for severe intractable depression or refractory mania. Yet ECT is not available in many places. Psychiatrists were not prepared to defend its use.

As psychiatrists we need to involve ourselves in controversies about the efficacy of treatments, but first we should stop to consider why some people in the antipsychiatry movement are so angry. They might be sad and frightened by their experiences, or disappointed and let down. They might have experienced terrible side effects. They might have felt helpless in our settings, which may have seemed like a factory set up for the doctors, not the patients. They might have felt that, in the pursuit of science, we forgot the basic role of the physician to provide hope, care, and understanding and to be there for the other. There may be many reasons why psychiatry's critics are angry, but we must not let that anger dissuade us from entering the public arena to demonstrate clearly that modern therapies are effective and are worth the money and effort.

Patients and their families are no longer passive consumers. They are now demanding, appropriately, to be part of the planning, governance (as I described with regard to the formation of CAMH's governing board), and evaluation of treatments that involve them. Clients are beginning to question the research agenda and want a role in determining which studies are being funded, and how they are being conducted. In the past, consumers were discouraged from seeking any type of employment in the setting of their treatment; now they're asking for jobs as part of their rehabilitation programs and asking to be peer counsellors. It is no longer appropriate for the psychiatrist to say that housing is not a key part in treating a patient with a chronic mental illness; patients are now requesting assistance with housing as a critical part of their therapy. The broader public is pushing toward a more holistic approach to the care of people who are ill. We owe it to them to listen.

People are asking for evaluations of the therapy they receive. In terms of evaluations, we can learn a great deal from our colleagues in Europe. The United Kingdom uses a star rating system for the trusts delivering care (there are four categories, from zero to three stars). Summary reports are available for each type of National Health Service (NHS) trust. Each one explains to local people and those responsible for leading and managing the trust how the trust has fared in the ratings. The ratings tables allow trusts to compare their performance against others, so they can share good practice and address weaknesses. The key targets and performance indicators are determined every year based on the accomplishments of the previous year and actual problems. What is done at the trust or hospital level can also be turned into accountability at the local departmental level.

The National Institute for Health and Care Excellence (NICE) was set up in 1999 to reduce variation in the quality of NHS treatments and care. NICE is an arm's-length body funded by the Department of Health. Its evidence-based guidelines help guide decisions about which medicines and treatments represent the best quality care and which offer the best value for money for the NHS. Its work is entirely based on independent committees of experts, including clinicians, patients, care providers, and health economists.

So there are NICE guidelines, for example, for the treatment of OCD, at times a severe and common psychiatric disorder (involving about 2% of the population). It is characterized by obsessions involving unwanted ideas, images, or impulses that repeatedly enter the person's mind (e.g., unrealistic worries about harm, such as being responsible for an accident, or the fear of contamination) and compulsions that are repetitive stereotyped behaviours (e.g., hand-washing) or mental acts (e.g., counting or repeating words in one's mind) driven by self-imposed rules that must be applied rigidly. Both obsessions and compulsions are unpleasant to the person and are felt by him or her to be irresistible.

The NICE guidelines start with behavioural and psychotherapeutic approaches: behaviour therapy (including exposure and response prevention) and cognitive behaviour therapy, then adding an SSRI (the evidence is that those with stronger serotonin blocking are most effective), and then, if necessary, using clomipramine, an older antidepressant that increases serotonin levels. What I like about this approach is how balanced it is—starting not with pharmacotherapy but with the least intrusive effective agent and then building on treatments as the clinical situation requires. This is also an evidence-based approach.

These guidelines help health care professionals in their work, but they do not replace their knowledge and skills. It is no longer acceptable to provide care purely on the basis of the physician's own theoretical stance; rather, treatment should be based on the patient's needs and the evidence that it works. On the other hand, we can never forget that humane care must include an understanding of the person and an appreciation for the human condition. Psychiatry is a science these days, but its practice remains an art.

Improved Treatments for Major Illnesses

Depression

We have powerful drugs for depression, but not surprisingly, they come with problems.

Some people don't respond even after four or five different medication trials, and it's impossible to predict in advance who will be affected in this way. Generally, the wait for a drug response can be very painful, and comes with risk when it can take six to eight weeks before you know if the medication will be effective. If the first drug doesn't work, it's essential to try again. A large US study, the STAR*D, showed that only about 33% of patients are in complete remission after one treatment trial but that the success rate can be doubled by sequential treatments of drugs from the same or a related class.[25,26,27]

SSRIs, though frequently effective, may have troublesome side effects. The most common one is a reduction of sexual drive. But the biggest concern is whether they can increase suicidal thoughts early in treatment, especially in young people. When all the studies were put into an FDA database, it was found that suicidal thoughts in young people doubled from 2 to 4%, according to Daniel Carlat of the Tufts University School of Medicine and author of an excellent commentary on the state of psychiatry titled, *Unhinged*.[28] None of the patients reporting an increase in such thoughts committed suicide. I have seen one youngster who I felt convinced was more actively suicidal on an SSRI, but it is really impossible to know, since as people begin to respond to medication they can become more activated, and this is generally a time of increased risk for self-harm. If an SSRI makes someone more agitated and causes poorer sleep before there is an antidepressant effect, risk of suicide has to be kept in mind.

The introduction of the SSRIs in the late 1980s represented an advance, since they are generally moderately effective, and for some individuals very effective; they have a reduced risk of suicide by overdose; and the side effects are more benign than the tricyclic antidepressants. But the tricyclics were powerful antidepressants (people were more likely to reach remission than just a reduction of their symptoms) and although they produced dry mouth, constipation, sedation, and weight gain, they did not have the same sexual side effects of the SSRIs.

Most of the new medicines the pharmaceutical companies have developed since 1990 are not much of an advance, except for the marketing outreach, which may have encouraged more people to accept treatment. We need new agents that act on the brain in unique ways. One potential compound is ketamine, an anesthetic that has been used as a horse tranquilizer and party drug, and which has been around since the 1960s. It was popular in the Vietnam War because anesthesia could be induced rapidly and briefly. It has a potential of treating depression rapidly—within hours instead of weeks. A single dose may last up to 10 days. Ketamine works by increasing the synaptic connections between brain cells, which are depleted in people with depression. Because of ketamine's side effects, other drugs that act in this way are being developed and tested. One of these drugs, called GLYX-13, has already been tested in two large groups of people. A small study conducted by investigators at the National Institute of Mental Health showed that after a single infusion of AZD6765, another drug that acts like ketamine, one-third of people with treatment-resistant major depressive disorder had a significant decrease in symptom scores. Unfortunately, the response was brief.

Agomelatine is a newer drug, developed in Europe and with some excellent qualities. It acts as an agonist for melatonin receptors (i.e., activating), and as an antagonist for serotonin receptors; it is different from other antidepressants in these qualities. In placebo controlled trials it has been shown to have an antidepressant effect with a low profile of side effects, including sexual side effects. It may be useful in restoring the sleep wake cycle and does not have an associated withdrawal syndrome. Agomelatine has been on the market in Australia but not in North America.

Other drugs that may work in novel ways are being studied, for example, developing new nerve cells in the hypothalamus or by decreasing inflammation. Early in 2013, Andrew Miller and his colleagues at Emory University found that a medication that inhibits inflammation, infliximab, is useful for depressed subjects, who have elevated rates of C-reactive protein. The neurogenesis and inflammation fields have great potential for both elucidating the pathways to depression and the development of novel treatments.

Another option for treatment-resistant depression is to augment the antidepressant medications with a thyroid hormone or lithium. Harvey Stancer and Russell Joffe were both interested in the role of thyroid hormone (triiodothyronine, or T3), and the literature suggests it's effective. Lithium, which enhances the movement of serotonin across nerve cells, can also act as an antidepressant augmentation strategy.[29]

In the last 20 years, investigators have been studying whether focused external stimulation of the brain with magnetic field pulses can be successfully used for people with treatment-resistant depression. Jeff Daskalakis, at CAMH and the University of Toronto, has demonstrated that about 40% of patients improve with transcranial magnetic stimulation (rTMS). Results from a double-blind, multicentre controlled trial of rTMS show that it is safe and effective in patients with major depression.

Several therapies use electricity to help reorient the brain. Electroconvulsive therapy is the most effective acute treatment we have for resistant severe depression and mania. Deep brain stimulation (DBS) is another. In this case, wires are surgically implanted into specific regions of a patient's grey matter (often into a deep brain region called cingulate gyrus 25) to excite the neurons with electronic pulses, providing a more long-term effect. DBS in itself will not ultimately be the mainstay for treating depression but may lead to the development of more specific medications, improving understanding of the pathways in the brain.[30] For example, it is believed that the inhibitory neurotransmitter GABA is being activated in these stimulation treatments.

Possibly the greatest improvements for treating depression in the last two decades have been in the addition of psychotherapies tailored to specific problems. Patients undergoing Marsha Linehan's dialectical behaviour therapy (DBT), for instance, are asked to make a verbal pledge to change their behaviour, to act opposite to the way they feel when an emotion is inappropriate. In studies in the 1980s and 1990s, researchers at the University of Washington and elsewhere tracked the progress of hundreds of patients with borderline personality disorder at high risk of suicide who attended weekly dialectical behaviour therapy sessions. These patients made far fewer suicide attempts than similar patients who did not get DBT. They were admitted to hospital less often and were much more likely to stay in treatment. Hopefully, we will see other creative investigators develop therapies for people not helped by our current treatments.

Schizophrenia

The antipsychotic drugs have truly revolutionized the treatment of psychosis. They don't just sedate; they also target the core symptoms of schizophrenia, like hallucinations and delusions. However, the early antipsychotics caused severe neurological side effects, including the potentially irreversible tardive dyskinesia (a movement disorder). Then, starting in 1993, came the so-called atypical antipsychotic drugs like Risperdal, Zyprexa, Seroquel, and Abilify. In the 1990s, there was real excitement at the idea that these drugs were more effective than the older ones and caused fewer neurological side effects. Some clinical investigators believed that the newer drugs were targeting the so-called negative symptoms of schizophrenia: social withdrawal, subtle cognitive changes, and apathy. However the CATIE trial (Clinical Antipsychotic Trials of Intervention Effectiveness) and other large studies have demonstrated that the new antipsychotics were no more effective or better tolerated than the older drugs. Unfortunately, in large studies such as these, we find that a high proportion of patients have stopped their medicines because of intolerable side effects rather than poor symptom management—which we know is a precursor to relapse.[31]

The second-generation antipsychotic drugs have serious side effects of their own, namely a risk of increased blood sugar, elevated lipids and cholesterol, and weight gain. They can also rarely cause tardive dyskinesia, though the risk is thought to be significantly lower than with the older antipsychotic drugs.

We need antipsychotic medication with a new mechanism of action, perhaps on other brain receptors such as the glutamate receptors, which may play a role in the known dopamine abnormalities. We need an improved understanding of the specific cognitive deficits that occur in schizophrenia and to then develop agents that target these deficits. Although drugs can relieve delusions and hallucinations, people with schizophrenia still have a whole range of cognitive problems that impair their quality of life. These include problems with attention and memory, which particularly affect the planning and organization required to achieve a goal. Researchers are now attempting to develop a new generation of compounds that target these problems. They are investigating the social deficits in autistic disorders for clues to the underlying mechanisms, hoping that this might lead to a family of compounds that are prosocial and would increase social behaviour. Some neuropeptides look promising in this regard.

More research is needed, but unfortunately the drug industry has cut back on its research into mental illness. Two recent reports published in the journal *Science Translational Medicine* state that drug development for major psychiatric disorders such as schizophrenia, depression, or bipolar disorder is virtually at a standstill. This has largely occurred because of stringent regulations and approval processes for drugs in the mental illness area. In 2011, for example, UK-based pharmaceutical giants GlaxoSmithKline and AstraZeneca both announced they were cancelling research into new antidepressant drugs. As Dr. Zul Merali, president of the University of Ottawa's Institute of Mental Health Research, told CTV'S *Canada AM*, "The costs have been going up and up and the number of drugs actually being approved for clinical use are not increasing in parallel. So it's a high-risk investment for the pharmaceutical industry," one which they are no longer prepared to take.[32]

Novel ways to fund much-needed research into mental illness have to be found. The answer may lie in the world of global health. In the 1990s, there was virtually no research into potential cures or vaccines for major infectious diseases that kill millions of people in the developing world. The pharmaceutical industry had promising leads but believed that there was no sense in developing and testing these compounds because there were no profits to be made in poor countries. As it turned out, there was another way: public-private partnerships (P3s). The private sector donated intellectual property and expertise, while public groups like the Gates and Rockefeller Foundations put up the money. Over the last 15 years, a number of P3s have emerged to tackle the diseases of the poor, and one of the biggest successes so far is a promising new vaccine for malaria. If P3 can be successful for neglected diseases in the developing world, perhaps this approach can be applied for the also neglected area of mental health?

Humane Treatment of Addictions

People in all cultures have used psychoactive substances over thousands of years. For a variety of reasons, our current societies have decided that some of these drugs are purely legal (e.g., alcohol, nicotine), some are legal with a doctor's prescription (e.g., Demerol,

Ritalin), and some are illegal (e.g., ecstasy, cocaine). In Canada the level of use of illegal substances varies from time to time, as do the preferences for the particular agents. Alcohol and tobacco remain the most commonly used drugs, with the highest overall health and social impact. Looking at Ontario, about 80% of the population have used alcohol at some time in the past year, 20% tobacco, 14% cannabis, and 2% cocaine.[33] Of those using, only a minority become addicts—in Ontario, 6% for alcohol and 1.2% for cannabis. Similarly, although 65% of Ontarians have gambled in any one year, only about 1 to 2% are moderate to severe problem gamblers. Recent research has put the prevalence of addiction worldwide at about 40 million people, most of them injection-drug users.

Illegal drugs are, in a public-health sense, far less of a problem than nicotine and alcohol. Worldwide, 250,000 people die each year from illegal drugs, a fraction of the 2.3 million people who die every year from alcohol, or the 5.1 million people who die from tobacco annually.

Drugs, illegal or not, are not always addictive. In fact, most people who use drugs do not become addicted. The question becomes: Who is at risk? Some people tell us that, from their first drink in adolescence, they knew they would never be able to control their drinking; they turn out to have a strong genetic predisposition to addiction. Others display a gradually evolving pattern most often related to the attempt to control a whole variety of negative feelings—sadness, loneliness, guilt, anxiety. Strong cultural contributors are apparent as well. The businessman who reduces his level of "stress" with a drink after a busy workday may later need two and then four drinks to have a relaxing effect. Clinicians have long been aware that patients with certain types of psychiatric illnesses, including mood, anxiety, and personality disorders, are more likely to become addicts. Alcohol, cocaine, and opiates initially relieve negative feelings but are terrible antidepressants in the long run and only worsen the underlying problem. Posttraumatic stress disorder has been known to lead to drug and alcohol dependency because of the need to reduce the terrors, even if only for a few hours. Some people with schizophrenia have anhedonia, an inability to feel pleasure. For this group, the high of a stimulant such as cocaine is often welcomed. Cocaine and nicotine are often used by women with an eating disorder to reduce hunger and control weight. Certain personality disorders also raise the likelihood of addiction. Narcissistic patients, who constantly battle feelings of unworthiness, are frequently drawn to stimulants like cocaine that provide a fleeting sense of power and self-confidence. People with borderline personality disorder, who struggle to control their impulses and anger, often resort to drugs and alcohol to reduce their intolerable moods.

Whatever the route, for a small minority of users, addiction becomes a disease, not a choice. Evidence shows that the use of substances creates changes in the brain in the reward centres and the neurotransmitter dopamine. Dr. Nora Volkow, director of the National Institute on Drug Abuse in the United States, has shown in several brain-imaging studies that people addicted to such drugs as cocaine, heroin, and alcohol have fewer dopamine receptors in the brain's reward pathways than do nonaddicts. Dopamine is a neurotransmitter critical to the experience of pleasure and desire, and creates signals in the brain promising positive feelings. Volkow's other research has shown that addicts have blunted reward systems in the brain, and that for them everyday pleasures don't come close to the powerful reward of drugs.[34]

Drug use changes the brain. Primates that aren't predisposed to addiction will become compulsive users of cocaine as the number of dopamine D2 receptors declines in their brains. One way to produce such a decline, Volkow has found, is to place the animals in stressful social situations. The American Society of Addiction

Medicine recently declared addiction to be a brain disease, basing its conclusion on findings like this.

Yet for every $1 spent on harm reduction programs targeting illicit drugs, $25 is spent on law enforcement. The main antidrug strategy worldwide is to try to control supply in a bid to drive up prices and make drugs less accessible. It has become clear that enforcement is costly and ineffective. Imprisoning drug suppliers and dealers can cut supply and increase prices, but the effect doesn't last for long. Putting drug users in jail is expensive and has no impact on overall drug use. Specific, immediate, and brief sentences, with mandated drug testing of offenders, works better to reduce drug use and associated crime. Overall, though, the enforcement strategy is not working well.

What does work? A team led by John Strang of the National Addiction Centre in London recently reviewed policies on drug and alcohol abuse.[35] The results the panel found were mixed at best. The research on decriminalization is modest or poor—but at least it keeps cannabis users away from other illegal drug markets. Prevention is only modestly effective: family-based or parenting programs work better than school-based and mass media programs.

What works best is treatment, intervening early with those who misuse drugs or alcohol. There is good evidence, for example, that opioid substitution with drugs like methadone or buprenorphine reduces mortality, heroin use, crime, HIV, and hepatitis infections. Residential rehabilitation programs seem to produce good results, but the quality of the research is mediocre. Rehab is also expensive, though less expensive than prison.

The concept of harm reduction rests on the premise that much of the harm is not because of the drugs themselves but because of the consequences of the unregulated manufacture and trade of drugs. Harm reduction seeks to reduce drug-related harm without requiring an immediate end to drug use, which is so difficult for many addicts. Harm reduction programs enjoy broad public acceptance; in Ontario, for example, 60% of adults support safe, supervised drug injection. That level of acceptance rises if these facilities increase drug users' contact with health care providers and social workers. Insite (Canada's heroin maintenance program in Vancouver) is one of hundreds of harm reduction programs delivered by Canadian health practitioners and community agencies over the past 20 years, many of which were equally controversial when first introduced. These include needle exchange programs, methadone and other replacement therapies, and even the nicotine replacement strategies recommended by family doctors for smokers struggling to quit. In short, the research shows that when it comes to illicit drugs, public-health measures work better than criminal sanctions. Stop treating them as criminals. Just treat them.

Mental Health Advocacy

We were always taught that as physicians we are the advocates for our patient's individual health. None of us would want it any other way when we are ill. However, psychiatrists today also need to be the advocates for the collective health and well-being of all patients. Healers involved in the HIV/AIDS pandemic two decades ago provide examples of how this can be achieved. Most psychiatrists, on the other hand, have defined their role as exclusively focusing on the individual patient. We need to change this behaviour. As psychiatrists we must maximize our ability to communicate our expert opinions on the most important and pressing issues relevant to public health. This includes being public advocates in fighting discrimination, and supporting policies that promote well-being and restoration of health.

We need to campaign for more money for mental illness. The overall burden of mental illness and addictions is more than one and a half times that of all cancers and more than seven times that of all infectious diseases, according to a groundbreaking report from the Institute for Clinical Evaluative Sciences and Public Health Ontario, *Opening Eyes, Opening Minds*, in October 2012.[36] Funding remaining at 7% of the health care budget is a disgrace for our country.

The most potent force for change lies in the developing alliance between the profession and an aware and knowledgeable community. This partnership of profession and community is actively combating stigma, and arguing for a fair share of health care resources and improved funding for research. We need to continue to build these alliances to secure mental health its fair share of public money for research and treatment.

Our problems sound daunting, but the future for our field looks brighter than it has in decades. The advances in neurobiology and the psychosocial sciences are recreating the ferment of 100 years ago, when Freud first described the unconscious and the spirochete organism was found to be the cause of syphilis. Now, a century later, we are exploring the effects of catastrophic experience on the human organism. We are finally able to acknowledge the profound neurobiological and psychological consequences of violence and trauma, and to provide better care for people with posttraumatic stress syndrome. The sciences of genetics, imaging, and cognitive neuroscience will soon provide physicians with the capacity for an entirely new range of clinical decisions based on a precise knowledge of the subtypes of illness.

These advances will permit the prescription of biological treatments specific to the individual, which some fear will erode the psychosocial role in understanding and care. It doesn't have to. In fact, if we think it through, the opposite may happen. The ability to know more about the biology of the individual will make it possible to identify psychosocial factors causing or inhibiting disease with greater precision. Progress in genetics, in other words, will not erase the significance of external factors, but rather may make us more aware of them. But this will happen only if the profession itself is capable of fusing science with care.

The new science driving psychiatry will impose a cost, as all massive changes do. But if we are thoughtful in our approach, we can capitalize on this astounding progress. We have to keep emphasizing that our patients will need, more than ever, the attentive presence of a healer. No matter how sophisticated the scientific tools are, we must always rely on our own humanity.

CHAPTER 26
To Be a Leader

I have always defined myself as a clinical psychiatrist with a strong academic bent, though I've actually spent most of my 40-year career leading and managing institutions at the forefront of the mental health revolution in Canada. Particularly during the last 10 years of my career, I became more interested in management and executive leadership issues than the psychiatric ones reported in my profession's journals and conferences.

As I grew in my leadership role, I confronted challenges at each of the three organizations I led. I had some successes and made my mistakes. I tried to learn from each experience, and the lessons I learned might be valuable for other managers of health care institutions.

Leadership Is about Vision

Leaders imagine a better tomorrow. To be effective they must communicate that vision to the people in their organization. That can be a complex job, especially in a large organization. Leaders need to draw a convincing picture, see possibilities, and develop new ways of perceiving. For example, mental illnesses and addictions can be considered separate conditions and be treated as such, in separate silos—or they can be considered to overlap. We could simply accept mental illness and addictions as the "poor orphan" of the health care world, or we could question this assumption. We could assume that all or most people with schizophrenia will have to be in a hospital for life, or we can look at the problem from another vantage point.

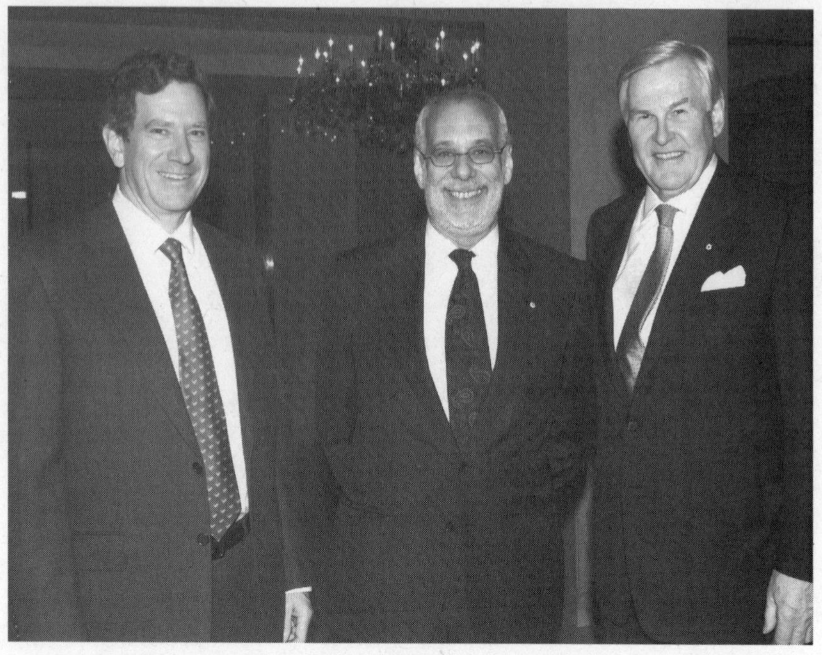

Board chair Jamie Anderson and the Honourable Michael Wilson.

My vision as a leader was different for each of the three institutions I led, largely because the contexts were so different. At Toronto General, I focused on strengthening psychiatry within a general hospital and improving scholarship. At the General, financial levers were helpful in driving home the message. At the Clarke, I focused on what would become my mantra, *Fusing science with care,* but I ran into trouble when key members of my team disagreed and tried to move General Psychiatry and close the ER. I had not been successful in communicating and instilling my vision. At CAMH, we had no choice about the merger but, serendipitously, the diversity of the founding partners stimulated the development of a broad vision—mental health and addictions on par with other medical illnesses—a vision that appealed to the underdog in all of us. Three institutions, three visions. Yet I never wavered from my fundamental values—respect for patients, excellence in care, high standards, and accountability—or from my mantra, *Fusing science with care.*

Leadership Is about Strategy

Leaders need vision, but the leader must also articulate a clearly defined strategy for implementation if the vision is to come to life. One must constantly consider the future, and think about where the organization should ideally be and the various possibilities for getting there. "What if" questions should be asked every day, not just every three years as required by the board.

A leader must also be prepared to push the team to revise a strategy, even a good one. Your innovation might be replicated by others around the world, as Toronto General's day hospital program for anorexia and bulimia nervosa was. An approach might be supplanted by new approaches—as the asylum was emptied once new medications erased psychosis. A treatment might reach the natural end of its lifespan, as daily psychoanalysis on the couch did once we realized it was not as effective as the focal therapies (cognitive behaviour therapy, interpersonal psychotherapy, dynamic therapy) in treating mental illness.

A leader should evaluate the broad landscape and incorporate changing trends into strategic planning. Leaders of all organizations have to do this, but for a major health care institution in Canada, the landscape is particularly complex. I used to keep a list of factors to consider on my desk, so that I would take them into account regularly:

- Population changes such as aging and immigration. (Aging has effects on depression, dementias, and neurological illnesses. Canada receives 250,000 new immigrants each year, within a population base of only 34 million, with implications for refugees with posttraumatic stress disorder, and effects of culture and language on illness and the meaning of illness.)

- Changes in religious practice and the family, which relate to coherence of community and its effects on the course of illness.
- Increasing income disparities and how illness is managed, both with and without resources, even in a largely publicly funded system.
- Ready availability of new knowledge.
- Cost controls and new funding opportunities.
- Changes in accountability.
- Changing roles of consumers relative to providers.
- Health promotion and prevention. (For example, can we develop new ways of preventing the lowered self-worth that occurs in female adolescents, and can this protect them from other problems in early adulthood?)
- The changing face of illness. (For example, HIV was first unknown, then fatal; now it is a chronic illness. Bulimia has emerged in the last 35 years.)
- New evidence regarding treatments. (We know a lot more about treating borderline personality disorders than we did 20 years ago, and that includes the harmful effects of hospitalizations and regressive psychoanalytic techniques compared with the benefits of dialectical behaviour therapy, individually and in groups.)
- New methods of delivering treatments (e.g., video).
- Evolving roles of various members of the health care team. (Are physicians with their unique training and expertise doing what only they themselves can do, or can others take on many of their current functions?)

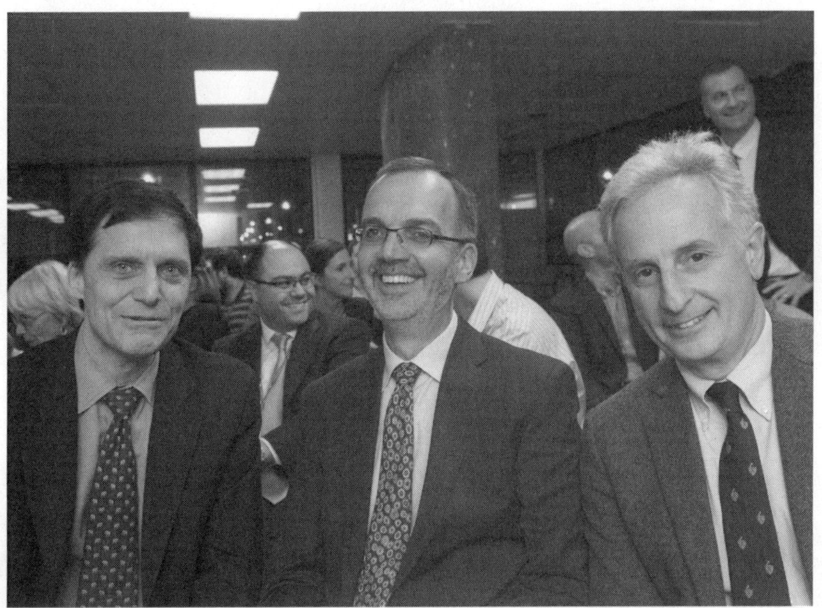

The three physicians in chief of CAMH: Benoit Mulsant, Trevor Young, and David Goldbloom. Courtesy CAMH Archives.

- Evolution of the hospital. (Hospitals have become larger and more regionalized, but far less treatment occurs here—less and less of the overall care will take place in the hospital over time.)
- Alternative medicines. (At a time when the science base for Western medicine's pharmacotherapy has never been stronger, what are we missing? Can interventions be developed as an adjunct to Western practices? Yoga, exercise, massage, which can lower blood cortisol levels, and meditation are going to be much more important to mental health care; how and where will they be delivered? In a hospital that has strong departmental lines, there are currently no positions for yoga therapists.)

Changes in the external landscape alter functions inside the hospital. If we provide better community support to enhance the lives of people with chronic severe illnesses, what is the role of the mental hospitals and what is our strategy for dealing with these changes?

Changes in the legal system may also alter practices in the hospital. In Ontario, mentally ill people who break the law are required to be admitted to a mental hospital "forthwith," often before our other patients, who may be suffering more severe illness and have urgent needs. This ruling has led to a doubling of CAMH's forensic population (85% of whom have schizophrenia) over its first decade of existence and created an important question for our strategy: Do we want to see forensic patients be the dominant group in mental hospitals? Los Angeles County Jail is the largest inpatient mental health provider in the United States. Is it desirable to have all of these patients sequestered on the basis of behaviour in places that may not have the best rehabilitation programs for psychosis or concurrent disorders? Would it be better to place those with minor offences in the regular mental health stream? How can we reinvent this program to take advantage of newer understanding and treatments?

In assessing the landscape, we had to consider other mental health organizations as well. During my time at CAMH, we formed a strong partnership with several umbrella groups in the community mental health sphere (including the Canadian Mental Health Association and the Ontario Federation of Community Mental Health and Addiction Programs). Together we became an exceptionally effective group for defining policy on these issues in Ontario. The first time we met with the then minister of health, George Smitherman, he turned to me and said, "What are you doing here with them?" I took his surprise as a compliment that CAMH had aligned itself with community partners. We also partnered with groups as diverse as the Workplace Safety and Insurance Board, general hospitals, the courts, and societies such as the Schizophrenia Society and the Mood Disorders Association of Ontario.

To be a leader in the health care world these days, one can't remain in an ivory tower. Listening to outside stakeholders is crucial to long-term success of the organization. We had not attended to this at the Clarke. At the Clarke in the 1990s, we had a kind of hubris: we knew we were right, and the fact is, we did many good things at that time, but we didn't check often and thoroughly enough how others saw us change, or determine what they needed from us. The Clarke had little local, community support and therefore was more vulnerable. This is one of the reasons there was no protest when the CAMH merger was proposed a few years later.

Leaders Define Culture

To implement vision and strategy, you have to work on culture: culture reflects a blend of attitudes, beliefs, and behaviours that, when combined, either create momentum or impede progress and cause poor morale. A strong culture flourishes with a clear set of values and norms that actively guide the way a group operates. Culture is evident every day in an organization. The conversations going on in various meetings or even just in the café all reflect a culture. And a nurse taking a patient for coffee, then reading the newspaper rather than talking or listening to the patient, says something about our culture.

Each culture I worked in was distinct. The Toronto General was a can-do culture. The attitude was: we're the best and we'll get it done. There were processes, but things happened quickly and efficiently. The Clarke and CAMH were never like that.

They seemed to require endless discussions and processes before action. I studied the Donwood group carefully because it was action-oriented but also patient-oriented. These were the major differences early on: some of the Donwood staff came from a personal addiction experience. Donwood did not have an academic affiliation, likely because of the modest operating scale, and its laudable response was in focusing its limited resources on treatment while not adding the functions, however vital and rewarding, of education and research. It wanted to connect with people; it was a small group, and the leaders were clear on their values. On the other hand, they came to the CAMH enterprise with a rather naive view of the value of medications.

Many people at Queen Street felt disempowered by the multi-year history of working for government, but we hoped they would want to feel passionate about their work and would want to remove the mind-numbing bureaucracy that slowed any momentum. As it turned out, some people were happy to see the bureaucracy go, whereas others preferred the status quo. Overall, the addictions clinicians were the most eager to improve the client experience.

To develop the culture for CAMH, the senior team focused on behaviour. We asked people to define the problem and come up with their own solutions. Many of our clinical staff were concerned about the weight gain and potential for diabetes that patients on the new antipsychotic drugs were developing. Clinicians were encouraged to come up with approaches to assess patients' metabolic state, to educate them, and to improve their diet and exercise regimens. Among many other creative solutions, they changed foods in the vending machines, replacing chips and candy with healthy snacks. By encouraging staff to feel effective and successful, we saw results for the patients and enhanced morale for the staff.

Nothing reinforces behaviours more than success. Once we had defined a specific problem, we had people work with the clinical

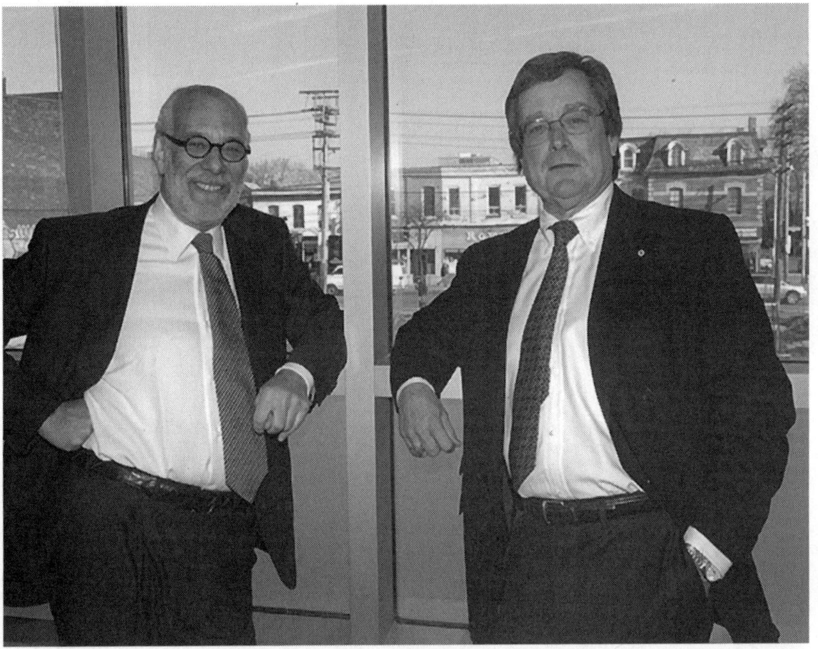

Paul Garfinkel with the outstanding board chair and leader, Paul Beeston. Courtesy CAMH Archives.

teams to develop and apply exemplary behaviours. When these behaviours had been clearly defined, they could be incorporated into performance reviews, and criteria for hiring and promoting. I felt strongly that people tend to do what's measured and rewarded, though I also learned how time-consuming and expensive this process can be. We developed key indicators for all aspects of our programming and reviewed these regularly, focusing on those not measuring up to expectations. For example, early on, concerns were expressed about the high levels of restraint being applied to inpatients—these could be mechanical, chemical (antipsychotic medicines), or the use of seclusion. We looked to other institutions for best practices, set up special teams, broke down the ingredients for success and for problems, and provided regular feedback. This led to positive results, with staff feeling effective and a huge reduction in the use of restraints.

In trying to change behaviour, we encountered significant roadblocks. The people at CAMH, for instance, were too anxious about making mistakes. To some degree, the fear of error at CAMH came from me and my medical training. I was taught to believe there were serious consequences to an error. But I also became more inhibited about failing after the difficulty I had with the early CAMH board and the publicity surrounding it, and then the reaction to the decision to hire and then de-hire one academic physician. Unfortunately, this became a public episode for which, as a new organization, we were not adequately prepared. Some of my fear of making mistakes also came from feeling that psychiatry was an underdog relative to other medical fields and having to prove myself in this new endeavour. The fear of error on the Queen Street side came from being run by government. Staff were taught never to make the government look bad. Indeed, in the early 1980s, one ward was built because of a single patient who was making embarrassing headlines for Queen's Park. The COO Jean Simpson and I had to be very active in the first years of the merger. One day I got a phone call from a senior executive at CAMH; he asked whether it was okay to send flowers to a grieving staff member! It was a long time before talented clinical directors were no longer too inhibited to make decisions.

That kind of attitude is hard to change. What I've learned from this is how important values are to a group. Doing it again, I would spend much more energy on using values as a filter to hire and evaluate staff.

In creating the right culture for an organization, the right people are essential. In a health care setting, recruitment is a critical task. Really talented people are in short supply. The work is difficult, and people are being asked to do more, often with less. When

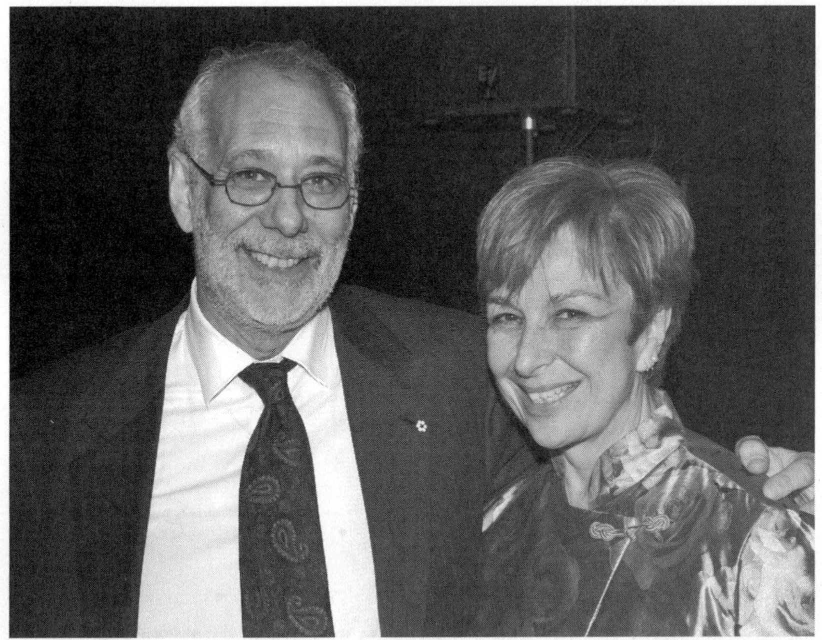

Paul Garfinkel celebrating with his successor, Catherine Zahn, in 2009.

an individual is hired, the organization may be making a 35-year commitment. It is important to get it right, and there are so many ways to get it wrong. Recruitment has often relied on gut feelings. An employer may hire someone because that person has similar traits or has a "name," or simply because of availability, or even because the person is actually very good, though not in the area being recruited for. Or the process may be rushed—"Let's hurry it up; we need the new person immediately!"

In hiring, we often think about how we feel about a person, based on an overall assessment or evaluation of the other, from the features we observe. Psychiatrists can feel they are good at assessing people, but our clinical assessment is not the same as a job interview. Recruiting people for a job requires one to identify the specific skills needed to help the organization meet its strategic directions. I learned this lesson the hard way. At Toronto General, I was good at recruiting highly talented people, but I just wanted the best. If we needed a good inpatient psychiatrist but an excellent person for outpatients was available, I hired that person anyway. It was a scattered approach. We had no disasters, but it didn't promote teamwork; some people were unhappy in their roles, underperformed, and left early. It is important to hire for the job, not hire the star and hope that he or she will somehow fit in.

It's a good idea to incorporate a mix of internal and external appointments in an organization. Internal appointments signal that loyalty to the organization is rewarded, but external ones ensure new and fresh ways of doing things. When recruiting externally, it is critical to assess attitudes and values. Skills can be learned, but values are more difficult to change. Real problems will develop if an organization is based on a model that fuses science with humane care but then recruits "stars" who believe only in the science side. Stars can be hired, but only if they adopt the values of the group, otherwise they wreak havoc. Despite their individual potential, people who do not share the values and culture of the organization should not be recruited.

Many organizations bring in managers who have no direct experience with the business in question. Sometimes it is seen as beneficial to have fresh eyes applied to difficult problems. In my experience, there was an advantage in being the leader of a group and having content expertise; that is, having worked in hospitals, and having had responsibility for very sick people and for worrying about which patients were sent home from the ER—these experiences had an impact on later discussions and decisions in the boardroom.

Academics do not always make good managers. They may have been excellent clinicians or scholars, but it doesn't necessarily follow that they are right for the new role. They may not be prepared to give up the old role; some just add the new title and feel they can do the job with a minimal time commitment. Physicians who were trained in an older model of individualism or who were exposed to role models who disparaged teamwork may have particular difficulties in this regard. These problems may be compounded by ill-defined job descriptions, inadequate management training, and a lack of mentoring or coaching in the new role.

Teambuilding is essential in a health care setting. Some teams work naturally and some don't. I found that the Toronto General group was the most team-like that I experienced, at least in its first five years. We were clear on the goals, we were results-oriented, and conflict was open. We could be vulnerable with each other, and the senior staff felt accountable to each other, not just to me. The Clarke and CAMH, however, were different. The teams achieved results but never felt accountable to each other. Highly ambitious, capable people in these circumstances can, and did, accomplish a great deal, but more could have been accomplished in an atmosphere of mutual accountability and trust.

Teams fail for various reasons. Sometimes they never jell. People may stay in their self-protective compartments; departments may function as if they are autonomous, rather than working for the overall well-being of the organization, or at times even undermine others. Some teams fail to deal with individual competition and conflict directly. Here, the responsibility has to lie with the leader. A lack of consensus about overall goals stifles productivity. Some organizations make everything important, which means that nothing really is.

By the time I got the job at CAMH, I knew that a value of teamwork was crucial to the implementation strategy and vision. The executive leadership team worked diligently to become a team at CAMH: using retreats and endless discussions of how we individually scored on the Myers-Briggs Type Inventory, and what this meant for working together. We held social events and tried to learn about each other. We had many occasions to get together and discuss our roles versus that of middle managers. We also focused on ways to motivate the managers, who in many ways were the key to our success. These efforts made a huge difference to how we functioned together.

Leadership Is about Maximizing the Evaluation Process

I have always believed that evaluation is more than about the job. It's a chance once a year to talk in a more formal way than we might in the daily bustle. It's a chance to have a proper discussion of the person's evolution and satisfaction with not only the day-to-day aspects of the position but also their future prospects. In my experience, people don't think about the future enough. We think too much about the immediate moment or one step ahead. It is important to take stock at least once a year: *How am I progressing toward my larger goals?* People might then make decisions about their career based on what they believe they will feel as they are older. You may not always succeed in your goal, but in taking an opportunity that presents itself, you are less likely to feel regret.

Studies on regret have found that there is a significant age effect: young people regret their poor behaviour (drinking, saying the wrong thing); as we get older we regret actions not taken and missed opportunities.[1] High achievers often let anxiety about their performance compromise their progress—they don't want to look bad or stupid. To achieve continued success, we must open ourselves up to new learning experiences that may make us feel uncertain at best and incompetent at worst. We have to remind ourselves that those feelings are temporary and a prelude to greater

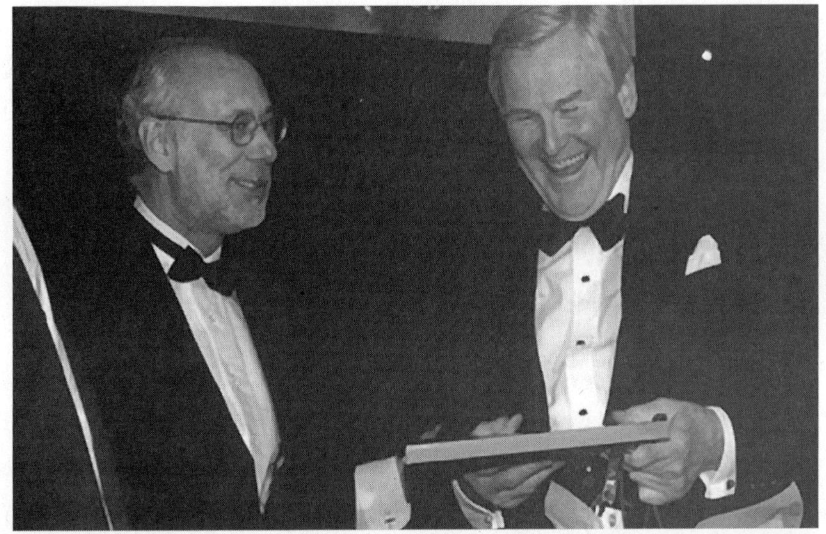

Paul Garfinkel with the Honourable Michael Wilson at an awards banquet in 2002. Wilson has done more than anyone in Canada to open the doors of business and community to better understanding and care for people with mental illness. Courtesy CAMH Archives.

professional ability. I had a rule for myself with each new job: I had to feel really frightened by the stretch involved or it was not a new job for me. Good people may avoid stressful opportunities because of the image they wish to preserve. Personal growth may be sacrificed. So, in staff evaluations, I've always emphasized the person—his or her satisfaction, growth, and life plans.

Feedback on performance is essential in these reviews, and it is important that feedback not be hindered by common problems:

- If there was no plan of the year's goals in advance, it is hard to measure the success of the goals.
- If the goals are measured but there are no competencies, the evaluation will be too general. The performance has to be relevant to the job description also. If the clinical

director published five excellent papers, that is admirable, but it may not be what is required of a clinical director.

- Feedback has to be timely to be an effective motivational tool. Some behaviours that help you succeed can also get in your way. Managers who received timely feedback had significant improvements in performance compared with those who did not receive feedback or who received feedback a year after assessment, according to Harvard's psychological theorist on motivation and achievement, David McClelland. The feedback should reflect comments made throughout the year. Also, the performance has to be measured. If we are not measured on our leadership style, our impact on people, or our emotional intelligence, there is no content for change.
- When there is a departmental structure, senior managers must have incentives to connect meaningfully across departmental lines. I made performance bonus compensation dependent on the effectiveness of these connections at CAMH.

Although this type of annual performance review is very useful, there is great value in periodically doing a 360, that is, anonymous ratings by peers, supervisors, and colleagues. For those of us who are clinicians, it might include patients as well. When done appropriately, these 360 reviews are especially illuminating. I relied on them for my senior teams and found them informative when my performance was appraised in this way.

Leadership Is about Character

Certain leadership qualities or skills can be developed, such as thinking strategically, creating a compelling vision, recruiting the right people, instilling values in an organization, and evaluating people in a timely and effective manner. But in the end, leadership is about character.

If you ask people what qualities are important in a leader, some would say intelligence. It helps somewhat to be smart, but by the time you are in health care and becoming a leader, everyone is smart.

Successful leaders are self-aware; they know their strengths and weakness and what kinds of situations and people push their buttons. They know how their feelings affect them, and they know what influences how they behave with other people and in their workplace. They know how deadlines affect them and they adjust accordingly. They are self-confident and interested in how others evaluate their performance. They like to enter into discussions about their performance and how they might improve. They can be candid about themselves. This type of reflection also involves knowing one's values and goals—*Am I doing this for the money, the status, to have an impact, or some other reason?* Self-awareness also involves knowing one's own physiology and susceptibility to illness and stress.

The concept of emotional intelligence (EI) is useful in this regard. Daniel Goleman thought of it as the ability to integrate thinking and feeling to make optimal decisions.[2] EI involves a series of competencies; according to Daniel Goleman and his colleague Richard Boyatzis, these can be clustered around four main areas: (1) self-awareness, (2) self-management, (3) social, and (4) relationship management.[3]

How the leader presents to the group is important. It took me months at Toronto General before I realized that saying good morning on the elevator, or chatting with an administrative assistant, was noted by all and had an impact on the entire group. I used to swim at the Queen Street pool during the last decade of my career—it was convenient to go at noon when it was open to staff, and I could go door to door in an hour. But I would schedule

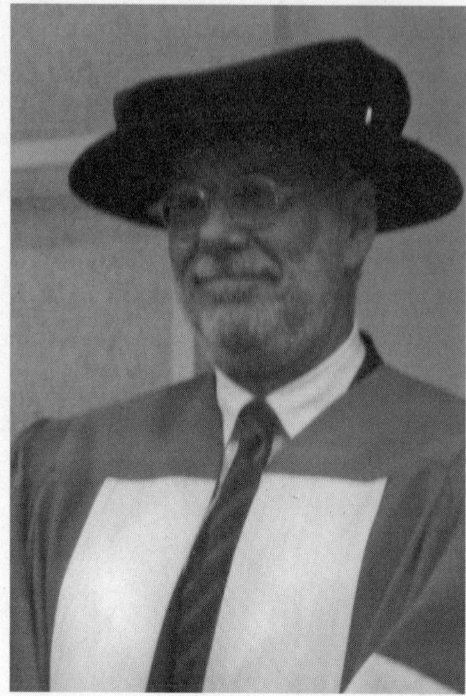

Paul Garfinkel receiving an honorary Doctor of Science from his alma mater, University of Manitoba, in 2012.

an hour and a half because the five-minute walk each way took me 15 minutes. I connected with clients, family members, buskers, and employees, and learned a great deal every day. People saw my genuine interest in them and the hospital.

Successful leaders must be able to enter into noncompetitive relationships with coworkers and to enjoy vicarious success. A good leader enjoys the growth and strength of close colleagues. Leaders have to maintain confidence in their own leadership, and display a resilience or hardiness to survive a wide variety of criticism and competitive envy. In this regard, leaders must distinguish between reactions to them as people and reactions provoked by them as symbols of authority. Other important psychological capacities include tolerance for ambiguity and the ability to make decisions with incomplete information.

Leaders have to maintain confidence in their own leadership, without being narcissistic. Years after I left Toronto General, I read Jim Collins's book *Good to Great*. It resonated deeply with my own experience with leadership.[4] Collins and his team studied a group of elite companies that made the leap to great results and then sustained those results for at least 15 years. They compared these 11 companies with a control group of companies that did not have excellent results over time, and they made empirical deductions directly from the data. Several principles explain the difference.

Collins and his team found overwhelming evidence that outstanding leadership and the ability to build superior executive teams were the two essential and foundational prerequisites for remarkable corporate performance. With regard to leadership, he found two characteristics that predicted this extra success: fierce determination and personal humility. If there is one thing all good leaders share, it is an intense drive, what I have thought of as "focused preoccupation." Collins emphasized that successful leaders are motivated to achieve, but not by the external trappings of salary and prestige. Their motivation is evident in their passion for the work and commitment to the organization. The motivation is accompanied by an optimism that, while not blind, can face the setbacks that invariably occur. Such leaders cannot tolerate mediocrity and will exert every effort to produce great results.

Collins also noted that humility is important in high-achieving leaders: they credit others or the team or good fortune for success, but when things don't go well, they accept the blame. They don't have to be the star. Many leaders cling to every morsel of fame and credit; they have a hunger and, like many people who have narcissistic personalities, that hunger is never sated. More humble leaders feel they have done a great deal and received recognition along the way; now it's time to put others in the spotlight.

Looking back, I can see that I had some very good leadership qualities, and many things to learn. I have always been highly motivated and conscientious, and have cared deeply about the endeavours I was connected to. I have always been reflective and tried to learn from others, and from my own errors. I liked being around strong people, and I enjoyed others' success.

I had to learn not to jump in and fix things. It was better to hold back more often and let a situation evolve. I developed more awareness of others' and respect for them and their abilities and roles. Considering my medical school training, this took some work, but I learned I could be part of a team.

I learned when and how to delegate, and to not just pretend to turn something over to others while retaining control. People are often reluctant to delegate because of a fear it won't be done to their standards. Sometimes they are afraid of letting colleagues look good. This wasn't my problem. I felt that their success enhanced us all. Once I delegated something, I learned to disengage from the temptation of inspecting the process or finding out if it was being done "my" way. We would agree on the expected outcomes, and I became able to let go.

I listened to others. I didn't get caught in a bubble surrounded by people who were there to please; people could speak frankly to me. And, finally and importantly after the 1980s, I didn't believe that some people should be put on a pedestal while others are denigrated. I kept in mind that I was the steward of a larger, noble enterprise, one that belonged to all and especially to our patients.

My problems were in the self-management realm. A few times a year I would blow, usually when someone was ignorant and obstructive and self-protective of personal gain or turf. Interestingly, these episodes occurred almost always when I was ill, often with a respiratory infection or flu-like illness that caused some clouding of consciousness, affecting my ability for self-control. At one meeting, I called someone a "turkey." Not my finest moment, and one that I regret. I like to think I improved, but this trait didn't entirely disappear with age or with success. But more often than not, I came to be able to put the angry email away for 48 hours before deciding whether to send it.

The cliché is true: it is lonely at the top. This is especially hard for new CEOs. In one survey, 61% of new CEOs say loneliness and the lack of feedback impaired their performance.[5] When the buck stops with you, it can be daunting to consider whether you are making the wisest decision based on the limited information you have. To overcome the isolation, CEOs need to find people they can trust and who can hold up the mirror to them. Jean Simpson played this role for me until her retirement. It is rare for it to be someone on the leader's management team; most often it becomes someone on the board or a peer CEO or former executive outside the company who has experience with a similar organization. The leaders in the aforementioned study of CEOs overwhelmingly said they find boards a fruitful source of feedback and support; 96% said they could speak honestly with certain directors about their performance and the impact of their decisions, and 59% cited the board as their most helpful source of feedback. I was so fortunate that I had such individuals on the CAMH boards. Herb Solway and Paul Beeston were always available to provide advice, support, and criticism as needed. Beeston was an outstanding board chair who knew a great deal about stars, leadership, and teams from his many years with Major League Baseball and the Blue Jays. He did everything asked of him and more. He initially professed to not being a fundraiser by comparing himself to Cecil Fielder (a home-run hitter): "Cecil Fielder doesn't steal bases." Once Beeston became involved and saw the need, Cecil Fielder stole bases.

A partner or spouse that understands both you and the organization is hugely valuable. People always have job frustrations, but a key support is someone to confide in, a close friend or a spouse. Even having one person you can vent to who cares is often enough. But if there is loneliness at the top, it suggests that many CEOs are so busy they don't have that one person or they are not people to open up, even to their closest partner. Barbara Dorian was a huge support during the CAMH years, both because of her nature and because of her level of understanding of the enterprise and the people. The lack of balance in one's life during the CEO years is one I always actively fought, but only partially successfully. I was very connected to Barbara in my later years, and to my kids, my brothers, a few friends, and also swimming. I missed out on other things—theatre, hobbies, and a different type of activity in the broad community. There is a price for everything. One of the biggest problems I had was when there was no time to think. I used to say that through the 1970s I could think about anorexia nervosa, or people more broadly, and I enjoyed it and it was time well spent. This type of time disappeared in the last 20 years of my career. A study of CEOs by researchers from the London School of Economics and Harvard Business School demonstrates this issue. In a typical 55-hour work week, CEOs spend an average of just six hours working alone. Most of their time is spent in meetings, at business meals, and on phone calls and conference calls, with much of the rest devoted to miscellaneous activities ranging from travel to personal appointments. This is exactly my experience, except I sequestered about 8 to 10 hours of a long week to treating patients. I didn't want to lose my clinical skills. After all, I knew I would be a doctor long after I stopped being a manager.

CHAPTER 27
On Endings

It's hard to leave a job you love. It's tempting to keep going. After a while, you know the business and the people in it. The prestige, power, and compensation are seductive. If you're the CEO of a hospital, you can feel you're having an impact at a broad level, which is a great feeling, and very different from a physician helping an individual in an office. It's heady to think you are influencing the next generation, placing people in different roles and providing them with new experiences so that it has a ripple effect 10 to 15 years later. And frankly, being a CEO can often be fun: people invite you to the right events, everyone in the room is aware of you, and they think you are funny and smart—but, of course, only as long as you are in the job. It's hard to leave a job, and especially one such as mine.

I have always thought that the university's 10-year rule for chairs and senior jobs was perfect. It permits you to bring in the changes you desire, and you still have time to see the results begin to take shape. The real effects of your term are apparent about five years after you've left the position. I realized that I had had my kick at the can; the organization would become quite different over the next decade. That too felt right; things have to move. I stayed two years beyond that limit (CAMH didn't have a formal term for me). The job was so satisfying, such a pleasure, and I wanted to see the approvals for the second phase of our redevelopment while I was still in office.

In 2004, in the middle of my term at CAMH, I got a call from my physician alerting me to an abnormal result on a routine blood test. While I experienced no symptoms, a biopsy confirmed that I had cancer and I was quickly admitted for surgery. I was 59, older than my mother was when she died. Because both my parents had died so young, I had lived my adult years knowing that death can come at any time and often far too soon. Having a cancer at 59 was not really surprising, but it was jarring. This was real. Because I am so conscientious, all I could see was what bad timing this was: my family and work obligations were still great. My successor had not been selected, the redevelopment was in flux, and many of the issues regarding standards and programming had not yet jelled. But of course it is a type of narcissism to believe that only I could usher in or solidify these changes; organizations suddenly lose leaders for a variety of reasons and many do well. The reality is that I was frightened that I would die, or more specifically, that I would no longer be.

My first bout with cancer left me feeling quite positive. Yes, there was the threat that it would return, but there was also a sense of mastery. I could beat it, and maybe I was no longer 30, but I could carry on successfully. I could feel that my body still worked, that my mind was sharp. I did experience some fatigue, but every doctor I saw said this was part of the recovery from cancer and a stressful job. After the second episode almost four years later, though, I was exhausted. I needed a nap every afternoon, and I became fatigued readily. A question-and-answer period after a dinner speech would leave me feeling depleted and at times irritable. I found I had less patience for some colleagues; I was less giving of myself. I could no longer be at a meeting and push for a cause, even for the most noble of enterprises. From age 60 to 64, I was faced with decline, mainly a decline in energy. There was real sadness in this. I just couldn't go on. I had previously known that my time at CAMH was coming to an end, but until that point it had been my choice. Now the choice was being taken from me, not by the board, but by my body.

I had no choice but to retire.

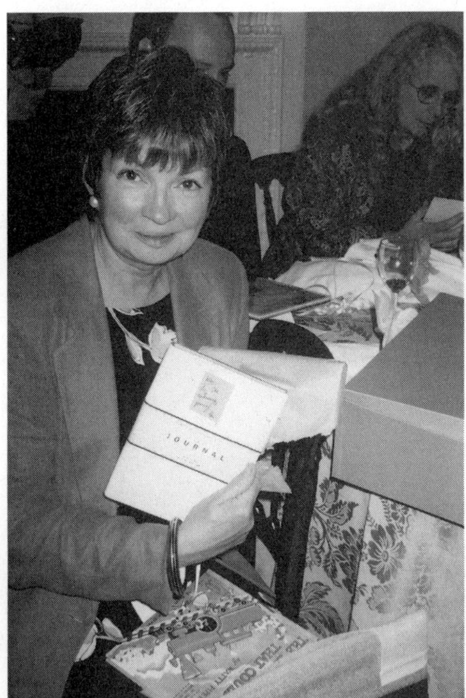

CAMH chief operating officer Jean Simpson at her retirement party in 2005. Simpson played a leading role in ensuring the success of CAMH in its early days.

I stepped down in December 2009, 12 years after I got the job as CEO of CAMH. I felt that I had done what I wanted to do and more at CAMH, which made it so much more natural to go. I knew that the board could choose my successor from a number of excellent people, which showed how far we as an organization had come. When the board selected such an accomplished person as Dr. Catherine Zahn, I was happy with the decision—she is a very capable leader.

Shortly after I retired, Barbara and I flew to our place in Italy for a long visit. When I came home, I returned to seeing patients three days a week and doing some teaching and writing. If this sounds like a decent week, it was about 40% of my previous workload. I had to get used to finishing at 5 or 6 p.m. and having a free

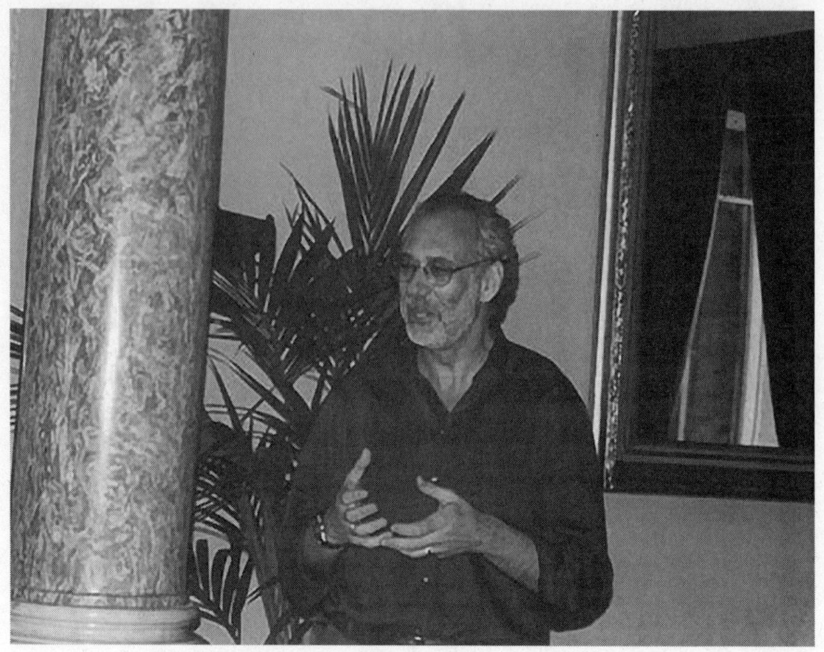

Paul Garfinkel, lecturing in Italy, in 2002.

evening during the week. I could now have a personal trainer, do tai chi, read in a variety of fields, or see movies when I wanted to.

My new life gave me time to think about the sharp line we still draw between mental and physical illnesses. After a time of much uncertainty and anxiety for me, my recovery from the surgery was uneventful, and I enjoyed what psychiatrists call secondary gain: flowers, fruit baskets, cards, and many visits by friends and family. In fact, the worst thing that happened was being yelled at by a nurse; the noise and laughter generated by my many visitors during my recovery period was proving disruptive to the ward, and my guests were asked to leave.

While hospitalized, I did not have to worry about my job, my relationships, or my home. My employer, the Centre for Addiction and Mental Health board, emphasized that my health was

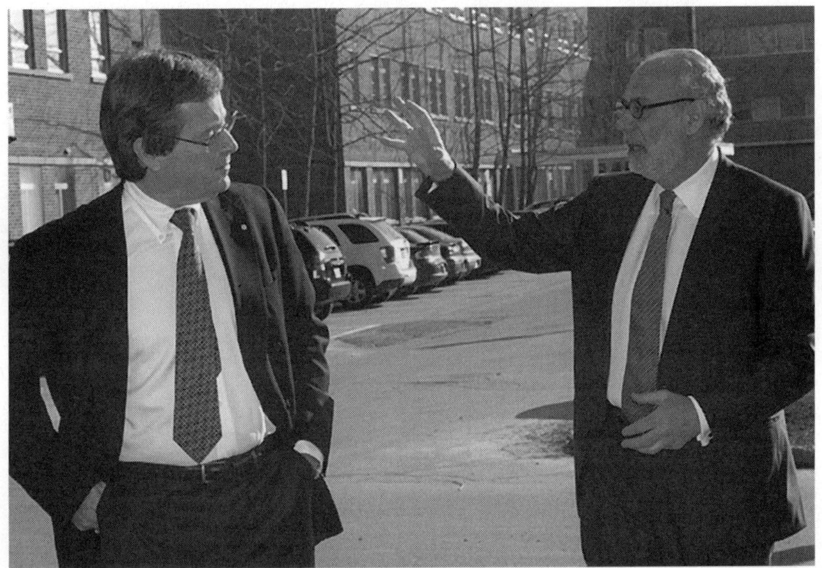

Paul Garfinkel and board chair Paul Beeston on the grounds of the asylum. Beeston has been an outstanding leader of the Toronto Blue Jays and an advocate for CAMH at many levels. Courtesy CAMH Archives.

the number one priority; my family were supportive and available throughout; and my home was waiting for my eventual return. I can tell you that this is not the way it would have happened if I had had an episode of psychotic behaviour or an addiction to prescription painkillers.

To start with, there are no blood tests for these conditions: unlike cancer, the funding for mental health and addiction problems is a fraction of that for physical illnesses. This means these problems are not researched as widely and, as such, diagnostic tests are not nearly as evolved. All we have to rely on are the symptoms, which are often extremely varied. Were I hearing voices or incapacitated by anxiety, I might not realize that I was sick, nor would I have the insight to recognize changes in my behaviour that are problematic. Instead of offering help, those around me would more

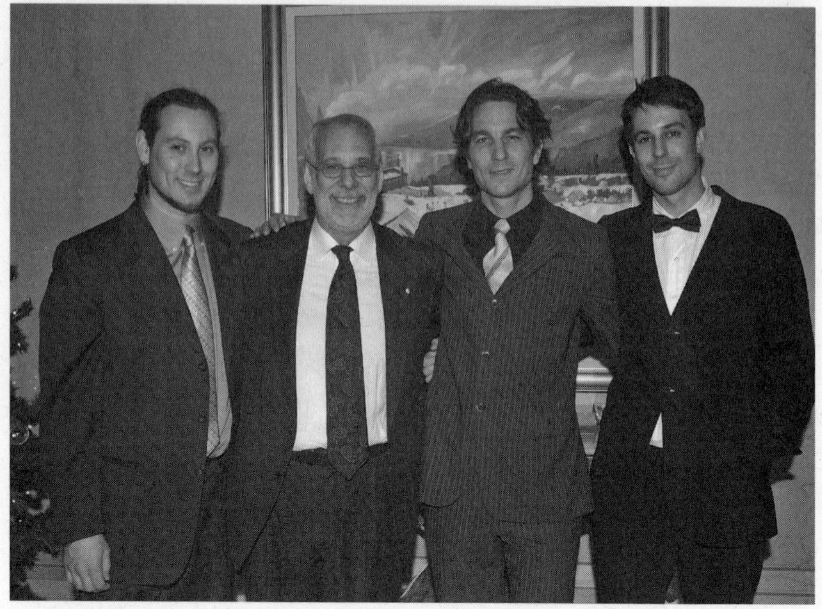

Paul Garfinkel and Steve, Jonathan, and Joshua at Paul's retirement dinner in December 2009.

likely ostracize me, as my behaviour would trigger feelings of discomfort and avoidance in them.

Of course, if I am fortunate to have someone close to me recognize my symptoms, I might get assistance. But there is a real possibility I will alienate the very people who are prompting me to seek treatment. If my work is slipping, or I make a habit of being late or forgetful, word will get to my employers, who may think that I just can't handle the pressure anymore, and my colleagues will gossip behind my back, speculating on my ability to work.

If I did have the ability, courage, and support to get help, the help I need may not be available. We all agree it's completely unreasonable for anyone to wait a year for a hip replacement, yet the average wait times for mental health and addiction services

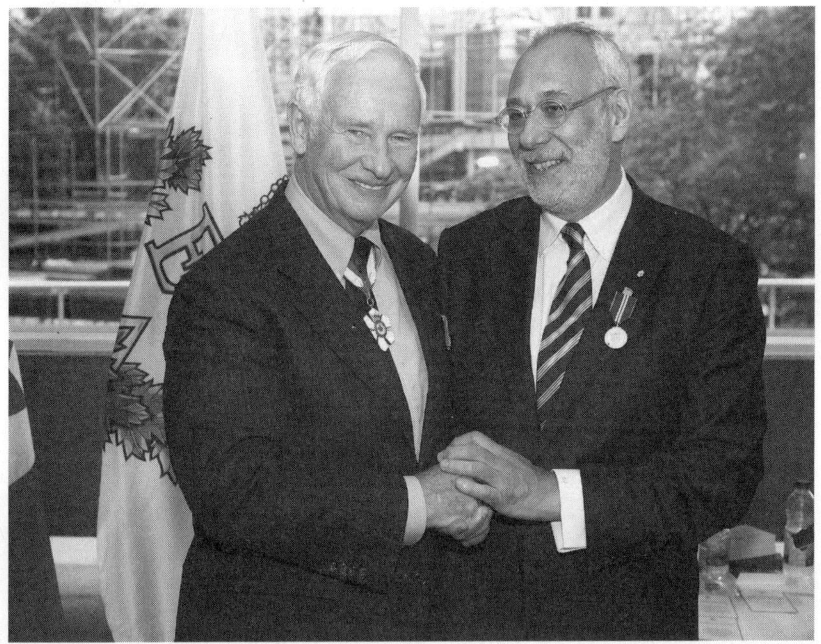

Queen's Diamond Jubilee Medal presented by Governor General David Johnston.

isn't measured in years but in lifetimes. Most people who need care never receive it.

Had I managed to access care, it would probably be in a sub-optimal clinical setting, designed not as a place to regain my health but more as a detention centre or prison. And the people treating me might blame me for my illness, claiming schizophrenia is the family's fault or that my addiction is a result of my moral weakness and shows how selfish I am. Visitors would be rare: 65% of the patients in the Queen Street mental hospital in the late 1990s received no visitors at all.

Finally, imagine that I was indeed fortunate to get help and am progressing well with my treatment. By this time, my employer no longer wants me, my family may not want me back home, and my friends and colleagues have gone on without me, my name only coming up in conversations about how the last CEO "lost it" and "went off the deep end." I can assure you, throughout this entire ordeal, no one will send me a card and the word "fruitbasket" will only be used by a former friend to describe what became of me.

The difference between my real situation and what could have happened to me is not simply that one illness is in the mind and the other in the body. The overriding difference here can be distilled to one word: "stigma." Stigma on the part of family members who are embarrassed, friends who run away, employers who care only about the bottom line, and health care workers who remain intensely judgmental in the face of contrary scientific evidence. A CAMH study from 2005 notes that half of Ontarians say they wouldn't socialize or want to work beside a person with schizophrenia, and 46% say they believe people use mental health issues as an excuse for bad behaviour.[1]

The stigma that has afflicted mentally ill patients since ancient times must be eradicated. We have improved somewhat—there is much more public discussion of mental illness—and yet mentally ill people who were once in asylums are now back on the street, or in jail, some with good support, many without. It's telling that the largest mental health provider in the United States by number of inpatient beds is the Los Angeles County Jail, as mentioned earlier. Wherever they are, people with mental illnesses still face a huge burden of discrimination. The prejudice they face affects their sense of self, and many people say it can be more debilitating than the illness itself. Stigma is so serious that one US Surgeon General called it the "most formidable obstacle to future progress in the arena of mental illness and health."[2]

Journalists Scott Simmie and Julia Nunes have chillingly described stigma in their book *The Last Taboo: A Survival Guide to Mental Health Care*.[3] "Dogs must be kept on a leash" a sign outside

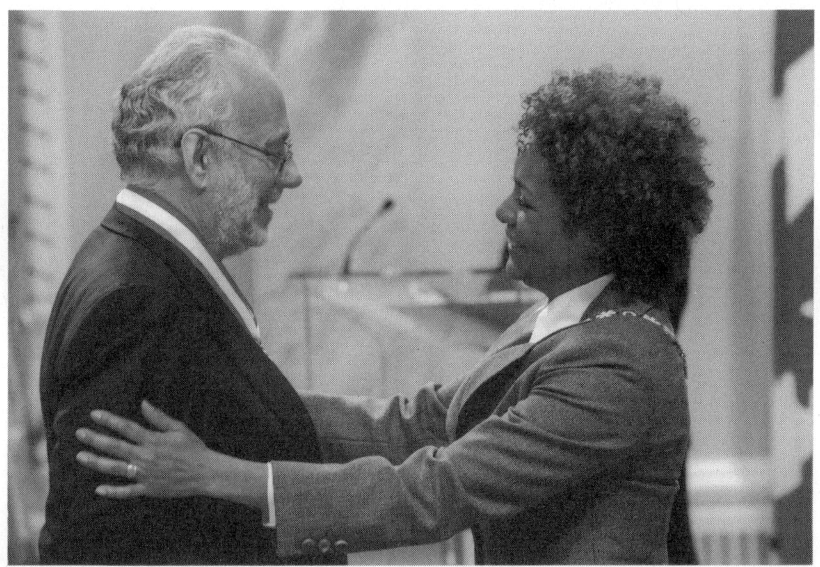

Becoming an Officer of the Order of Canada, with a presentation by Governor General Michaëlle Jean, in 2010.

a mental institution read; it was marked up to read "Nuts must be kept on a leash." It stood for a year in public view. No one made an effort to remove it. Simmie and Nunes and journalist Sandy Naiman (of Psych Central) have asked, imagine what would have happened if the word "dogs" had been replaced by the word "blacks," "Jews," or "gays"?[4] The act would have been described as a hate crime; the sign would have been removed immediately.

During the last decade of my leadership career, I had a vision of what it might be like at our new Queen Street facilities once we have truly wiped out this problem. Instead of visiting hospital wards, I will pop into one of our new condos for treating people with addiction, women who've been abused, or people with major mental illness. As one does on ward rounds, I'll stick my head into a patient's room and notice the personal belongings, smiling faces in framed photographs, a bedspread, and lots of flowers. I'll move on

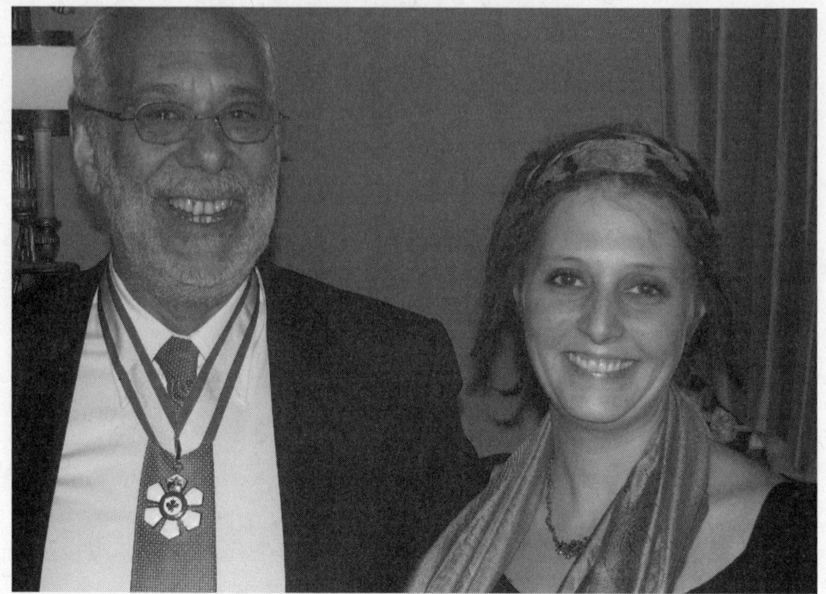

Paul Garfinkel with his step-daughter, Lindsay, after receiving the Order of Canada.

to the next room, where one of our clients is discussing a graded and dignified return to work with her employer. And, as I make my way to the last room in the unit, drawn in by the laughter and animated chatter, I'll squeeze myself into a room where the patient is surrounded by a dozen visitors—and surprise even myself by saying, "Shh ... you're too noisy ... keep it down." I yearn for the day I can say this.

My life's work has been directed toward the fulfillment of this vision. But as long as social attitudes, policies, and funding continue to lag behind the enormous progress in the art and science of psychiatry, little will change. I'm hoping this book will contribute to a greater understanding of mental illness, and to ridding it of its stigma.

I have been a part of an ongoing process to pull our profession and our patients out of the darkness of discrimination and stigma. It is essential for psychiatrists to recognize that it is the process, the journey, that counts. It is never just about getting there but also how we get there that matters. This belief was hugely important as I came to understand that the issues affecting the mental and physical well-being of people and their treatment, service needs, income, education, and especially opportunity continue to widen. These factors were and are critical to the illnesses I was studying and the very people I wanted to help. Fighting to remedy them is a never-ending process.

It has been a privilege to contribute to the huge effort to bring patients and the practice of psychiatry out of the dark. I often think of the Talmudic advice to leave the world a little better than you found it. I came into medicine with a concern for the underdog and have always believed that disadvantaged people are deserving of care and attention. I've learned so much from my patients over these last four decades. I was fortunate to find something I truly enjoy that has great meaning for me.

So much remains to be done. I urge my fellow psychiatrists to not sit on the sidelines but to jump into the fray. Too much is at stake, too much that matters in our world. If we as a profession speak out often to support our patients, in every forum and especially the public one, then perhaps that day will come in my lifetime when people with mental illness are treated like anyone else who is suffering and in pain.

• • •

Sir William Osler said it wonderfully:

> I have had three personal ideals:
>
> One, to do the day's work well and not to bother about tomorrow.
>
> The second ideal has been to act the Golden Rule, as far as in me lay, toward my professional brethren and toward the patients committed to my care.
>
> And the third has been to cultivate such a measure of equanimity as would enable me to bear success with humility, the affection of my friends without pride, and to be ready when the day of sorrow and grief came, to meet it with the courage befitting a man.[5]

ENDNOTES

1. Author Pierre Berton wrote a haunting report for the *Toronto Daily Star* on January 6, 1960, republished in the *Star* in 2013, www.thestar.com/news/insight/2013/09/20/huronia_pierre_berton_warned_us_50_years_ago.html.
2. Roy Porter, the British social historian of medicine, put it this way: "The asylum was not instituted for the practice of psychiatry[,] rather the practice was developed to manage its inmates." Porter R, *Madness: A Brief History* (New York: Oxford University Press, 2002), 100.
3. Those in the Muslim world during the Middle Ages leaned toward the belief that madness was divinely inspired and therefore mad people should be treated accordingly, with respect and kindness. Consequently, they were among the first to build asylums for the mentally ill—in Baghdad in the 700s; later in Cairo and Aleppo. Despite their belief in a divine origin of their patients' issues, the therapies, in addition to baths and medication, presaged today's music therapy and occupational therapy, accompanied by dancing, concerts, and fine food. On recovery, the patients of Cairo were said to have been discharged with a small bag of gold to help insulate them from society's economic stresses.

   The oldest mental hospital in the English-speaking world, the Priory of St. Mary of Bethlehem, founded in 1247, was later known as Bedlam (as a short form of "Bethlehem"). It became a toponym for uproar and confusion. Its inmates were restrained with chains for the first 300 years of its history. Not until the late 1700s were they considered to be patients, classified as either curable or incurable, and even then, they were deemed to be a source of amusement: for a penny, the public could peer into their cells and laugh at their antics.

   Before 1800, medical supervision in an asylum was not required in any country, and when it was present, it did not mean that care was good. This was changed in Britain with a series of laws in the 1820s. Alexander FG and Selesnick ST, *The History of Psychiatry* (New York: Harper and Row, 1966), 62.
4. Bleuler E, Die Prognose der Dementia praecox (Schizophreniegruppe), *Allgemeine Zeitschrift für Psychiatrie und psychischgerichtliche Medizin* 65 (1908): 436–64.

Chapter 2: Falling for Psychiatry

1. The University of Manitoba had a medical school since the Manitoba Medical College was incorporated in 1884 as the first such school west of the Great Lakes. It was reorganized in 1919 as the Faculty of Medicine of the University of Manitoba. It accepted about 75 students each year when I attended.

   A psychiatry department had been formed in the early 1950s. It was still being led by its first chair, Dr. George Sisler, when I was a student. Sisler, originally from Winnipeg, had studied at the University of Manitoba and then in Kentucky before returning home; he remained chair until 1975. He was followed by Dr. Harry Prosen and later Dr. William Bebchuk, Dr. Samia Barakat, and Dr. Murray Enns.
2. Recruitment into psychiatry is a complex process, depending on attitudes of medical students, the image of psychiatry, doubts about the effectiveness of psychiatric treatments, and especially poor opinions of peers and faculty about psychiatry. Psychiatry still receives a small proportion (5%) of the students graduating in medicine. Psychiatry still seems so different from other parts of medicine, and decisions regarding career choice have to be made early on, shortly after students have selected medicine. Often the undergraduate experience is on inpatient wards, where the students are exposed to the sickest people—again emphasizing the difference from other parts of medicine. Also, for a time, psychiatry was selected by medical students interested in the whole person and the humanities; as family medicine changed and became more of an accepted specialty, it siphoned off some of the students who previously selected psychiatry. Low levels of status and compensation also contribute to this; what the students' role models—the senior clinicians—think and say have a great bearing on career choices.
3. The first superintendent, Dr. Alvin Mathers, later became the provincial psychiatrist and then dean of medicine in the 1930s.
4. I came away from the PI with a very positive impression of psychiatry, not only because of the patients but also because of the leadership. Dr. John Varsamis held seminars for the psychiatry residents who were studying for their fellowship exams. He took a shine to me and invited me to attend those seminars, which I did. He had a magnificent way of helping psychiatry residents understand the academic literature so they could incorporate and implement it in their relationships with patients. This was

something I endeavoured to replicate years later when I held study groups for residents.

The chief of service for the women's unit where I first worked was Dr. Nona Doupe. Nona Wright was born in Northamptonshire, England, the daughter of a successful shoe merchant. While a medical student, she met a young Canadian, Dr. Joseph Doupe, who was studying at Queen Square. They married and returned to Winnipeg, where he became director of clinical research at the medical school. Nona raised the children and worked part time in public health. Joe had diabetes, and he held the popular view of the time that he would die regardless of his treatment. So he did not seek medical attention beyond Nona's varying his insulin doses. When Lisa, their youngest daughter, was about 10 years old, Joe became blind from diabetes. He encouraged his wife to "get a career." Nona identified psychiatry as her choice and in the mid-1950s did her residency at the University of Manitoba.

By the early 1960s, she had begun working at the PI, where I encountered her in 1968. Nona was always kind and patient with me. Far from neutral with her patients, she expected them to work as hard as she did in effecting their recovery. After a decade at the PI she switched to Winnipeg's Victoria General Hospital and private practice. There she was encouraging to her patients, and they loved her. A practical woman, she emphasized hope and the therapeutic alliance. She died at the age of 73 in 1986. Nona always said that her great accomplishment at the PI was getting curtains for the women's unit. Moore T and Doupe J, *Bedside Physiologist* (London: Associated Medical Services/Hannah Institute for the History of Medicine, 1989), 57, and personal communication with Lisa Doupe, 2010.

5. Bobby's and all the patients' names have been changed to protect confidentiality. At times, personal identifying details have also been altered.

Chapter 3: A Profession Split

1. We have since learned that abstract and unconscious defences are real and valuable to each of us: they help maintain an equilibrium by decreasing the distress of conflict, which could be between our sense of our external world, our relationships, our emotions or drives, and our conscience. The Grant Study has shown that there is reliability between different raters in assessing the defences people use. Vallaint G, *Triumphs of Experience, The Men of the Harvard Grant Study* (Boston: Belknap Press, 2012).

2. The terms "patient" and "client" are used interchangeably in this book. Traditionally, people using psychiatric services have been called "patients"; many physicians still prefer this term. It has been criticized as implying suffering and passivity—that is, treatment is done to them. For many people, the term "client" implies a more active participation in the treatment. Some patients prefer one term over the other. Others prefer to be considered as consumers, survivors, or users. I like to ask the person which term they prefer, "patient" or "client."
3. Jacob Moreno was a Romanian-born psychiatrist who grew up in Vienna. He graduated from its medical school in 1917 and later moved to New York. He had begun to work with the prostitutes while in Vienna, in groups. He introduced such terms as "psychodrama"—referring to a structured, directed, and dramatized acting out of a patient's personal and emotional problems, with the goal of self-realization.
4. Nathan Ackerman and Canada's Nate Epstein were proponents of family therapy. Salvador Minuchin, an Argentine-born physician, developed structural family therapy, which addresses problems within a family by charting the relationships between family members, or between dyads in a family. The therapist tries to disrupt dysfunctional relationships within the family, to cause them to settle back into a healthier pattern. I attended a meeting on anorexia nervosa in 1976 where Minuchin was chiding the rest of us (about 40 who specialized in the problem had been invited to Bethesda by the National Institute of Mental Health) on not following his simple but effective methods.
5. Eysenck HJ, The effects of psychotherapy: an evaluation, *Journal of Consulting Psychology* 16 (1952): 319–24.
6. Since ancient times we have known that some people behave in strange ways, imagine things that are not there, or think in ways that make no sense to the ordinary person. Hippocrates described clinical states that resemble psychosis, and problems with impulse control and depression in the fourth century BC. The Babylonian Talmud described bulimia (literally "hungry as an ox"). We knew also that some people had extremes in moods. In the Old Testament, Saul suffers from depression, probably with manic episodes, and ultimately commits suicide. King Nebuchadnezzar experienced severe depression with a delusion that he had become a wild beast.

   The ancient Greeks and Romans knew, or suspected, that mental illness may have had a physical source. But these views changed completely in medieval Europe. Christian priests blamed mental illness on sin and immorality, demonic possession and witchcraft, along with overwork. They framed mental illness as a moral issue, either a punishment for sin, or a test of faith and character. They endorsed various therapies—fasting and praying, exorcism or immersion in cold water, the same punishment for suspected witches. People who were mad became the objects of ridicule, even after they were sequestered away in jails, madhouses, or poorhouses for their own safety. At times, they were sent back to their hometowns, or sent away to roam the countryside, where they would be looked after by pilgrims or merchants. Sometimes they were put on ships that were sailing for distant ports.

By the end of the 17th century, Enlightenment thinkers shifted their view of mental illness. They were less likely to view madness as a moral issue and more as a physical phenomenon. The mentally ill were treated like wild animals. Instead of roaming the countryside, as they had done for generations, many of them were sent home to be abused, restrained, put in stocks, and even brutally tamed by their own family members. Because of the shame and stigma attached to mental illness, many people hid their mentally ill family members in cellars, caged them in pens, or put them under the control of servants. See Porter R, *Madness: A Brief History* (New York: Oxford University Press, 2002).

7. Pinel, a physician, became very interested in mental illness after the suicide of a friend. One of Pinel's students, Jean-Étienne Esquirol, put his ideas into place, notably the therapeutic community: patients and staff lived as a community of members in the asylum, including eating their meals together. He felt this isolation of patients from family and friends would be beneficial to improvement.
8. Grosskurth P, *The Secret Ring: Freud's Inner Circle and the Politics of Psychoanalysis* (Reading, MA: Addison-Wesley, 1991).
9. Freedman L, *The Lives of Erich Fromm: Love's Prophet* (New York: Columbia University Press, 2013).
10. Luhrmann TM, *Of Two Minds: The Growing Disorder in American Psychiatry* (New York: Alfred A. Knopf, 2000), 186.
11. In the 19th-century, scientists used the scientific method to transform understanding of the human body. Gregor Mendel set the stage for the new science of genetics, and independent of this, Charles Darwin changed thinking by describing how evolution came about. Just earlier, in the

1840s, Ignaz Semmelweis insisted on the washing of hands by medical staff, and this reduced the fevers of childbirth, and deaths. British surgeon Joseph Lister 20 years later proved the principles of antisepsis for wound infections.

Louis Pasteur linked microorganisms with disease and developed vaccines for rabies and anthrax. Robert Koch cofounded bacteriology and discovered the tubercle bacillus and the cholera bacillus. Claude Bernard set the stage for physiology when he described the principle of the equilibrium of the body's internal environment. As so often happens, these developments in the sciences were accompanied by practical achievements, such as the ability to measure blood pressure, the development of the stethoscope, blood transfusion, anesthesia, and, a few years later, the first use of X-rays.

12. Fichtner PS, *Historical Dictionary of Austria* (Lanham, MD: Scarecrow Press, 2009), 327.
13. Miller A, The lobotomy patient—a decade later: a follow-up study of a research project started in 1948, *CMAJ* 96 (1967): 1103.
14. In 1914, Dr. Joseph Goldberger restricted prisoners' diets to induce pellagra, which he suspected were caused by vitamin deficiencies, not infectious diseases, as was then believed. This work was followed by a nomination for the Nobel Prize. In the early 1940s, the Harvard biochemist Edwin Cohn injected Massachusetts prisoners with cow blood as part of an experiment sponsored by the US Navy. In the 1950s Albert Sabin's studies on the new polio vaccine were partly conducted on prisoners in Ohio.

The Japanese in the 1930s and 1940s conducted a number of studies on the Chinese, including germ-warfare experiments after they invaded Manchuria. Most widely known are the many examples of Nazi experimentation on Jews, the mentally ill, gays, and Gypsies. They were especially interested in scientific "management" of the races—eliminating the "unfit" and improving the Aryan people. It was an easy step from this horrible research on people who can't refuse to sterilization by society rule, the practice of eugenics (widely promoted in North America before the Nazi era), restricting immigration, and euthanasia for involuntary groups considered to be inferior. These are instances that can be mistakenly justified by serving the greater societal good: the individual is deemed to be less important.

15. Shorter E, *A History of Psychiatry: From the Era of the Asylum to the Age of Prozac* (New York: Wiley, 1997).
16. Eisenberg L, Were we all asleep at the switch? *Acta Psychiatrica Scandinavica* 122 (2010): 89–102.
17. Carrere R, Psychoanalysis conducted at reduced frequencies, *Psychoanalytic Psychology* 27 (2010): 153–63.
18. Medawar P, "Victims of Psychiatry," *New York Review of Books*, January 23, 1975, 21.
19. To Thomas Szasz, mental disorders were either brain illness or "problems in living," to be analyzed in terms of social rules and role playing. Psychiatry to him should involve a private contract between two people, replacing state coercion. These views gained considerable popularity in academic circles.

Chapter 4: The Clarke Institute

1. Reprinted in Greenland C, C.K. Clarke: A founder of Canadian psychiatry, *Canadian Medical Association Journal* 95 (1966): 155–60.
2. Weir Mitchell S, 1894 address. See Shorter E, *A History of Psychiatry*.
3. Jones had been eager to leave the United Kingdom—he had come under great criticism for living with a woman who was not his wife and for talking too openly about sexuality with youngsters at a school where he consulted.
4. Clarke was anti-Semitic, anti-Irish, and anti–"ethnic minorities," and he displayed these qualities in his correspondence and in notebooks he produced on "Cottage Life." He also commissioned a caricaturist, "Will Frost" (apparently a *nom de plume*). These all showed him to be more anti-Semitic than the norm for his time and social group. For example, he maintained that children of Jewish immigrants belong to "a very neurotic race," a certain proportion of whom were therefore "mental defectives" who "should be kept for several days under inspection, and the weaklings weeded out remorselessly." Connor JTH, *Doing Good: The Life of Toronto's General Hospital* (Toronto: University of Toronto Press, 2000), 198. CAMH archives, C.K. Clarke fonds: ink and colour cartoon/caricature illustrations with text/captions drawn for Clarke, *c.*1915-20, by "Will Frost." Included is Clarke's story, "A Day on the Meston [*sic*] Golf Links," about Clarke and Dr. C.M. Hincks. Clarke published an edited version in *Saturday Night* magazine, December 25, 1920. C.K. Clarke in *Bulletin of the*

Ontario Hospitals for the Insane 8 (April 1915): 103-8; CNCMH *Quarterly Magazine*.

5. Lifton RJ, *The Nazi Doctors: Medical Killing and the Psychology of Genocide* (New York: Basic Books, 1988).
6. Farrar became very influential in American psychiatry through his editorship of the *American Journal of Psychiatry*, a position he held for more than 30 years. He used to go to the American Psychiatric Association annual meetings with two suitcases: one for his clothes and one empty, which he filled with manuscripts to take back for publication.
7. Shorter E, "C.B. Farrar: A Life," chap. 3 in *TPH: History and Memories of the Toronto Psychiatric Hospital, 1925–1966*, ed. E. Shorter (Toronto: Wall & Emerson, 1996), 86, citing "Joan Farrar's Notebook, Farrar Private Archive" (95n112), now held by the University of Toronto Archives.
8. Peter, Stokes Aldwyn's oldest child, has written a lovely description of his father. In part it reads:

> [Along with his] considerable academic achievement and robust activity in sports (cricket and rugger) to the extent that he won a scholarship to Jesus College in Oxford University … his science studies and related achievements at Oxford turned him toward medicine … and King's College Hospital (where he met a young and beautiful nurse, Margaret, my mother, and courted her on the squash courts), the Maudsley/Institute of Psychiatry, Mill Hill Hospital during the war years (1939–1945) and then again the Maudsley.
>
> Aldwyn married Margaret Agnes FitzGerald in 1934, a change that must have required considerable fortitude because of her staunch Catholicism … One great source of interest and happiness for the young couple was a traveling fellowship that took them to Norway, an experience upon which they reflected many times. During the war years and the "blitz of London" my father remained at Mill Hill, London, but sent the rest of the family to stay with relatives. My father sailed for Canada in 1947 … He arrived in Toronto in February, without warm clothes or boots, and found it "perishing cold."
>
> Soft-spoken, somewhat shy, ever courteous and respectful of others, my father Aldwyn could sometimes surprise and impress

audiences in his teaching and public presentations. Careful, thoughtful preparation was the key.

His colleagues may well remember Dr. Aldwyn Stokes as teacher, physician, distinguished professor and champion of psychiatry. My siblings and I will have softer memories, and remember him for thousands of blessings which he delivered daily as head of family and loving father, considerate and kind to the very end.

9. It was this work by Stokes and Gjessing, and then the latter's son, Lieve, that stimulated Harvey Stancer's interest in mood disorders as a type of periodic illness.
10. Provincial legislation to amend the name of the Ontario Psychiatric Research Institute to the Clarke Institute of Psychiatry is found at 2nd Session, 27th Legislature, Ontario, Bill 58, 12–13 Elizabeth II, 1964; and 3rd Session, 27th Legislature, Ontario: Bill 161, 12–13 Elizabeth II, 1965.
11. It opened as the Provincial Lunatic Asylum but by 1871 had changed its name because other asylums were being built and "lunatic" was no longer an acceptable term. It was the Asylum for the Insane, Toronto, until 1907, when it became the Hospital for the Insane, Toronto. From 1919 to 1966 it was called the Ontario Hospital, Toronto. In 1966 the name became the Queen Street Mental Health Centre, until it became part of CAMH in 1998.
12. Dr. Charlie Roberts, a Newfoundland-born and Dalhousie-trained psychiatrist with administrative experience, was brought in by the board as executive director in 1965 to manage the closure of the Toronto Psychiatric Hospital and the opening of the Clarke. He had previously been at the Verdun in Montreal; by 1969 he was appointed chair of psychiatry at the University of Ottawa. On his departure, Robin Hunter took the role not only of psychiatrist-in-chief but also director of the Clarke, as well as retaining the chair of the university department.

Chapter 5: My Early Years

1. This was a job taken on in the mid-1970s by Abe Miller, who had been at the Queen Street asylum. Miller took a six-month crash course in psychiatry when in the military. This plus his two subsequent years of military service and a postwar residency year resulted in his being appointed to the faculty, and to the staff of the Toronto Psychiatric Hospital in

1948. He joined the Queen Street staff in 1956. John Court, personal communication.

2. May PR, *Treatment of Schizophrenia: A Comparative Study of Five Treatment Methods* (New York: Science House, 1968).
3. The Hincks was named after Dr. Clarence Hincks, a Toronto-educated, practising clinician who was born in 1885. He was close to C.K. Clarke and worked in the outpatient department of the asylum after the departure of Ernest Jones. He played a major role in founding the Canadian National Committee for Mental Hygiene, in 1918. He was an outstanding fundraiser and was responsible for securing a large grant from the Rockefeller Foundation that enabled the completion of the Toronto Psychiatric Hospital.
4. Soon after the gun episode, a buzzer system was installed, but it was several years before the ER was moved to the ground floor, then many years more before there was a proper setup, in terms of both privacy and security.

   Guns weren't the only problem. During off hours, we often had trouble locating patients' charts. They might be in medical records waiting for the typing pool to turn dictation into records, or in a doctor's office (or not), or on the ward, or signed out to a social worker. Those were the days before electronic records, and each file—there was only one per patient—was stuffed with sheets of hand-written notes, some of it illegible. At times, this breakdown in communications was a real problem. We'd have to treat a patient without knowing the background because we couldn't wait any longer. Sometimes there was money involved. In the 1980s, a certain Mr. Beverly died, leaving $3 million to the Clarke in gratitude for having been seen once in the ER many years earlier. Mr. Beverly's chart could not be located, and there were no surviving relatives to help. As a result, almost every physician took credit, in hopes of claiming the use of the donated funds. Rakoff, by then the Clarke's director, used the money for a unique type of visiting professor program and to start the foundation.

Chapter 6: Training Takes Its Toll

1. Valko R and Clayton P, Depression in the internship, *Diseases Nervous System* 36 (1975): 263–69.
2. Koran L and Litt I, House staff well-being, *Western Journal of Medicine* 148 (1988): 97–101.

3. Garfinkel PE and Waring EM, Personality, interests and emotional illness in psychiatric residents, *American Journal of Psychiatry* 138 (1981): 51–55.
4. Garfinkel PE, Steiner BW, and Hunter RCA, The processes of psychiatric residency training: II. trainees who drop out, *Canadian Psychiatric Association Journal* 19 (1974): 201–6.
5. Rueve M and Welton R, Violence and mental illness, *Psychiatry* 5 (2008): 34–48.
6. US Department of Justice, Bureau of Justice Statistic, National Crime Victimization Survey, 2000 (ICPSR 22921).
7. In 1999, Drs. Christine Dunbar, Mike Bagby, Barbara Dorian, and I conducted a survey of Ontario's psychiatrists to learn more about their experiences. The results of this survey are described later in the book. As part of the study, Christine Dunbar interviewed a subgroup of the doctors Ted Waring and I had studied during their residencies in the 1970s. Quotations from some of these interviews are provided in this book, while protecting the anonymity of the psychiatrists.
8. Luhrmann, *Of Two Minds.*
9. Pasnau RO and Russell AT, Psychiatric resident suicide: an analysis of five cases, *American Journal of Psychiatry* 132 (1975): 402–6.
10. Garetz FK, Raths ON, and Morse RH, The disturbed and the disturbing psychiatric resident, *Archives of General Psychiatry* 34 (1976): 445–50.

Chapter 7: Depression: Beginning in Research

1. It was renamed by Moldofsky the Psychosomatic Medicine Unit (PMU), when Stancer moved his office up to the 11th floor to work with Emmanuel Persad on the newly created Mood Disorders Unit.
2. Milrod D, A current view of the psychoanalytic theory of depression: with notes on the role of identification, orality, and anxiety, *Psychoanalytic Study of the Child* 43 (1988): 83–99.
3. Bowlby J, The making and breaking of affectional bonds: I. aetiology and psychopathology in the light of attachment theory, *British Journal of Psychiatry* 130 (1977): 201–10.
4. Schildkraut J, The catecholamine hypothesis of affective disorders: a review of supporting evidence, *American Journal of Psychiatry* 122 (1965): 509–22.
5. Garfinkel PE, Warsh JJ, Stancer HC, and Godse DD, CNS monoamine metabolism in bipolar affective disorder evaluation using a peripheral decarboxylase inhibitor, *Archives of General Psychiatry* 34 (1977): 735–39;

Brown GM, Garfinkel PE, Warsh JJ, and Stancer HC, Effect of carbidopa on prolactin, growth hormone and cortisol secretion, *Journal of Clinical Endocrinology and Metabolism* 43 (1976): 236–39; Garfinkel PE, Warsh JJ, Stancer HC, and Sibony D, Total and free plasma tryptophan in patients with affective disorders: the effects of a decarboxylase inhibitor, *Archives of General Psychiatry* 33 (1976): 1462–66; Garfinkel PE, Warsh JJ, Stancer HC, Godse DD, Brown GM, and Vranic M, The effect of a peripheral decarboxylase inhibitor (carbidopa) on monoamine and neuroendocrine function in man, *Neurology* 27 (1977): 443–47.

6. Schildkraut's paper caused a huge splash, and yet subsequent studies have not proven his ideas. There are some supportive data: in the 1990s, it was shown that lowering serotonin has a strong negative effect on people with a family history of depression—it has no effect on healthy volunteers. Ecstasy (MDMA) acts simultaneously as a stimulant and a hallucinogen. It increases the release of serotonin and dopamine, and the individual may then experience increased energy and euphoria. A few hours later, there is a decrease in serotonin levels, and this is associated with the crash, often a low mood or even depression. People who have impulsively committed suicide consistently have lower levels of brain serotonin. But overall the results have not supported the original hypothesis.

   Although the monoamine hypothesis has not been well supported by research over the last 30 years, one area has consistently shown research evidence, and that relates to dopamine in mania. There is evidence that the prefrontal cortex in people with mania is overactive, just as it is when people are on cocaine or amphetamine. Under these circumstances, cells die off because of oxidative stress, an area that Trevor Young of the University of Toronto has been studying. That is, free radicals are not being cleared, which results in damage to DNA and RNA. We know this is important in a variety of brain disorders, such as Parkinson's disease and tardive dyskinesia. Antipsychotics can help control the level of dopamine in the brain and reduce the drastic mood swings that occur with the disease.

   At the same time as this research was being conducted, the whole field of neuroscience was being turned upside down. We had always been taught that no new nerve cells could emerge in adults; neurones formed during childhood, and that was all you ever had. This proved false. A neuroscientist, Fred Gage, of the Salk Institute for Biological Studies in La Jolla, in the late 1990s showed that mice, and later human adults, have some immature nerve cells and that these can be induced to become mature. Physical exercise can enhance the growth of new brain cells, especially in the hippocampus that controls memories, and is linked to parts of the brain that regulate emotion.

What has been discovered is that being able to grow new nerve cells in the hippocampus is a crucial factor for depression. Scientists have developed methods of stressing mice so that they develop severe symptoms, not exactly like human depression but with some overlapping features. These behaviours are associated with a reduction of hippocampal nerve cells. It is also possible to have mice develop in enriched environments, and this produces the opposite effect: adventurous, rapid-learning, and active animals. Strikingly, they have a large increase in new cells of the hippocampus. Aimone JB, Deng W, and Gage FH, Adult neurogenesis: integrating theories and separating functions, *Trends in Cognitive Sciences* 14 (2010): 325–37.

7. René Hen, a neuroscientist at Columbia University, has studied the effects of various antidepressants, electroconvulsive therapy, and mood stabilizers like lithium: all increase nerve cell growth in the hippocampus. What Hen's team discovered was that mice that were "depressed" changed their behaviour when given Prozac—they became adventurous and active. When the development of new hippocampal brain cells was blocked by X-rays, Hen and his team found, the benefits of the Prozac were eliminated. The drug seems to need the birth of new brain cells in the hippocampus to work. Santarelli L et al., Requirement of hippocampal neurogenesis for the behavioral effects of antidepressants, *Science* 301, 5634 (2003): 805–9.

   Another line of research into the mechanisms of depression links it to inflammation. Most of the evidence here comes from three sources: First, a significant subgroup of depressives has an elevation in blood levels of markers that indicate inflammation. Elevated levels of C-reactive protein, a marker of inflammatory disease, appear to be associated with increased risk of depression and psychological distress according to a study of over 70,000 Danes in 2012. The direction of this association remains unclear; that is, do the inflammatory molecules affect some of the transmitter substances and receptors in the brain that determine our state of mind and regulate our mood or does depression trigger an inflammation?

A second line of evidence is that inflammatory diseases such as rheumatoid arthritis, colitis, and lupus erythematosus are associated with elevated rates of depression (beyond those of other illnesses). Inflammation is thought to also play a role in heart disease and Parkinson's disease, which have high rates of depression. The third line of evidence relates to the treatment of patients with inflammation-producing drugs (cytokines, proteins made by immune cells that govern responses to foreign antigens): very high rates of depression have been reported. Andrew Miller and his colleagues at Emory University found that a medication that inhibits inflammation, infliximab, is useful for depressed subjects, but only those with the elevated rates of C-reactive protein. Wium-Andersen MK, Ørsted DD, Nielsen SF, and Nordestgaard BG, Elevated C-reactive protein levels, psychological distress, and depression in 73,131 individuals, *JAMA Psychiatry* 70, 2 (2013): 176–84; Copeland WE, Shanahan L, Worthman C, Angold A, and Costello EJ, Cumulative depression episodes predict later C-reactive protein levels: a prospective analysis, *Biological Psychiatry* 71, 1 (2012): 15–21.

Chapter 8: Changing Fields: Anorexia Nervosa

1. Morton R, *Phthisiologica: Or a Treatise of Consumptions* (London: S. Smith and B. Walford, 1964).
2. Lasègue C, De l'anorexie hysterique, *Archives General de Medicine* 385 (1873); reprinted in *Evolution of Psychosomatic Concepts: Anorexia Nervosa, a Paradigm*, ed. RM Kaufman and M Heiman (New York: International Universities Press, 1964), 141–55.
3. Gull WW, The address in medicine delivered before the annual meeting of the BMA at Oxford, *Lancet* 2 (1868): 171; Gull WW, Anorexia nervosa (apepsia hysterica, anorexia hysterica) (1873), published in the Clinical Society's Transactions, vol. 7, 1874, 22.
4. Allbutt TC, "Neuroses of the stomach and of the other parts of the abdomen," in *System of Medicine*, ed. TC Allbutt and HD Rolleston, 386–409 (London: Macmillan, 1910).
5. Theander S, Anorexia nervosa: a psychiatric investigation of 94 female cases, *Acta Psychiatrica Scandinavica* 214 (Suppl) (1970): 1–194.
6. This and the following quotation are from Garfinkel PE, "Hilde Bruch, a seeker of truth," in *Women Physicians in Leadership Roles*, ed. L Dickstein

and C Nadelson, 121–30 (Washington, DC: American Psychiatric Association Press, 1986).

7. And we began to use this technique and first published on this method with Harvey Stancer and Steve Kline in 1973.
8. Bruch H, Perils of behavior modification in treatment of anorexia nervosa, *JAMA* 230, 10 (1974): 1419–22.
9. Garfinkel PE, Moldofsky H, and Garner DM, "The outcome of anorexia nervosa: significance of clinical features, body image and behaviour modification," in *Anorexia Nervosa,* ed. R Vigersky, 315–29 (New York: Raven Press, 1977).
10. Weiner H, *Psychobiology and Human Disease* (New York: Elsevier Science, 1977).
11. Garfinkel PE and Garner DM, *Anorexia Nervosa: A Multidimensional Perspective* (New York: Bruner Mazel, 1982).
12. Rodin G, Daneman D, Johnston L, Kenshole A, and Garfinkel PE, Anorexia nervosa and bulimia in female adolescents with insulin dependent diabetes mellitus: a systematic study, *Journal of Psychiatric Research* 19 (1985): 381–84.
13. Garfinkel PE, Lin B, Goering P, Spegg C, Goldbloom D, Kennedy S, Kaplan A, and Woodside B, Bulimia nervosa in a Canadian community sample: prevalence and comparison of subgroups, *American Journal of Psychiatry* 152 (1995): 1052–58.
14. Garner DM and Garfinkel PE, Socio-cultural factors in the development of anorexia nervosa, *Psychological Medicine* 10 (1980): 647–56.
15. Becker AE, Burwell RA, Hamburg P, and Gilman SE, Eating behaviours and attitudes following prolonged exposure to television among ethnic Fijian adolescent girls, *British Journal of Psychiatry* 180 (2002): 509–14.
16. Akiba D, Cultural variations in body esteem: how young adults in Iran and the United States view their own appearances, *Journal of Social Psychology* 138 (1998): 539–40.
17. Lee S and Lee A, Disordered eating in three communities in China. *International Journal of Eating Disorders* 27 (1999): 317–27.
18. Pinhas L, Toner BB, Ali A, Garfinkel PE, and Stuckless N, The effects of the female ideal of beauty on mood and body dissatisfaction, *International Journal of Eating Disorders* 25 (1999): 223–26.
19. Eisler I, Dare C, Russell GFM, Szmukler G, le Grange D, and Dodge E, Family and individual therapy in anorexia nervosa: a 5-year follow-up, *Archives of General Psychiatry* 54, 11 (1997): 1025–30.

20. Garfinkel PE, Moldofsky H, and Garner DM, The heterogeneity of anorexia nervosa: bulimia as a distinct subgroup, *Archives of General Psychiatry* 37 (1980): 1036–40.
21. Garfinkel PE, Lin B, Goering P, Spegg C, Goldbloom D, Kennedy S, Kaplan A, and Woodside B, Purging and non-purging forms of bulimia nervosa in a community sample, *International Journal of Eating Disorders* 20 (1996): 231–38.
22. Sontag S, *Illness as Metaphor* (New York: Farrar, Straus and Giroux, 1978).
23. Keys A, Brožek J, Henschel A, Mickelsen O, and Taylor HL, *The Biology of Human Starvation*, 2 vol. (Minneapolis: University of Minnesota Press, 1950).
24. Garfinkel PE, Brown GM, Moldofsky H, and Stancer HC, Hypothalamicpituitary function in anorexia nervosa, *Archives of General Psychiatry* 32 (1975): 739–44.
25. Farquharson RF and Hyland HH, Anorexia nervosa: the course of 15 patients treated from 20 to 30 years previously, *Canadian Medical Association Journal* 94 (1966): 411–19.
26. Kaplan AS and Strasberg K, Chronic eating disorders: A different approach to treatment resistance, http://pro.psychcentral.com/2011/chronic-eating-disorders-a-different-approach-to-treatment-resistance/00338.html
27. Kaplan AS and Garfinkel PE, Difficulties in treating patients with eating disorders: A review of patient and clinical variables, *Canadian Journal of Psychiatry* 44 (1999): 665–670.

Chapter 9: What Are You Doing in a Mental Hospital?

1. Allan Kaplan was hard-working, organized, and fun. He was a welcome addition to the group and later proved a leader in developing educational programs and research. He went on to hold the first Loretta Anne Rogers Chair in Eating Disorders and later to become vice-dean of Graduate and Life Sciences Education in the Faculty of Medicine.
2. Barbara Dorian held a Career Investigator Award from the Ontario Mental Health Foundation for her research before focusing on teaching in the clinical setting and program development at both Women's College and the Centre for Addiction and Mental Health.
3. The John David Eaton Building had just opened, and to help finance it, physicians had to pay an ongoing rental fee for their offices. They didn't like this because it increased their overhead costs to a much higher level than elsewhere in the city.

4. The barrier to Jewish physicians had broken down 15 years earlier when Calvin Ezrin was accepted for an internship at the General in the late 1950s.
5. da Silva J, Gonçalves-Pereira M, Xavier M, and Mukaetova-Ladinska EB, Affective disorders and risk of developing dementia: systematic review, *British Journal of Psychiatry* 202 (2013): 177–86.
6. Fang F, Fall K, Mittleman MA, Sparén P, Ye W, Adami H-O, and Valdimarsdóttir U, Suicide and cardiovascular death after a cancer diagnosis, *New England Journal of Medicine* 366 (2012): 1310–18.

Chapter 10: A Department with Crackle

1. Months before the merger was to occur, as incoming chair of the Medical Advisory Board, I was asked to chair the Medical Bylaws Committee. This is both an extremely tedious and essential task that I didn't always enjoy. Yet it provided great experience and an opportunity to see a merged organization form at very close range. Many of the issues we dealt with would have faced any large teaching hospital at the time: How would program and human resource planning occur? What were the range of procedures that nonphysicians might be able to take on? How do you begin to interest physicians in information technology? Can a birthing centre be introduced into obstetrics. And what about house staff fatigue and resulting errors? We also had an opportunity to be involved in the larger health care arena from a position of some influence.
2. Mergers disrupt networks, like the telephone system and how to order lab tests, and this really annoyed physicians, who like the familiar ways so they can focus on their central task: patient care. So if the pharmacy processes are new, or the records, or there's an audit, it becomes confusing, and fuses are short. How many hours were spent by a "forms subcommittee" harmonizing all the organization's forms? (But if you don't do it, there is chaos.) Then there is the issue of who sits on the various committees. Each committee was scrutinized, as if the whole merger depended on it, and the doctors always counted the number of doctors from each hospital on each committee to decipher the meaning and the implications.

   A key issue in this process was the speed of change. Consensus can never be reached on some issues, and I think we moved too slowly in some cases. There were duplicate committees (one at each site) over that first year, for pharmacy, nursing, records, infectious disease, and the ORs. Some were centralized more quickly—for example, planning, budget, credentials, audit, and research. But given the feelings of the day, we continued with two medical staff associations.

The hospital administration came up with incentives to consolidate where it made sense. Many department heads were won over by the plan to let them keep up to 50% of any savings through consolidation for approved projects that could enhance care, teaching, or research. Some exciting new developments emerged—an eye research institute, for example; there were very significant savings in merging laboratories and performing routine hematology at one site. Great plans evolved to enhance programs in primary care through family and community medicine. The Western began to enlarge its neuroscience program with a new MRI, and today it is a real force in neuroscience because of the merger.

Chapter 11: Crossing the Line

1. Stone A, "Where will psychoanalysis survive?" Keynote address to the American Academy of Psychoanalysis, December 9, 1995.
2. Gartrell N, Herman J, Olarte S, Feldstein M, and Localio R, "Prevalence of psychiatrist-patient sexual contact," in *Sexual Exploitation in Professional Relationships*, ed. GO Gabbard, 1070–74 (Washington, DC: American Psychiatric Press, 1989).
3. Carr M and Robinson GE, Fatal attraction: the ethical and clinical dilemma of patient-therapist sex, *Canadian Journal of Psychiatry* 35, 2 (1990): 122–27.
4. Twemlow SW and Gabbard GO, "The lovesick therapist," in *Sexual Exploitation in Professional Relationships*, ed. GO Gabbard, 71-87 (Washington, DC: American Psychiatric Press, 1989).
5. Kardener SH, Fuller M, and Mensh IN, A survey of physician's attitudes and practices regarding erotic and nonerotic contact with patients, *American Journal of Psychiatry* 130 (1973): 1077–81.
6. Epstein RS, Simon RI, and Kay GG, Assessing boundary violations in psychotherapy, *Bulletin of the Menninger Clinic* 56 (1992): 150–66, and Epstein RS, *Keeping Boundaries: Maintaining Safety and Integrity in the Psychotherapeutic Process* (Washington, DC: American Psychiatric Press, 1994).
7. Dorian BJ, Kaplan AS, and Garfinkel PE, Ensuring standards: the issue of accountability in academic psychiatry, *Annals RCPSC* 32 (1999): 422–26, and Garfinkel PE, Dorian BJ, Sadavoy J, and Bagby, RM, Boundary violations and departments of psychiatry, *Canadian Journal of Psychiatry* 42 (1997): 764–70.

8. Stone A, "Sexual exploitation of patients in psychiatry," in *Law, Psychiatry and Morality*, ed. A Stone (Washington, DC: American Psychiatric Press, 1989), 191–216.
9. Penfold SP, Sexual abuse by therapists: maintaining the conspiracy of silence, *Canadian Journal of Community Mental Health* 11 (1992): 5–15.
10. Quadrio C, Woman-centered perspectives on female psychosexuality, *Australian and New Zealand Journal of Psychiatry* 28 (1994): 478–87.

Chapter 12: A Patient Commits Suicide

1. World Health Organization, *World Report on Violence and Health* (Geneva: October 2002), www.who.int
2. Parker-Pope T, "Suicide rates rise sharply in US," *New York Times*, May 2, 2013.
3. Newer treatments, especially the antidepressant medications, might have reduced the suicide rate a little, but it's not clear. The highest risk for suicide is in the first few weeks after beginning medicine for depression. People often become mobilized before their moods really improve. This phenomenon is seen with the SSRIs, such as Paxil and Zoloft, just as it had been with the tricyclics and monoamine oxidase inhibitors years ago. I don't know if there is something new or different about some SSRIs when given to youth. But there are many people who are convinced that these drugs agitate a subgroup of young people. These concerns led the FDA to issue its black box warning. Psychiatrists must caution patients that these drugs can potentially lead to increased suicidal thoughts and behaviours, especially in children and young adults under the age of 25. The issue of antidepressant medication and suicide risk is not settled, as studies have not produced a clear picture to date. See Gibbons RD, Brown CH, Hur K, Marcus SM, Bhaumik DK, and Mann JJ, The relationship between antidepressant medication use and rate of suicide, *Archives of General Psychiatry* 62 (2005): 165–72.
4. Ruskin R, Sakinofsky I, Bagby RM, Dickens S, and Sousa G, Impact of patient suicide on psychiatrists and psychiatric trainees, *Academic Psychiatry* 28, 2 (2004): 104–10.
5. Goode E, "Patient suicide brings therapists lasting pain," *New York Times*, January 16, 2001.
6. Chemtob CM, Hamada RS, Bauer G, Kinney B, and Torigoe RY, Patients' suicides: frequency and impact on psychiatrists, *American Journal of Psychiatry* 145 (1988): 224–28.

7. Hendin H, Lipschitz A, Maltsberger JT, Pollinger Hass A, and Wynecoop S, Therapists' reactions to patients' suicides, *American Journal of Psychiatry* 157 (2000): 2022–27. All quotations in this passage are from this work.
8. Ibid, p. 2024.
9. Gitlin MJ, A psychiatrist's reaction to a patient's suicide, *American Journal of Psychiatry* 156 (*1999)*: 1630–34.

Chapter 13: Burdens and Satisfactions

1. Luborsky L, *Principles of Psychoanalytic Psychotherapy: A Manual for Supportive-Expressive Treatment* (New York: Basic Books, 2000).
2. Strupp HH, Hadley SW, and Gomes-Schwartz B, *Psychotherapy for Better or Worse* (New York: Jason Aronson, 1977).
3. Fiedler F, A comparison of therapeutic relationships in psychoanalytic, nondirective and Adlerian therapy, *Journal of Consulting Psychology* 14 (1950): 436–45.
4. Garfinkel PE, Bagby RM, Schuller DR, Williams CC, Dickens SE, and Dorian B, Predictors of success and satisfaction in the practice of psychiatry: a preliminary follow-up study, *Canadian Journal of Psychiatry* 46 (2001): 835–40.
5. Mckelvey RS and Webb JA, Career satisfaction among psychiatrists in Texas, *Southern Medical Journal* 88, 5 (1995): 524–30.
6. Kalman TP and Goldstein MA, Satisfaction of Manhattan psychiatrists with private practice: assessing the impact of managed care, *Journal of Psychotherapy Practice and Research* 7 (1998): 250–58. See also Leigh JP, Tancredi DJ, and Kravitz RL, The 4th wave of the Community Tracking Physician Study (CTS) in the US, *BMC Health Services Research* 9 (2009): 166. The authors found that 14% of psychiatrists were "somewhat" or "very" dissatisfied. The top two specialties that were positively associated with satisfaction were pediatric emergency medicine and geriatric medicine. The bottom two specialties that were negatively associated with satisfaction were pulmonary critical care medicine and neurological surgery. Psychiatry ranked 17th out of 42 specialties; child and adolescent psychiatry ranked considerably higher (9th). In this same US study, satisfaction was significantly and positively related to income and employment in a medical school but negatively associated with more than 50 work-hours per week, being a full owner of the practice, greater reliance on managed care revenue, and an uncontrollable lifestyle.

7. Lepnurm R, Dobson R, Backman A, and Keegan D, Factors explaining career satisfaction among psychiatrists and surgeons in Canada, *Canadian Journal of Psychiatry* 51, 4 (2006): 243–55.
8. Garfinkel PE, Bagby RM, Schuller DR, and Dickens SE, Predictors of professional and personal satisfaction with a career in psychiatry, *Canadian Journal of Psychiatry* 50 (2005): 333–41.
9. Torre DM, Wang NY, Meoni LA, Young JH, Klag MJ, and Ford DE, Suicide compared to other causes of mortality in physicians, *Suicide and Life-Threatening Behavior* 35 (2005): 146–53.

   Johns Hopkins University professor, Daniel E. Ford, led a study of suicide among over 1,200 physicians from the graduating classes of 1948 to 1964 at the Johns Hopkins University School of Medicine. "Suicide is the first or second leading cause of years of potential life lost for physicians because they commit suicide at a relatively younger age," Dr. Ford wrote. This risk is much higher in women than in men. The combined results of 25 studies suggest that the suicide rate among female doctors is 130% higher than that among women in general, while the rate for male doctors is 40% higher than that among men in general.

   As many as one-quarter of people who commit suicide are drunk when they die, according to autopsy studies and other evidence. This could contribute to the high rate of suicide among female physicians, since alcoholism is more common among female physicians than it is in the general population. Drug addiction has been linked to suicide in physicians. In one study, more than one-third of physicians who killed themselves were believed to have had an addiction at some time in their lives, double the rate of the control group. Drug use is more common among psychiatrists, anesthesiologists, and emergency physicians than it is among other doctors. They usually turn to drugs to relieve anxiety or other unpleasant feelings rather than seeking professional help.
10. Rich CL and Pitts FN, Suicide by psychiatrists: a study of medical specialists among 18,730 consecutive physician deaths during a five-year period, 1967–72, *Journal of Clinical Psychiatry* 41 (1980): 261–63.
11. Reprinted in Epstein R and Bower T, Why shrinks have problems, *Psychology Today*, July 1, 1997.
12. Hawton K, Clements A, Simkin S, and Malmberg A, Doctors who kill themselves: a study of the methods used for suicide, *QJM* 93 (2000): 351–57.

13. Vaillant GE, Sobowale NC, and McArthur C, Some psychologic vulnerabilities of physicians, *New England Journal of Medicine* 287 (1972): 372–75.
14. Bermack GE, Do psychiatrists have special emotional problems? *American Journal of Psychoanalysis* 37, 2 (1977): 141–46.
15. Deary IJ, Agius RM, and Sadler A, Personality and stress in consultant psychiatrists, *International Journal of Social Psychiatry* 42 (1996): 112–23.
16. Shailesh Kumar surveyed all practising psychiatrists in New Zealand. He found that while job satisfaction levels for the group were high, they experienced moderate to severely high levels of emotional exhaustion. Why job satisfaction remains high in the presence of burnout is not clear.

    Burnout is common in physicians, with surveys showing that 30 to 40% meet criteria. Psychiatrists and other mental health workers display comparable levels of burnout.

    Psychiatrists generally score highly on personal achievement, as in job satisfaction, in spite of adverse circumstances or feelings. Work environment–related factors most conducive to burnout have also been identified: inadequate administration, lack of social support, patients' and relatives' dissatisfaction with unrealistically anticipated therapy outcomes, and the impossibility of establishing informal relations with patients.

    Certain factors may trigger burnout in this already vulnerable group. Violence perpetrated by patients is one such factor. Despite the frequent occurrence, dealing with violent patients is stressful for all psychiatrists, no matter what their level of experience.

    McCranie EW and Brandsma JM, Personality antecedents of burnout among middle-aged physicians, *Journal of Behavioral Medicine* 14 (1988): 30–36, used a prospective design to examine personality traits of burnout among 440 physicians. These physicians had been given the Minnesota Multiphasic Personality Inventory before entering medical school and then were surveyed an average of 25 years later for symptoms of burnout. The study found that higher burnout scores were related to earlier MMPI scales measuring low self-esteem, feelings of inadequacy, dysphoria, obsessive worry, passivity, social anxiety, and withdrawal. There is other research showing that psychological well-being among physicians is related to high levels of support from an intimate relationship and lower levels of practice stress.
17. Garfinkel PE and Waring EM, Personality, interests and emotional illness in psychiatric residents, *American Journal of Psychiatry* 138 (1981): 51–55.

18. Garfinkel PE, Bagby M, Waring EM, and Dorian B, Boundary violations and personality traits among psychiatrists, *Canadian Journal of Psychiatry* 42 (1997): 758–63.
19. Garfinkel PE, Bagby RM, Schuller DR, Dickens S, Fitzgerald L, and Williams CC, Gender differences in the practice characteristics and career satisfaction of psychiatrists in Ontario, *Academic Psychiatry* 28 (2004): 310–20.
20. The high-regret group in our survey was almost entirely composed of men. Although women accounted for 44% of the respondents to the questionnaire, only 18% of those with regret in their career choice were women.
21. Frank E, McMurray, JE Linzer M, and Elon L, Career satisfaction of US women physicians: results from the Women Physicians' Health Study; Society of General Internal Medicine Career Satisfaction Study Group, *Archives of Internal Medicine* 59, 13 (1999): 1417–26.

Chapter 14: Science and Care

1. Ten years later, American psychiatry was still debating the case. Gerald Klerman, a prominent psychiatrist/psychopharmacologist of Cornell Medical College and New York Hospital said that depression should be treated with drugs. Alan Stone, a professor of law and psychiatry at Harvard, and a former president of the American Psychiatric Association, said it's not malpractice to provide therapy alone in a case like this. Klerman GL, The psychiatric patient's right to effective treatment: implications of Osheroff v. Chestnut Lodge, *American Journal of Psychiatry* 147 (1990): 409–18; Stone A, Law, science and psychiatric malpractice: a response to Klerman's indictment of psychoanalytic psychiatry, *American Journal of Psychiatry* 147 (1990): 419–27.
2. Fonagy P, Kächele H, Krause R, Jones E, Perron R, Clarkin J, Gerber A, and Allison E, *An Open Door Review of Outcome Studies in Psychoanalysis,* 2nd ed. (London: International Psychoanalytical Association, 2002). The comment is regarding psychoanalysis itself—dynamically oriented therapies have been shown to be effective, as described in this review and later in this book.
3. Giving anticoagulants to people with the heart arrhythmia atrial fibrillation to prevent strokes, for instance, was based entirely on clinical supposition and not supported by science. Putting heart-attack patients to bed for several weeks was another. More recently there has been a real effort to prevent heart disease with low-fat, high-carbohydrate diets; this was

related to the belief that since heart disease was associated with disturbed blood lipids and that there were fatty plaques in the arteries, diet could prevent this (not keeping in mind the effects of high carbohydrates). In early 2014, high sugar content of diets was found to be a strong predictor of later heart disease.

4. "Caring has gone out of medicine," a doctor in 1999 told Christine Dunbar when she interviewed our subjects in the Ontario survey. "The reason why it has happened is because caring doesn't pay. We as a society have made the decision that caring for another human being is something that is relegated to an eight-dollars-an-hour [salaried] new immigrant, and what he or she tries is quickly to get their kid into a technical school so that they can go and get some technical competence and become, let's say, a nuclear medicine technician, and then that generation tries to make their kid a radiologist. So at some level, this is across the spectrum, it's like, who cares for your relatives, who cares for the little children in society. We farm them off to daycares, including mine, where we pay the lowest wage in society. So I think at some level what we are seeing is the fact that we as a society have thought that regular interpersonal human caring is the lowest form of remunerable human interaction. The moment you introduce skill, so for example, CBT, may in the long run become more reimbursable because it's kind of technical and objective and you can quantify it more than perhaps other forms of therapy. And similarly, the guy who can do procedures makes more than the guy who can give a pill, and I think that's a larger social decision we've made."

Chapter 15: Return to the Clarke

1. James Papez had studied the effects of rabies virus in cats in the late 1930s, and based on this he proposed that there is an "emotion system" linking the cortex with the hypothalamus. In the 1930s, the researchers Heinrich Klüver and Paul Bucy demonstrated that damage to the amygdala in monkeys led to a constellation of symptoms, including lack of fear, hyperorality, blunting of emotion, and placidity as well as a tendency to neglect of infants by females.
2. As a physician, I was part of a self-regulating profession. We were not employees of the hospital. I did have some understanding of how boards operate. I had been president of the medical staff association at the Clarke

in 1980, and this gave me two years as a member of its board. I was also chair of the medical advisory committee at Toronto General as it was forming the Toronto Hospital, which put me on the board of that institution at a critical time.

3. Although Tremain never wanted recognition for himself, I wanted to honour him in 2000, so we named a staff recognition award after him. Now every year about 3,000 people vie for the honour of receiving a "Teddy," as the Tremain Awards are commonly called.
4. Fortunately for the science, the molecular biology lab did well, since one of their junior colleagues, Fang Liu, had matured to excellence. In 2012, "Dr. Liu and her team found that nicotine exposure can enhance binding between two types of brain receptors: a nicotinic receptor and a glutamate receptor. They identified the sites where the two receptors bind together. With this information, they were able to generate a protein peptide to disrupt the binding of the two receptors." (CAMH press release Oct. 22, 2012.) This peptide has the effect of reducing attempts to seek nicotine in animals and is now being tested as an antismoking medication that directly targets the relapse process.
5. Other disorders run in families too. Patrick Sullivan and his colleagues have summarized these as varying from about 0.37 for depression to 0.75 for bipolar disorder and 0.81 for schizophrenia. Sullivan PF, Daly MJ, and O'Donovan M, Genetic architecture of psychiatric disorders: the emerging picture and its implications, *Nature Reviews* 13 (2012): 537–51.
6. This type of approach is beginning to produce results, though not of the blockbuster variety but, rather, as more of a "niche-buster," with small, steady gains. At present there's really no way of knowing how an individual will react to a given antidepressant medication unless he or she has tried it before. In other words, it's often a long and difficult process of trial and error. Some people will have no side effects to whichever one is prescribed; others will have many side effects from that same drug. Moreover, what works for one person might not work for another. So finding a way to personalize drug prescribing would be valuable.
7. His team discovered an epigenetic modification of DNA (chemical changes to DNA) in humans in 2009. This flags genes to be turned "on"—signalling the genome to make a protein—or to be turned "off." It is this pattern that allows a neuron to use the same genome as cells from

other parts of the body but create a different and specialized cell. This line of research also pursues these changes in the major mental illnesses and in terms of early environmental stressors and their effects on genes. For example, a Canadian team investigated genome-wide alterations induced by early-life trauma in men and found that childhood adversity is associated with alterations in the promoters of several genes. See Labonté B et al., Genome-wide epigenetic regulation by early-life trauma, *Archives of General Psychiatry* 69, 7 (2012): 722–31.

8. The CAMH merger even further strengthened this remarkable genetics group. Rachel Tyndale is a top molecular geneticist in the genetics of addiction who has made important inroads into our understanding of nicotine addiction. The group as a whole, as it matured, became first rate—at, or near, the best anywhere.
9. The results of the inquiries into the genetics of psychiatry have produced intriguing but inconclusive results. We don't understand the pathways to develop the illnesses we're most interested in, but research is showing that genes may play a key role. Schizophrenia is a good example. Normally, there is cortical thinning in the brain that occurs with aging. In schizophrenia it is advanced and occurs earlier than for normal people. But a gene for BDNF (brain-derived neurotrophic factor) has been show to predict the drop off in grey matter. This gene might play a role in people with schizophrenia who are well early in life and then become ill in late adolescence. They may be vulnerable in other ways. Women who became pregnant during the Dutch famine in World War II, and women who got influenza during pregnancy, both have been shown to have increased risk of schizophrenia. Marijuana use may play a role in some people developing a form of the illness. We don't know whether marijuana use actually causes the disease for a small group, or whether people in the prodrome of the illness are more likely users. A British group led by the Institute of Psychiatry's Robin Murray believes marijuana causes schizophrenia.

   We now know that no single gene causes schizophrenia or bipolar illness. Multiple genes are involved, so now investigators have found a way to study a person's whole genomic profile with genome-wide association studies. These studies use silicone chips with over 1 million DNA probes on them to map the person's genome. Data from these probes can be processed by a laser and computer. But we still cannot answer the basic question of who will get a mental illness.

10. Kapur S, Remington G, Jones C, Wilson A, DaSilva J, Houle S, and Zipursky R, High levels of dopamine d2 receptor occupancy with low-dose haloperidol treatment: a PET study, *American Journal of Psychiatry* 153 (1996): 948–50. PET has also played a role in furthering the monoamine hypothesis of mood disorders. Jeffrey Meyer of Toronto has found that the enzyme that breaks down several of the important monoamines, MAO-A, is elevated in people with major depression; reduced levels of some 5-HT receptors also occur. Again, we don't know whether these are state or trait markers.
11. Volkow gave both groups a stimulant. Healthy people found it aversive, whereas addicts with low levels of dopamine receptors enjoyed it. The reward systems in drug addicts' brains may be blunted.
12. The principles of compensation could be changed to align with my values, just as the recruitment and promotion processes could be altered, and we did these important things over a prolonged first two years. With regard to funding, I argued to establish principles for how the pooled "overage" of the group's funds would be redistributed according to defined priorities. The overage was the money that came in beyond each person's anticipated "draw." Because this extra was due to the staff's clinical earnings, it was hard to say it belonged to the university or hospital. But I could argue for a compromise: that 50% of it belonged to the individual and 50% to the group, to be redistributed to emphasize quality in teaching and research. The university or hospital wouldn't keep a penny of it. In a large group, that 50% was a considerable amount to be distributed by them according to the principles—after the principles and priorities were defined I was not directly involved—so they were happy and I was happy.

Chapter 16: The Academy

1. Mary Seeman had a very distinguished career, becoming an Officer of the Order of Canada, and awarded an honorary doctorate of science by the University of Toronto for her work on women with schizophrenia.
2. The University Health Network is the renamed version of Toronto General Hospital and Toronto Western Hospital after they incorporated the cancer hospital Princess Margaret (and later the Toronto Rehabilitation Institute) into their organization.
3. Burke JD, Pincus HA, and Pardes H, The clinician-researcher, *American Journal of Psychiatry* 143 (1986): 968–75.

4. Boyer EL, *Scholarship Reconsidered: Priorities of the Professoriate* (Lawrenceville, NJ: Princeton University Press for the Carnegie Foundation for the Advancement of Teaching, 1990), 15–25.
5. Boyer EL, "The Scholarship of Engagement," *Bulletin of the American Academy of Arts and Sciences* 49, 7 (1996): 18–33.
6. Levinson DJ, with Darrow CN, Klein EB, and Levinson M, *Seasons of a Man's Life* (New York: Random House, 1978).
7. Roche GRT, "Much ado about mentors," *Harvard Business Review* 57 (1979): 14–28.
8. Kirsling RA and Kochar MS, Mentors in graduate medical education at the Medical College of Wisconsin, *Academic Medicine* 65 (1990): 272–74.
9. The retention of physicians is a tricky matter because they aren't the organization's employees and they can always get another job—in clinical practice or in another hospital or academic setting. Physicians have to want to be in this particular organization. Sometimes it's about status and gaining experience before they move on. But mostly it is feeling valued and respected for their role, whatever it may be. Doctors also like to be connected in some way to the board, CEO, or senior management and feel that their work is both interesting and appreciated. I have usually felt that most of my colleagues overemphasize the role of compensation. Compensation can serve as a disincentive if one's pay is significantly below that of other colleagues. But otherwise, people don't move about for minor differences in compensation. Physicians in Ontario who complain about compensation—and there are many—are those that haven't worked elsewhere.

Chapter 17: Who Do We Serve?

1. Results from the 2007 National Survey on Drug Use and Health: National Findings (Rockville, MD: US Department of Health and Human Services, Substance Abuse and Mental Health Services Administration, 2008).
2. For an excellent discussion of mental health reform in progressive countries see Shera W, Aviram U, Healy B, and Ramon S, Mental health system reform: a multi-country comparison, *Social Work Health Care* 35, 1–2 (2002): 547–75.
3. Robert Graham was a volunteer, as the chair of the Rideau Valley District Health Council, based in Smith Falls, Ontario, and the chair of the provincial association of District Health Councils.

4. Burns T, Rugkåsa J, Molodynski A, Dawson JK, and Vazquez-Montes M, Community treatment orders for patients with psychosis (OCTET): a randomised controlled trial, *Lancet* 81, 9878 (2013): 1627–33.
5. Crisp AH, Gelder M, Rix S, Meltzer H, and Rowlands OJ, Stigmatisation of people with mental illnesses, *British Journal of Psychiatry* 177 (2000): 4–7.
6. Grausgruber A, Schöny W, Grausgruber-Berner R, Koren G, Apor BF, Wancata J, and Meise U, "Schizophrenia has many faces": evaluation of the Austrian Anti-Stigma-Campaign, 2000–2002, *Psychiatrische Praxis* 36, 7 (2009): 327–33.
7. FitzGerald, James, *What Disturbs Our Blood* (Toronto: Random House, 2010).
8. Cassels C, Psychiatrists urged to fight stigma linked to mental illness, *Medscape Medical News*, October 20, 2011.
9. Thornicroft G, Rose D, and Kassam A, Discrimination in health care against people with mental illness, *International Review of Psychiatry* 19, 2 (2007): 113–22.
10. Gallop R, Lancee W, and Garfinkel PE, How nursing staff respond to the label "borderline personality disorder," *Hospital Community Psychiatry* 40 (1989): 815–19.
11. In Toronto one-quarter of patients were seen more than 17 times per year (in Ontario outside the cities, half were seen fewer than three times a year). One-quarter of Toronto psychiatrists (about 200) see fewer than 40 patients per year; they account for 6% of treatment of patients. And 50% of the high frequency patients are from upper-quintile income brackets.

    Despite all of this, this regular therapy did not cut the hospitalization rate or trips to the ER. What's more, the seriously ill patients who did go to the hospital for schizophrenia and depression didn't get proper follow up: only half were seen a month after discharge. For cardiac care patients, that figure is 99%. Kurdyak P, Stukel TA, Goldbloom D, Kopp A, Zagorski B, and Mulsant BH, Universal coverage without universal access: a study of psychiatrist supply and practice patterns in Ontario, forthcoming.
12. Deinstitutionalization is not without its risks, especially when it focuses on bed reductions and not on enhanced help in the broad community. When deinstitutionalization isn't done well, there is a significant rise in homelessness among the seriously mentally ill; we see more psychotic people in libraries and in bus and train stations. There are many more calls to the police, who have to be well trained to understand this population.

Substance abuse becomes common in people with chronic psychosis, and this is what is especially associated with violence among psychotic people when they are not compliant with ongoing medications. The vast majority of people living with mental health problems and illnesses are not involved with the criminal justice system. In fact, they are more likely to be victims of violence than perpetrators.

Deinstitutionalization has another important side effect. The people who are in the psychiatric hospitals are increasingly the "forensic" population. The forensic population are overwhelmingly people with schizophrenia, and sometimes they are people who have been unable to access the regular mental health system or for whom it has been inadequate—a study of the CAMH forensic population revealed that three-quarters of the patients were already in some contact with the mental health system.

What so many of these patients require is more rehabilitation for their chronic psychosis. They should be integrated with programs for psychosis so that the psychotic people within the forensics systems have access to the excellent ambulatory post-discharge programs that have been developed for others with chronic psychosis. And with modern risk assessments, it is possible to have many more of these patients treated from an ambulatory perspective.

The other big problem with deinstitutionalization is that we have passed on the problems to other parts of our society and, in this instance, back to the family; as I mentioned, in Ontario starting in the mid-1990s, there was a downloading of services from the province to the city and ultimately from the city to the family, largely to women who have borne the brunt of the family burden. Related to this has been the story of now aging couples who have great concerns as their dependent children are now middle-aged, and may have nowhere to turn once their parents die.

Chapter 19: Four Become One

1. In mid-2013 this group was disbanded because of changes in provincial regulation regarding how boards are selected.

Chapter 20: Managing a Merger

1. Bridges W, *Managing Transitions: Making the Most of Change* (Cambridge, MA: Perseus Books, 1991).

Chapter 21: The Asylum as Urban Village: There Is No Plan B

This chapter is largely derived from a collaboration with Frank Lewinberg, the outstanding urban planner of Urban Strategies and portions of it have appeared in *Spacings* magazine.

1. In 1888 the government had sold off 24 acres of the property to developers.
2. Crawford PK, "Asylum landscape," in *The Provincial Asylum in Toronto: Reflections on Social and Architectural History*, ed. E Hudson (Toronto: Toronto Region Architectural Conservancy, 2000).
3. British physician Dr. John Conolly, at the Hanwell Asylum in the early 1840s, followed the pioneering reformer William Tuke and the York Retreat, and Dr. William Ellis, his predecessor at Hanwell.
4. Brown T, Living with God's afflicted: a history of the Provincial Lunatic Asylum at Toronto, 1830–1911, PhD thesis, Queen's University, 1980.
5. At one point there was an attempt to close "999," Koziel says. C.K. Clarke recognized the importance of research if advances were to be made in the treatment of mental illness, but with the need to treat so many patients, this made spending time on research impossible. He advocated closing the hospital and treating the short-term patients in the new Toronto Psychiatric Hospital, opened in 1925 adjacent to Women's College Hospital (now Surrey Place Centre). The other more chronic patients requiring asylum would be moved to Whitby, as Queen Street by this time had been surrounded by the urban sprawl of Toronto. However, after World War I, with the continuing growth in the civilian population and the return of shell-shocked soldiers, the need for Queen Street remained.
6. The wall: A temporary wall was made of wood in 1851. It was thought that this wasn't durable or substantial. In 1860 an all brick wall was completed under the direction of the provincial architect Kivas Tully (he had designed Trinity College). He designed a 12- to 16-foot-tall brick wall that went all around the institution (it varied in height depending on the location). A big chunk of the south wall was missing so a rail line could go to the property and deliver coal, in the early 20th century. The south wall is the last remaining part of this 1860 wall. The front wall on the north side had two gates with ornamental wrought iron. The front wall was taken down in the late 1970s. There were farm gates on the west wall (the farming was just to the west of the buildings). Patients were utilized in both the 1860 and 1888 construction. It was done by the provincial

architects with stone masons supervising patients who were assisting the craftsmen.

7. In 1992 Australia announced a mental health policy that increased national and state funding for services. The goal was "a seamless set of relationships from inpatient ward to community support," and the policy framework included increased federal funding, priority for people with serious mental illness, enhanced consumer rights, and a strategy to involve general practitioners as providers of primary care (Shera, Aviram, Healy, and Ramon, Mental health system reform, 547–75). National government funding was provided on a matching basis to help the states shift care from institutions to a community-focused system. Of importance, the Australian reform included benchmarking to measure progress.

   In 1978 Italy passed a law phasing out its psychiatric hospitals. This law shifted care to community mental health centres and general hospital psychiatric units. The last psychiatric hospital there was closed in 1999. Care is focused in the community, as opposed to the general hospital, though there is more burden on families. Living arrangements shifted from the hospitals to residential care facilities with 24-hour staffing, or to light residential care.

   Italy has developed a system of social cooperatives that employ people living with mental illness. Some municipalities give contracts to these social cooperatives. For example, the social cooperatives have contracts with the municipality for parking tickets; they also book appointments and process X-rays for hospitals, do laundry for hospitals and nursing homes, and have an industrial cleaning service. Trieste has a tourist hotel and restaurant operated by social cooperatives where 40% of the employees are people living with mental illness (Steve Lurie, personal commincation, 2013).

   Social cooperatives do provide access to work for some people living with mental illness, but their benefit has not been well evaluated. Whether disadvantaged people make the leap to other competitive employment is not clear.

8. In the final analysis, the city and the neighbourhood approved the proposed development on the property, which held some 800,000 square feet in existing buildings, and allowed the construction of a new mental health and addictions hospital comprising 1,400,000 square feet plus an additional 1,300,000 square feet of non-CAMH buildings. We were able to increase developable space more than threefold—an amazing feat

in real estate terms—and it's a credit to the public process that CAMH committed to and never wavered from. The approved building massing approach allowed CAMH to determine the actual buildings when it needed them and was ready to design them, thus retaining the flexibility that had been an important policy of the vision.

9. The proposed buildings were defined in a general sense as masses, demarcated only by their height and their location within each block. The masses were generally kept low at the edges of the property, where they were adjacent to the existing neighbourhood fabric, and allowed to rise to 10 storeys in the centre of the property.

Chapter 22: DSM Dysfunction

1. The *Diagnostic and Statistical Manual* had been introduced by the American Psychiatric Association in 1952 to provide standardized diagnostic criteria for psychiatric disorders, for use primarily by clinicians. There had earlier been a recognized need to collect statistical information, at first as a standard international list of causes of death, so a classification of mental disorders was required; in 1880 in the United States, this classification consisted of seven categories: mania, melancholia, monomania (delusional disorder), paresis (caused by syphilis), dementia, dipsomania (craving for alcohol), and epilepsy. After World War II, the system was broadened; in 1948 the sixth edition of the World Health Organization's International Classification of Diseases contained a chapter on mental illnesses. But it lacked descriptions of chronic brain syndromes, transient situational disorders, and many personality disorders, and was felt to be unsuitable for American psychiatry, with its emphasis on outpatient-based analytic practice. So in 1951 the US Public Health Service commissioned work involving the American Psychiatric Association and the Veterans Administration to develop DSM, which for the first time was a glossary of definitions.

   DSM-I didn't have illnesses or disorders, but rather "reactions," as Adolf Meyer would have wanted. He thought mental disorders were actually reactions of the personality to psychological, social, and biological factors. DSM-I differed from the international classification in that it was more psychodynamically based and relied on the experiences of World War II veterans and outpatients, rather than those in mental hospitals. It included ill-defined terms such as "psychoneurotic reactions," which were "disorders of psychogenic origin or without clearly defined tangible cause or structural change." Schizophrenic "reactions" and "affective reactions" were also described as "disorders of psychogenic origin or without clearly defined tangible cause or structural change."

DSM-II, when it came out in 1968, maintained a similar causal bias and terminology, except the term "reaction" was dropped. It used the term "disease" carefully—only for mental retardation and organic brain syndromes—and it used "illness" only for manic depressive psychosis. There were a few improvements in DSM-II, such as recognizing the fluctuating nature of some clinical conditions. The "functional psychoses" were now classified under an awkward but more precise term "psychosis not attributable to physical conditions previously stated" (the beginning of a recognition that the actual causes of such illness as schizophrenia were not really known). Psychoanalysis was dominating American psychiatry, and it influenced the way the DSM classified illnesses. These diagnoses were based on theory, not on empirical studies, but it didn't really matter because, with some exceptions, the treatment was likely to be the same, regardless of the diagnosis. *American Psychiatric Association Diagnostic and Statistical Manual of Mental Disorders*, Washington, DC, 1952, reprinted in Freedman AM, Kaplan HI, and Kaplan HS, *Comprehensive Textbook of Psychiatry* (Baltimore: Williams and Wilkins, 1967), 584–89; *American Psychiatric Association Diagnostic and Statistical Manual of Mental Disorders* (DSM-II), Washington, DC, 1968, reprinted in Freedman AM, Kaplan HI, and Sadock BJ, *Comprehensive Textbook of Psychiatry*, 2nd ed. (Baltimore: Williams and Wilkins, 1975), 826–45.

2. Parker G, *A Piece of My Mind: A Psychiatrist on the Couch* (Sydney: Macmillan, 2012).
3. Patten SB, Major depression prevalence is very high, but the syndrome is a poor proxy for community populations' clinical treatment needs, *Canadian Journal of Psychiatry* 53, 7 (2008): 411–19.
4. If the symptom complex presented after the loss of a loved one, the diagnosis of depression previously was not made because it was believed that this was a normal response to such a loss. DSM-IV-TR, the revised DSM-IV, specifically recommended against diagnosing major depression in the bereaved when the symptoms are milder and of less than two months' duration. This is known as the "bereavement exclusion." (If the signs of depression are severe—the patient has thoughts of suicide, for example—major depression is supposed to be diagnosed.)

5. In the new version, the exclusion criterion has been replaced by two notations: a footnote at the end of the criteria that cautions clinicians to differentiate between normal grieving associated with a significant loss and a diagnosis of a mental disorder, and a note embedded within the criteria that reminds clinicians that major depression and bereavement can coexist.
6. Many of the problems we see exist on a continuum, and the extreme end of the continuum is serious and requires help. The DSM-5 has a diagnosis called "disruptive mood dysregulation disorder" that describes "children who exhibit persistent irritability and frequent episodes of behavior outbursts three or more times a week for more than a year." American Psychiatric Association, *Diagnostic and Statistical Manual of Mental Disorders*, 5th ed. (Arlington, VA: American Psychiatric Publishing, 2013). Parents might call them tantrums, but the DSM is referring to extreme hostility and outbursts beyond normal tantrums. It is much better to have this disorder included than what some had wanted: bipolar disorder in children. So this disruptive mood regulation disorder was a compromise. At the mild end of each of these conditions they blend with normal, but the extremes can be incapacitating and warrant treatment.
7. We are already seeing extremely high rates of diagnoses for ADHD in the United States. Alan Schwarz and Sarah Cohen have recently described a Centers for Disease Control and Prevention study (*New York Times*, March 31, 2013) that found that about 11% of children now receive such a diagnosis, there's been a 41% rise in such diagnoses in the past decade, and many or most (about two-thirds) of those diagnosed are put on medication. By contrast, the careful study described by the United Kingdom's National Collaborating Centre guidelines, published in 2009, described a more modest prevalence of 3.6% in boys and 0.9% in girls in the United Kingdom. Stimulant medicines (Ritalin, Concerta) are beneficial for kids with ADHD but do lead to problems—insomnia, anxiety, and addiction, for example. Even within the United States the rates vary widely by geography, with the highest levels in the southern states. What accounts for this?

   Some of this is fuelled by drug company advertising and media stories that enhance parents' worries. Some children are being medicated when they may have attachment problems or lack of adequate parenting; others are normal kids, just at the end of the continuum for activity and concentration. DSM-5 won't help this problem and probably will expand the numbers of ADHD cases, since it is changing the age requirement. DSM-5 also requires that symptoms merely impact daily activities, rather than cause impairment. Severe ADHD that goes untreated has been shown to increase a child's risk for academic failure and substance abuse, so an accurate diagnosis is extremely important. But are we contributing to overdiagnosing and overmedicating our children?

8. A further area of improvement in DSM-5 has been the diagnosis of autism, an area of great concern, since about 1 in 90 children are born with one or another form of this heterogeneous condition (the frequency of diagnosis has increased greatly, though whether it's because of improved diagnosis or an actual increase in the frequency of condition is not known). In the new criteria, Asperger's syndrome (in this context, a vague term for intellectual children with social problems and obsession with specific topics) and pervasive developmental disorder (an umbrella type of term for other disorders characterized by delays in the development of many basic functions, including socialization and communication) will be folded into the autism spectrum. This will permit more rapid diagnosis, which in the United States allows for more ready access to treatments. A study reported in 2012 of close to 5,000 people found that just 10% of children previously diagnosed would not meet the new narrower definition. Huerta M, Bishop SL, Duncan A, Hus V, and Lord C, Application of DSM-5 criteria for autism spectrum disorder to three samples of children with DSM-IV diagnoses of pervasive developmental disorders, *American Journal of Psychiatry* 169 (2012): 1056–64.

DSM-5 also started to do a really good job with personality disorders, but then this set of changes was voted down. The general criteria for personality disorder that were introduced into DSM-IV lacked an empirical basis and have been generally considered extremely nonspecific. In the fifth edition, the biggest change was the incorporation of personality dimensions (instead of categories)—this reflects what we generally see in patients, in that often traits are present along a continuum and in many people mixed types of personality exist. Humans are complex; we mostly cannot be simply categorized as having or not having this or that personality disorder. But after the vote was turned down, DSM-5 now lists both categories and dimensions in order to stimulate further research on this topic. In field studies involving interviewing large numbers of people with psychiatric diagnoses, borderline personality disorder had good reliability (over time and with different interviewers); other personality disorders either lacked reliability or insufficient numbers of people were interviewed to make valid conclusions. On the positive side, there is also new emphasis on impairment in "interpersonal functioning" (how the personality affects how the person relates to others—a spouse, partner, or boss, for example): it is not just the presence of certain features but the way life is hindered as a result.

9. Farahani A and Correll CU, Are antipsychotics or antidepressants needed for psychotic depression? A systematic review and meta-analysis of trials comparing antidepressant or antipsychotic monotherapy with combination treatment, *Journal of Clinical Psychiatry* 73 (2012): 486–96.
10. McCarthy LP and Gerring JP, Revising psychiatry's charter, document DSM-IV written communication 11 (1994), 147–92.
11. Brooks D, "Heroes of uncertainty," *New York Times*, May 27, 2013.

Chapter 23: Psychotherapy: The New Evidence

1. Beck AT, Rush AJ, Shaw BF, and Emery G, *Cognitive Therapy of Depression* (New York: Guilford Press, 1979).
2. Weissman M and Markowitz JC, *Comprehensive Guide to Interpersonal Psychotherapy* (New York: Basic Books, 2000).
3. Linehan MM, Rathus JH, and Miller AL, *Dialectical Behavior Therapy with Suicidal Adolescents* (New York: Guilford Press, 2006).
4. Kabat Zinn J, *Mindfulness Meditation for Everyday Life* (London: Piatkus Books, 2001).
5. Segal ZV, Williams MG, and Teasdale JD, *Mindfulness-Based Cognitive Therapy for Depression: A New Approach to Preventing Relapse* (New York: Guilford Press, 2002).
6. Smith ML, Glass GV, and Miller TI, *The Benefits of Psychotherapy* (Baltimore: Johns Hopkins University Press, 1980).
7. Weisz JR, Kuppens S, Eckshain D, Ugueto AM, Hawley KM, and Jensen-Doss A, Performance of evidence based youth psychotherapies compared with usual clinical care, *JAMA Psychiatry* 70 (2013): 750–61.
8. Abbass AA, Hancock JT, Henderson J, and Kisely S, Short-term psychodynamic psychotherapies for common mental disorders, *Cochrane Database of Systematic Reviews* 4 (2006): CD004687.doi:10.1002/14651858.CD004687.pub3.

9. Jones EE and Pulos SM, Comparing the process in psychodynamic and cognitive behavioral therapies, *Journal of Consulting and Clinical Psychology 61* (1993): 306–16.
10. Karl Jaspers, a German psychiatrist and philosopher of the first half of the twentieth century, developed phenomenology, where the patient's inner experiences are placed at the centre of clinical interest.
11. Paul McHugh of Johns Hopkins has repeatedly emphasized this over the past two decades. McHugh and his collaborator Phillip Slavney have highlighted the need to look at four models of psychiatric disorders: a disease perspective (what is wrong with the structure of the brain itself), a dimensional perspective, (how does a person's character cause difficulty) a behavioural perspective (what actions are problematic because they are reinforced), and a life-story perspective (what events in the person's life have contributed). They have written that a psychiatrist has to have knowledge and comfort in using several different perspectives (models of explanation or understanding) in order to grapple with the range of psychiatric problems seen in clinical practice and to use treatments appropriately. McHugh PR and Slavney PR, *The Perspectives of Psychiatry,* 2nd ed. (Baltimore: Johns Hopkins University Press, 1998).
12. Tsemberis S and Eisenberg R, Pathways to housing: supported housing for street-dwelling homeless individuals with psychiatric disabilities, *Psychiatric Services* 51 (2000): 487–93.
13. Bond G, Supported employment: evidence for an evidence-based practice, *Psychiatric Rehabilitation Journal* 27, 4 (2004): 345–59.
14. Strong social support may significantly improve recovery from both physical and mental illnesses. For example, Eugene Paykel of Cambridge has shown that onset and recurrence of depression are related to lack of social support. Paykel ES, Life events, social support and depression, *Acta Psychiatrica Scandinavica* 89 (Suppl 377) (1994): 50–58.

Chapter 24: What Makes a Good Psychiatrist?

1. Bhugra D, Sivakumar K, Holsgrove G, Butler G, and Leese M, What makes a good psychiatrist? A survey of clinical tutors responsible for psychiatric training in the UK and Eire, *World Psychiatry* 8 (2009): 119–20.
2. Montgomery K, *How Doctors Think: Clinical Judgment and the Practice of Medicine* (New York: Oxford University Press, 2006).

3. Holmes OW Sr, *The Writings of Oliver Wendell Holmes*, vol. 9 (Cambridge, MA: Scholastic and Bedside Teaching, 1891), 275.
4. Frank J, *Persuasion and Healing: A Comparative Study of Psychotherapy* (Baltimore: Johns Hopkins University Press, 1993).
5. Osler W, *Aequanimitas: With Other Addresses to Medical Students, Nurses, and Practitioners of Medicine*, 3rd ed. (Philadelphia: R. Blackiston's Son & Co., 1932) (originally published in 1905).
6. Stewart M, Brown JB, and Donner A, The impact of patient-centred care on outcomes, *Journal of Family Practice* 49 (2000): 796–804.
7. Chen P, "Can doctors learn empathy?" *New York Times*, June 21, 2012.
8. Truax CB and Carkuff R, *Toward Effective Counseling and Psychotherapy: Training and Practice* (Chicago: Transaction Publishers, 1976).
9. Some studies show that empathy drops after just one year of medical school. Others have found that it's most pronounced during the third year, a time when the class is moving to patient care; this is when empathy is most essential. Hojat M, Vergare MJ, Maxwell K, Brainard G, Herrine SK, Isenberg GA, Veloski J, Gonnella JS, The devil is in the third year: a longitudinal study of erosion of empathy in medical school, *Academic Medicine* 84, 9 (2009): 1182–91.
10. Neumann M, Edelhauser F, Tauschel D, Fischer MR, Wirtz M, Woopen C, Haramati A, and Scheffer C, Empathy decline and its reasons: a systematic review of medical students and residents, *Academic Medicine* 86 (2011): 996–1005.
11. Women have higher empathy scores than men. Students going into internal medicine, family medicine, pediatrics, obstetrics, gynecology, and psychiatry showed greater empathy than those entering specialties such as surgery, pathology, and radiology. Empathy scores are also associated with ratings of clinical competence in medicals students.
12. Another area of value related to the study of empathy has been self-psychology, which for the last 40 years has been associated with the seminal work of Heinz Kohut. Kohut, an Austrian-born psychoanalyst, moved to Chicago in 1940, where he was a traditional Freudian analyst, but he broke with Freud to develop the field of self-psychology. Kohut studied narcissistic personality disorder. People considered to have this disorder suffer less from internalized conflicts in a modern, less repressive society but experience problems with identity and have a sense of meaninglessness

and interpersonal difficulties. Kohut believed that these people had problems evolving largely from early experiences and in analysis required an "accurate empathy." He shifted a part of psychoanalysis away from the interpretation of internalized conflict and toward the empathic stance of the analyst. Strozier CB, *Heinz Kohut: The Making of a Psychoanalyst* (New York: Farrar, Straus and Giroux, 2001).

13. From the other side of the coin, many physicians miss empathic "opportunities." We can see this with oncologists, who were video-recorded speaking with their patients. When emotions were expressed by the patients (e.g., statements such as "I've got nothing to look forward to") they were often overlooked by the physicians. The oncologists responded only 22% of the time. In contrast, three-quarters of the time they chose instead to discuss some other aspect of medical care, such as a change in therapy. Other studies have confirmed this finding. Morse DS, Edwardsen EA, and Gordon HS, Missed opportunities for interval empathy in lung cancer communication, *Archives of Internal Medicine* 168 (2008): 1853–58.
14. Luhrmann, *Of Two Minds*.
15. Wu AW, Folkman S, McPhee SJ, and Lo B, Do house officers learn from their mistakes? *JAMA* 265 (1991): 2089–94.
16. Chen P, "The bullying culture of medical school," *New York Times*, August 9, 2012.

Chapter 25: Restoring the Public Trust

1. Psychiatry's image takes a hit when psychotic patients commit violent crimes. As I write this, Canada is cracking down harder on mentally ill people who break the law. One significant driver is the highly publicized accounts of violent actions by mentally ill people. When a patient who was not taking his medications beheaded a passenger on a bus in Western Canada, people got scared—and at times like this, many people blamed psychiatry for not preventing the awful murder. Although psychiatrists are capable of conducting good risk assessments these days, people with schizophrenia sometimes go off medication and get addicted to drugs, whether being followed, or not, in the poorly funded side of the community mental health system. Then terrible things can happen. But bear in mind that the mentally ill account for just 4% of violent crime; they are much more likely to be the victims of crime. Even with excellent funding and follow up, we will never get 100% accuracy because we are dealing

with human beings; we have to strive to 100%, but we don't want to lock up many ill people who won't commit crimes. This part of dealing with psychotic people would be helped by better medicines that people stay with, or by more use of injectible antipsychotic drugs.

2. Halter M, Perceived characteristics of psychiatric nurses: stigma by association, *Archives of Psychiatric Nursing* 22 (2008): 20–26.
3. Freidson E, *Profession of Medicine: A Study of the Sociology of Applied Knowledge* (Chicago: University of Chicago Press, 1970).
4. Simpson J, *Chronic Condition: Why Canada's Health Care System Needs to Be Dragged into the 21st Century* (Toronto: Penguin Books, 2012).
5. Professions in general are characterized by (1) ownership of a specialized body of knowledge and skills, which defines the field of competence and the scope of potential clients, including the demarcation from other professions; (2) holding a high status in society (both through financial and other rewards); (3) being granted autonomy (and thereby power) by society, for example, in recruiting and excluding members; and (4) being obliged, in return for the above, to guarantee high-quality standards in providing services (being "professional") and following ethical rules. Katschnig H, Are psychiatrists an endangered species? Observations on internal and external challenges to the profession, *World Psychiatry* 9, 1 (2010): 21–28.
6. Nordt C, Rössler W, and Lauber C, Attitudes of mental health professionals toward people with schizophrenia and major depression, *Schizophrenia Bulletin* 32 (2006): 709–14.
7. Seeman M, Psychiatry in the Nazi era, *Canadian Journal of Psychiatry* 50 (2005): 218–25.
8. Colaianni A, A long shadow: Nazi doctors, moral vulnerability and contemporary medical culture, *Journal of Medical Ethics* 38 (2012): 435–38.
9. Beauchamp T and Childress JF, *Principles of Biomedical Ethics*, 5th ed. (New York: Oxford University Press, 2001).
10. Woollard RF, Addressing the pharmaceutical industry's influence on professional behaviour, *Canadian Medical Association Journal* 149 (1993): 403–4.
11. Hodges B, Interactions with the pharmaceutical industry: experiences and attitudes of psychiatry residents, interns and clerks, *Canadian Medical Association Journal* 153 (1995): 553–59.
12. Waud DR, Pharmaceutical promotions: a free lunch? *New England Journal of Medicine* 327 (1992): 351–53.

13. McCormick BB, Tomlinson G, Brill-Edwards P, and Detsky AS, Effect of restricting contact between pharmaceutical company representatives and internal medicine residents on posttraining attitudes and behavior, *JAMA* 286 (2001): 1994–99.
14. Chakrabarti A, Fleisher WP, Staley D, and Calhoun L, Interactions of staff and residents with pharmaceutical industry: a survey of psychiatric training program policies, *Annals* (Royal College of Physicians and Surgeons of Canada), 35, 8 (Suppl) (2002): 541–46.
15. Appelbaum P, "Throw them out?" *Psychiatric News*, July 5, 2002.
16. Harris G, "Top psychiatrist didn't report drug makers' pay," *New York Times*, October 3, 2008.
17. Friedman RA, "A call for caution on antipsychotic drugs," Nytimes.com, September 24, 2012.
18. Kessler RC, Chiu WT, and Walters EE, Prevalence, severity, and comorbidity of twelve-month DSM-IV disorders in the national comorbidity survey replication (NCS-R), *Archives of General Psychiatry* 62 (2005): 617–27.
19. We could open up time for the sickest in society if we stopped routinely seeing patients once a week. Instead, we should see patients as frequently as their clinical state requires. For example, once a patient feels somewhat better, he or she might be fine with a visit every two or four weeks, instead of once a week. When the patient is in a crisis, two or three appointments may be required, but again these decisions should be individualized. We can stop seeing people on a regular basis—as long as we can assure them that if they need to see us, we will make time for them. The key issue is to see that patients receive the treatment they need, not the same standard treatment a doctor provides no matter what the problem, and whether it's an antidepressant or psychodynamic therapy. In other words, psychiatrists have to be much better at tailoring treatments to the patients' needs rather than to their own.
20. Frank JR, ed., *The CanMEDS 2005 Physician Competency Framework: Better Standards, Better Physicians, Better Care* (Ottawa: Royal College of Physicians and Surgeons of Canada, 2005).
21. Mental Health Commission of Canada, *Changing Directions, Changing Lives: The Mental Health Strategy for Canada* (Calgary: Mental Health Commission of Canada, 2012).
22. Ibid, p. 42.

23. Ibid.
24. Lurie S, Why can't Canada spend more on mental health? *Health* 6 (2014): 684–90.
25. Warden D, Rush J, Triuedi MH, Fava M, and Wisniewski S, The STAR*D Project results: a comprehensive review of findings current, *Psychiatry Reports* 9 (2007): 449–59.
26. Because of these issues, switching from one antidepressant to another is common and generally occurs early in treatment (about 70% of the time within days). However, it was even more common when the older tricyclic antidepressants were used than in the current SSRI era, largely because of intolerable early side effects (sedation, dryness, weight gain).
27. Of course, the next step also involves the very thing I was interested in 40 years ago: predicting who will respond to which treatment. The diagnoses themselves offer little more than we already know: we do need genome studies coupled with brain imaging, and hopefully this will add to our ability to predict response and get us to the era of biological markers.
28. Carlat D, *Unhinged: The Trouble with Psychiatry; A Doctor's Revelations about a Profession in Crisis* (New York: Free Press, 2010).
29. Less strong evidence exists for an extended release form of methylphenidate. Recently, evidence has shown that adjunctive therapy with atypical antipsychotics has the potential for beneficial antidepressant effects in the absence of psychotic symptoms. In particular, aripiprazole (Abilify) has shown efficacy as an augmentation option with standard antidepressant therapy in two large randomized, double-blind studies.

    Calcium channel blockers affect the movement of calcium into the cells of the heart and blood vessels, relaxing the blood vessels and increasing the supply of blood and oxygen to the heart. They are generally used to treat high blood pressure, irregular heartbeat, and angina. Some calcium channel blockers (e.g., verapamil) are also being studied for use in the treatment of bipolar disorder as mood stabilizers. One reason for the interest in this application is that these drugs are safer for use during pregnancy than lithium or any of the anticonvulsants commonly used to stabilize moods and treat mania.
30. Helen Mayberg, an enquiring neurologist at Emory University, previously worked at the University of Toronto as the first Sandra A. Rotman Chair in Neuropsychiatry. Working with Professors Andres Lozano and Sidney Kennedy, she showed that treatment responders often have reduced

activity in subgenual cingulate gyrus 25, whereas some nonresponders don't. Mayberg found a high rate of positive mood changes during electrical stimulation to this specific brain area in patients resistant to antidepressant therapy. This stimulation requires serotonin to be effective.

31. Berkowitz RL, Patel U, Ni Q, Parks JJ, and Docherty JP, The impact of the Clinical Antipsychotic Trials of Intervention Effectiveness (CATIE) on prescribing practices: an analysis of data from a large Midwestern state, *Journal of Clinical Psychiatry* 73 (2012): 498–503.
32. CTV News, "Big pharma pulling back from mental health drug research: studies," October 29, 2012, http://www.ctvnews.ca/health/health-headlines/.
33. Adlaf EM, Demers A, and Gliksman L, eds., *Canadian Campus Survey 2004* (Toronto, Centre for Addiction and Mental Health, 2005).
34. Kalivas PW and Volkow ND, The neural basis of addiction: a pathology of motivation and choice, *American Journal of Psychiatry* 162, 8 (2005): 1403–13.
35. Strang J, *Recovery-Orientated Drug Treatment: An Interim Report* (London: National Treatment Agency for Substance Misuse, 2011).
36. This high burden is largely because of three factors: the emergence of these conditions early in life, the conditions' prolonged durations, and their relatively high prevalence. The early onset of mental illness and addictions coincides with a time of major life transitions, such as completion of high school, transition to higher education, entry into the workforce, and marriage.

    According to a study released by CAMH in 2006, the estimated total economic cost attributable to mental illness and substance abuse in 2000 was about $33.9 billion per year in Ontario; approximately 85% ($28.7 billion) is due to productivity losses and the remaining ($5.2 billion) is related to direct costs, $2.1 billion of this to mental health treatment programs. The cost of substance abuse was higher, at $3 billion, because of the higher costs of law enforcement.

    In 2012 Canada's Mental Health Commission issued its first mental health strategy report and recommended an increase in the proportion of social spending that is devoted to mental health by two percentage points from current levels; a need to identify current mental health spending that should be reallocated to improve efficiency and achieve better mental health outcomes; and a need to engage the private and philanthropic sectors in contributing resources to mental health.

Chapter 26: To Be a Leader

1. Gilovich T and Husted Medvec V, The experience of regret: what, when, and why, *Psychological Review* 102, 2 (1995): 379–95.
2. Goleman D, *Emotional Intelligence: Why It Can Matter More than IQ* (New York: Bantam Books, 1995).
3. Goleman D, Boyatzis R, and McKee A, *Primal Leadership: Learning to Lead with Emotional Intelligence* (Cambridge, MA: Harvard Business School Press, 2001).
4. Collins, JC, *Good to Great: Why Some Companies Make the Leap ... and Others Don't* (Toronto: HarperCollins, 2001).
5. Immen W, "The downside of success: loneliness and stress," *Globe and Mail,* January 12, 2012.

Chapter 27: On Endings

1. Adlaf E, Goldbloom DS, and Garfinkel PE, unpublished data.
2. United States, Public Health Service, Office of the Surgeon General, *Mental Health: A Report of the Surgeon General* (Rockville, MD: National Institute of Mental Health, 1999).
3. Simmie S and Nunes J, *The Last Taboo: A Survival Guide to Mental Health Care in Canada* (Toronto: McClelland and Stewart, 2001).
4. Naiman S, "Comments on day two: the toxic word—"stigma"—ban it!" Coming out Crazy blog, *PsychCentral,* June 12, 2012, http://blogs.psychcentral.com/coming-out-crazy/discuss/11484/.
5. The Sir William Osler quotation is from "Remarks at a farewell dinner address in New York," May 20, 1905, later published in Osler, *Aequanimitas,* 473.

ACKNOWLEDGEMENTS

I've written this book over four years after retiring from my role as CEO of The Centre for Addiction and Mental Health (CAMH). During this period, I have gone back to "my first love": treating patients. I've really enjoyed the process of writing this book, alternating my clinical work with time spent reflecting on my experiences several days each week, punctuated by more intense bursts of writing while I took several weeks here and there to be in Italy.

This process has permitted me to recollect and, in fact, relive some experiences, and for some events it has helped provide a type of "working through" that had not happened previously with the busy everyday of work and home life. I also wrote this book in an attempt to help understand some of the events I've lived through, and I hope some of this may generalize for others and their experiences. I especially wanted my family to understand why I did some of the things I did. I realize how privileged I am to have had this experience.

Many people helped me through this project. Early drafts of my writing were reviewed and critiqued by Tessa Wilmot and Lisa Schmidt. Sarah Scott of Barlow Book Publishing provided valuable organizational and editorial comments and then guided me through each step of the publishing process. Sarah assembled a capable team: Barbara Berson and Judy Phillips were excellent editors. Geri Savitz-Fine and Zoja Popovic fact-checked the manuscript. Tracy Bordian led the production team. Luke Despatie designed both the interior and cover of the book. Kyle Gell typeset the book. Liz Milroy was helpful in organizing the endnotes and photographs.

I am grateful that several colleagues made useful comments on portions or drafts of the book: Gary Rodin, David Goldbloom, Christine Dunbar, Jean Simpson, and Shitij Kapur. John Court, the very capable archivist at CAMH, made many contributions as he reviewed drafts and discussed the early history of the asylum in Toronto. Stuart Yudofsky of Baylor College of Medicine provided the photograph of Hilde Bruch. Simone Rodrigue was always available for administrative support.

I was most fortunate to have been provided support for this project by the University of Toronto, The Centre for Addiction and Mental Health, and the CAMH Foundation.

Barbara Dorian played a significant role in seeing this manuscript to completion—she was able to inspire, debate, critique, and, in the latter stages, edit my writing.

Much of the content of this book I have learned from my patients. I am so grateful to have been allowed into their private worlds as their psychiatrist.

Paul Garfinkel, O.C., M.D.
September, 2014

Index

Note: Page numbers in *italics* refer to photographs; PG is Paul Garfinkel

D

E

F

M

N

ABOUT THE AUTHOR

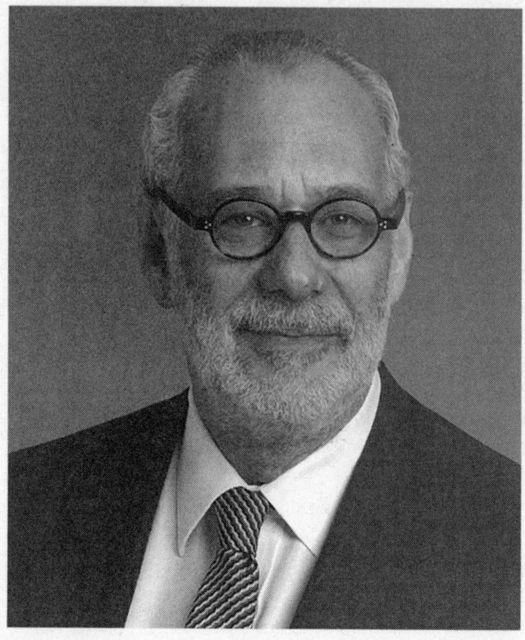

Paul Garfinkel, MD, is currently professor emeritus in the Department of Psychiatry at the University of Toronto, and staff psychiatrist at the Centre for Addiction and Mental Health (CAMH). He has been chief of psychiatry at Toronto General Hospital, chair of psychiatry at the University of Toronto, and president and CEO of the Clarke Institute of Psychiatry. In 1997, he was appointed chief executive officer of CAMH and held this position until 2009. Garfinkel is the author and editor of nine books on eating disorders. He has received many honours for his work, including fellowship in the Royal Society of Canada, and has been recognized as an Officer of the Order of Canada.